FOOD FIGHT

FOOD FIGHT

The Inside Story of the Food Industry,
America's Obesity Crisis,
and What We Can Do About It

KELLY D. BROWNELL, PH.D.
AND KATHERINE BATTLE HORGEN, PH.D.

Contemporary Books

Chicago   New York   San Francisco   Lisbon   London   Madrid   Mexico City
Milan   New Delhi   San Juan   Seoul   Singapore   Sydney   Toronto

Library of Congress Cataloging-in-Publication Data

Brownell, Kelly D.
     Food fight : the inside story of the food industry, America's obesity crisis, and what we can do about it / Kelly Brownell and Katherine Battle Horgen.
        p.   cm.
     Includes bibliographical references and index.
     ISBN 0-07-140250-0 (alk. paper)
     1. Obesity—United States.   2. Nutrition—United States.   3. Food industry and trade—United States.   4. Food habits—United States.   I. Horgen, Katherine Battle.
II. Title.

RA645.023B76   2004
616.3'98'00973—dc21   2003053081

1 2 3 4 5 6 7 8 9 0 AGM/AGM 2 1 0 9 8 7 6 5 4 3

ISBN 0-07-140250-0

Interior design by Nick Panos

This book is printed on acid-free paper.

*To my wife, Mary Jo, and our children, Kevin, Kristy, and Matt,
and to my parents, Arnold and Margaret Brownell, each of whom has
loved and supported me.*
KDB

*To my parents for giving me an education, to my husband for giving me
support, and to my daughter for giving me hope in the future*
KBH

CONTENTS

ACKNOWLEDGMENTS

Many people have contributed to our work and thinking, and we are grateful to them one and all.

Our greatest source of intellectual stimulation comes from our students, colleagues, and friends at the Yale Center for Eating and Weight Disorders. This lively, fiercely intelligent, and warmly supportive group led by Marlene Schwartz, herself a tireless advocate for improving the food environment, brings us inspiration and joy. Andrew Geier deserves special thanks for suggestions on the title.

Colleagues at Yale have been instrumental in sharing expertise with us and have been most helpful in enriching our thinking. Peter Salovey, Edward Zigler, Robert Sternberg, and Paul Bloom in the Department of Psychology; Michael Graetz at the Yale Law School; and the late James Tobin from the Department of Economics stand out in this regard.

We thank the research assistants who have worked with us over the years. Julia Kasl, Melissa Napolitano, Jennifer Hoffman Goldberg, Jumi Hayaki, Molly Choate, Alyse Behrman, Sophie Woolston, and Sarah Goldblatt have helped collect information from all corners of the world.

Trusted and very helpful colleagues gave us feedback on chapters as they were prepared. We drew heavily from their work to create *Food Fight* and are grateful for their specific input as this book was being produced. We thank Steven Blair (Cooper Institute), Russell Pate (University of South Carolina), Kenneth Warner (University of Michigan), Simone French (University of Minnesota), Anthony Sclafani (Brooklyn College), David Ludwig (Harvard Medical School), Barry Popkin (University of North Carolina), James Hill (University of Colorado), Rogan Kersh (Syracuse University), James Morone (Brown University), Douglas Besharov (American Enterprise Institute and University of Maryland), Michael Jacobson (Center for Science in the Public Interest), Marion Nestle (New York University), Anna Puglia (Branford High School), and Thomas Wadden (University of Pennsylvania). We are also deeply appreciative for the guidance and support of our agents Marilyn Allen, Robert Diforio, and Coleen O'Shea, who quickly became colleagues and friends.

We have friends and family members to thank for feedback and for help with collecting information. These include Kevin Brownell; Matthew Brownell; Steve, KieAnn, and Chase Brownell; Mary Jo Brownell; Jay Horgen; Jane and Joe Battle; Bob and Brooke Tanner Battle; and Clovis and Bett Battle Pitchford. Specials thanks go to Seth and Robin Ersner-Hershfield and to Kristy Brownell and Greg Nobile for their knowledge of modern culture.

Two final groups deserve special note. The first are our mentors and closest colleagues for providing guidance in so many ways. G. Terence Wilson, David Barlow, Albert Stunkard, and Thomas Wadden top this list.

And finally, we are most grateful to our spouses and children, who endured hours of work beyond imagination. Their understanding and support for our research and writing are appreciated more than they can know.

FOOD FIGHT

PART 1

BIOLOGY MISMATCHED WITH THE MODERN WORLD

1

BIG FOOD, BIG MONEY, BIG PEOPLE

It came quickly, with little fanfare, and was out of control before the nation noticed. Obesity, diabetes, and other diseases caused by poor diet and sedentary lifestyle now affect the health, happiness, and vitality of millions of men, women, and, most tragically, children and pose a major threat to the health care resources of the United States. Most alarming has been the national inaction in the face of crisis, the near-total surrender to a powerful food industry, and the lack of innovation in preventing further havoc.

The Centers for Disease Control and Prevention (CDC) labels the obesity problem an "epidemic."[1] Within the United States, 64.5 percent of Americans are either overweight or obese, with the number growing. For many reasons, some obvious and some not, the increase in overweight children is twice that seen in adults.

Other nations are in hot pursuit. Country after country follows the American lead and grows heavier. Overconsumption has replaced malnutrition as the world's top food problem.[2] From Banff to Buenos Aires, from Siberia to the Sahara, the world need only look to America to see its future. There are now clinics for obese children in Beijing.

Similar to a new virus without natural enemies, our lifestyle of abundant food and inactivity faces little opposition. Quite the contrary, powerful forces push it forward, spreading the problem to all segments of the population. These forces are woven so tightly into our social systems (economics, health care system, even education) that change seems almost beyond imagination. Despite talk of an obesity crisis, government reports, and Presidents pushing exercise, obesity is increasing in all races, ages, income groups, and areas of the world.

> In the United States, obesity now contributes more to chronic illness and health care costs than does smoking.[3]

The picture with children is sad. Projecting ahead to their adult years, today's children face a life of serious health problems and severely impaired quality of life.[4] Children are targeted in a relentless way by the food companies. Institutions such as schools that would like to protect children instead must sell soft drinks and snack foods to function.

While writing this chapter, one of us (KB) visited his brother, wife, and three-year-old niece. This girl, the daughter of educated, successful, health-conscious parents, ran by, so a quick interview was conducted.

"What's your favorite breakfast?"
"I like Buzz Lightyear" was her reply.
"Where do you like to go out to eat?"
"I like to go everywhere," she said.
"What's your most favorite place of all?"
"McDonald's," she answered.

It is easy to blame parents, but they face off every day with an environment that grabs their children and won't let go. Children and the parents who raise them do not get what they deserve—conditions that support healthy eating and physical activity. The environment wins in most cases, and we have an epidemic to show for it.

By any definition, we face an emergency.

The reasons for this growing problem are simple and complex at the same time. People eat too much and exercise too little, but this easy truth masks a fascinating dance of genetics with modern lifestyle. Economics, breakthroughs in technology, how our nation thinks about food, and, of course, the powerful and sophisticated food industry, are all actors in this tragic play. Our environment is textured with risk. It intersects with genes in a way that makes an obese population a predictable consequence of modern life.

Some individuals have the biological fortune or the skills to resist this risk, leading to arguments that weight control is a matter of personal responsibility. Choices people make are important, but the nation has played the willpower and restraint cards for years and finds itself trumped again and again by an environment that overwhelms the resources of most people.

The cost of inaction will multiply human suffering, place our nation at a strategic disadvantage, and have a massive impact on health care costs.

> One-fourth of all vegetables eaten in the United States are French fries.[5]

Biology Overwhelmed

Picture yourself a child, rather a zygote. Your father's sperm penetrates your mother's egg, unleashing a cascade of biological events. What you will eat later in life, your upper and lower limits for body weight, and how your physiology responds to being sedentary have been partially fixed.

The lives of your ancestors, dating back many thousands of years, reside in your genes. Unpredictable food supplies and looming starvation were their everyday realities. Those who adapted ate voraciously when food appeared, stored energy (as body fat) with extreme efficiency, survived later scarcity, and contributed to the gene pool from which you draw your DNA.

Married to this food biology are genes related to physical activity. Extreme exertion was once required to hunt and gather food. The body

functioned optimally with bouts of heavy activity punctuated by periods of rest needed to conserve energy.[6] Modern culture has removed
strenuous exercise.

You are an exquisitely efficient calorie conservation machine. Your
genes match nicely with a scarce food supply, but not with modern living conditions. As a child, you are about to be broadsided by a "toxic"
environment. Your body is unprepared for the plummeting need to be
physically active and cannot anticipate the impending confrontation
with Big—Big Gulp, Big Grab, Big Mac, Biggie Fries, Big everything.

If you could speak with your ancient ancestors, they would explain
that people eat a lot when food is abundant, particularly foods high in
fat, sugar, and calories, a fact proven by scientists thousands of years
later.[7] These foods provide quick energy but more important, are optimal for storing energy.

As you breathe for the first time outside the womb, your genes are
mismatched with modern conditions. The environment is distorted
beyond your body's ability to cope. It will pound you with inducements
to eat, make exertion unnecessary, and do little to defend you against
diseases that most threaten you.

Good fortune may bring you parents who are committed to healthy
eating. They keep junk food out of the home, have healthy foods available, and teach you good nutrition. But then you go to play groups,
birthday parties, and school. You see billboards, watch TV, go to
movies, and travel the supermarket aisles where your favorite Disney
and Nickelodeon characters are linked with sugared cereals, snack
foods, and ice cream. Your parents now face Goliath.

At its peak, the 5 A Day fruit and vegetable program from the National Cancer Institute had $2 million for promotion. This is one-fifth the $10 million
used annually to advertise Altoids mints.[8] In turn, the Altoids budget is a
speck compared to budgets for the big players—$3 billion in 2001 for Coca-
Cola and PepsiCo combined just for the United States.[9]

If you are a typical child, you will be introduced early to fast foods,
snack foods, and soft drinks. Your tiny fingers might have grasped baby

bottles bearing soft drink company logos.[10] Television connects you with some of Madison Avenue's brightest minds, hence you may recognize Ronald McDonald before you can speak. You will like the silly rabbit, Fred and Barney, the leprechaun, the friendly captain, the clown, and the pitcher with a smiling face. You see them thousands of times each year and see nothing similar for apples or carrots.

You may start to weigh too much, not a surprise given your diet. You eat too many calories, too much sugar, and too much fat, but have too few fruits and vegetables and too little fiber. Your weight, diet, and inactivity each increase your risk for very bad diseases, but nobody thinks of this—you're just a kid.

If you are very overweight, you could develop Type 2 diabetes before age ten. Kids like to feel grown up, so here is a chance—this disease used to be called Adult Onset Diabetes. You could have a heart attack, be blind, or need coronary bypass surgery before age twenty-five.

Not every child will develop this way. Some will (a) have a protective biology that keeps them from gaining weight despite what they eat; (b) not be interested in food; (c) be active enough to stay thin; or (d) want to resist the environment. Even when added together, however, these groups represent a minority of the population.

As you develop into a typical child, you would have every right to ask those in charge:

"Why do you let this happen to me?"
"Why do you ignore this obvious crisis?"
"Why don't you protect me from the food companies?"
"Are corporate profits more important than my health?"
"Why must schools feed me fast food, snack foods, and soft drinks?"
"Why don't my national leaders do something?"

The Toxic Environment

Biology comes undone when confronted by modern eating and exercise conditions, what we call the toxic environment.[11] *Toxic* is a powerful word, but powerful language is needed to describe the situation.

Names we give our food say it all: Double Whopper with Cheese, Super Supreme Pizza, Bacon Double Cheeseburger, Colossal Burger, Double Decker Taco Supreme, and Extreme Gulp. Chicken requires a "bucket." Food is

- available 24 hours per day
- accessible in restaurants, machines, and stores as never before
- sold in places previously unrelated to eating (gas stations, drugstores)
- cheap
- promoted heavily and, in some cases, deceptively
- designed by food technologists to taste really good and keep people coming back for more

The second half of the energy equation, physical activity, has also been affected in disastrous ways. Few children walk or bike to school; there is little physical education; computers, video games, and televisions keep children inside and inactive; and parents are reluctant to let children roam free to play.

The American landscape has been altered in profound ways. Cheeseburgers and French fries, drive-in windows and supersizes, soft drinks and candy, potato chips and cheese curls, once unusual, are as much our background as trees, grass, and clouds. We now take notice when food isn't there. Gas stations *without* a mini-market look old-fashioned and unappealing.

American spending on fast food has increased eighteenfold since 1970.

The world of fast food is only one of many changing influences but may be the most dramatic. In his book *Fast Food Nation*, Eric Schlosser notes that American spending on fast food went from $6 billion to $110 billion annually in the last thirty years. He states:

Fast food is now served at restaurants and drive-thrus, at stadiums, airports, zoos, high schools, elementary schools, and universities, on cruise ships, trains, and airplanes, at K-Marts, Wal-Marts, gas stations, even at hospital cafeterias. (p. 3)[12]

Fast food is high in fat, calories, and sugar; low in fiber; and nearly devoid of fruits and vegetables beyond fried potatoes.

> McDonald's has 30,000 restaurants in 118 countries, serving 46 million people (not each year, month, or week, but each *day*). Back in 1996, McDonald's opened a new restaurant every three hours.[13]

Food, not just fast food, is everywhere. Think of the modern drugstore. The items you need, like pain relievers, bandages, cough remedies, and vitamins, not to mention the pharmacy, are in the rear of the store, requiring you to pass through aisles of items you did not intend to buy. Many people gravitate naturally to the center aisles, home to a large collection of candies and foods. When you leave the pharmacy and walk back along the far aisle, notice what you encounter.

Children are valuable consumers, affecting billions of dollars in sales each year. Food marketing directed at children, almost exclusively for unhealthy foods, is as sophisticated as marketing gets. There are books, advertising journals, and conferences describing how to best market to children. It is no surprise that we have a nation of children consuming record amounts of sugar, soft drinks, fast foods, and snack foods.

In a *New York Times* article on snack foods in schools, Nicole Talbott, a student from Fremont High School in California, said:

Lunch for me is chips, soda, maybe a chocolate ice cream taco. Every day, just about the same thing. That's all I like to eat—the bad stuff.[14]

Nicole is not unusual. We have created for Nicole and her peers a terrible food environment. Her generation uses *supersize* as a verb. She would stand out much more if she had a healthy diet.

The vignette of a child wanting soda, chips, and ice cream has a cute side, but cute fades quickly when we consider that the diseases children face later in life, such as heart disease, cancer, stroke, and diabetes, could be developing right here, right now.[15] The environment does little to help Nicole eat healthy and be active.

Accessibility of bad food is coupled with a key economic reality: unhealthy food is cheap. It is also convenient, fast, packaged attractively, and tasty. Healthy foods are more difficult to get, less convenient, and more expensive. If you came from Mars and knew nothing but this about a country, an epidemic of obesity is exactly what you'd predict.

This confluence of declining physical activity and an altered eating environment, both in toxic proportions, has created a human crisis.

The Double Meaning of Big Food

Food is big, but so are the companies making and selling it. Massive agribusiness companies control a surprising amount of the food chain, raising grave concerns with issues such as dwindling genetic diversity in plants and farm animals, resistant strains of bacteria resulting from the overuse of antibiotics, and undue influence on the nation's nutrition and agriculture policy.[16]

Once food becomes products, other powerful business interests enter the scene. Huge companies like Nabisco, Frito-Lay, Pillsbury, Betty Crocker, and Post Cereals are in turn owned by bigger companies. Figure 1.1 shows only a partial list of brands owned by a few of the major players in the food industry.

A consequence of this consolidation is that enormous power and influence rest in the hands of a few companies. Their presence in Washington, D.C., is visible and felt in many ways, some more obvious than others. What crops get subsidized, which commodities get shipped to schools through the National School Lunch Program, what foods get emphasized in the food guide pyramid, and whether soft drinks are permitted in schools are a few places where political influence can affect the national nutrition environment. There are many, many cases where business interests conflict with public health. People deserve to know how and when this occurs and the impact it has on them and their children.

Kraft*	General Mills	PepsiCo	ConAgra
Nabisco	Betty Crocker	Pepsi	Armour
Post Cereals	Pillsbury	Frito-Lay	Knott's Berry
Oscar Meyer	Big G Cereals	Mountain Dew	Farm
Maxwell House	Yoplait	FruitWorks	Brown 'n' Serve
Jell-O	Bisquick	Aquafina	Bumblebee
Good Seasons	Old El Paso	Tropicana	Chef Boyardee
Country Time	Columbo	Gatorade	Chun King
Breyer's	Häagen-Dazs	Dole Juice Drinks	Healthy Choice
Kool-Aid	Green Giant	Quaker	Hebrew National
Tombstone Pizza	Pop Secret	Aunt Jemima	Peter Pan
Breakstone	Lloyd's Barbecue	Cracker Jack	Van Camp's
Stove Top	Jeno's	SoBe	Wolfgang Puck's
Toblerone	Nature Valley	Rice-a-Roni	Act II
DiGiorno	Progresso		Crunch 'n'
Louis Rich	Gold Medal		Munch
Philadelphia			Orville
Cream Cheese			Redenbacher's
Baker's Chocolate			Banquet
			Butterball
			Country Pride
			La Choy
			Libby's
			Marie
			Callender's
			Hunt's

*Kraft itself is owned by Philip Morris

Figure 1.1 Big Food (Partial List of Brands Owned by Leading Companies)

The word *big* applied to the food industry conjures up images of Big Oil, Big Energy, Big Tobacco, and so on. The public image of such industries is that a small number of giant companies led by ruthless executives control an entire industry and manipulate the political system, finances, and public opinion in self-serving ways that damage the public's interests. You may draw your own conclusions about whether the food industry deserves this label.

> Just two soft drink brands (Coca-Cola and PepsiCo) sell more than 70 percent of the carbonated beverages in the world, providing the majority of the fifty-two gallons of soft drinks consumed annually by the typical American. Ten to 15 percent of all calories consumed by America's teenage girls are from soft drinks.[17]

Attack Biology or the Environment?

The mismatch between biology and the environment might be solved in several ways. Letting evolution catch up to the environment is one possibility, but this could require thousands of years.

Fooling or overriding biology might be a solution. Clever scientists might find a drug that switches off the evolutionary need to store energy, counteracts desires to eat, or makes foods we now crave uninteresting. Children may one day be inoculated against measles, mumps, rubella, and obesity.

No such advance is even remotely on the horizon. Even if this dream came true and one could remain thin despite poor diet and inactivity, the diet and inactivity themselves would be harmful.

Changing the environment is the obvious place to begin. The deteriorating environment is the clear cause of the obesity epidemic and must be the basis for its remedy. Attacking a problem by considering its causes is logical and leads squarely to a public health imperative—prevention.

Prevention is appealing for several reasons:

1. With obesity the nation's most common major chronic health problem, vast numbers of people could benefit.
2. Children are the logical focus when a disease begins early in life. Food preferences, eating habits, and, possibly, brand

loyalties take shape in childhood, so the best opportunity for creating healthy habits may exist in the early years.

3. Obesity is very difficult to treat, and most people who lose weight do not keep it off.[18] The most optimistic estimates are that 25 percent of people lose weight and maintain the loss, often requiring many tries. This lack of success combines with the very high cost of treatment to make most approaches cost-ineffective. We will never treat this problem away.

4. The nation has a long history of supporting prevention to protect its children. Child safety seats, childproof medicine bottles, warnings on toys that are choking hazards, immunization requirements, and the prohibition of tobacco sales to children are examples. Such programs show good return on investment. Improving diet and physical activity and preventing obesity rival any of these programs in importance to public health.

Investing in Children

The United States invests wisely in children in some ways (such as immunizations) and poorly in others. Failure to invest in improving diet, physical activity, and body weight raises interesting parallels with failures to invest in early education.

> According to McDonald's, "Ronald McDonald can be found in every McDonald's market around the world—and speaks twenty-five languages, including Cantonese, Portuguese, Russian, Tagalog, Papiamento, and Hindi."[19] Ronald McDonald is the second most recognized figure in the world, topped only by Santa Claus.[20]

James Heckman, Nobel Prize–winning economist at the University of Chicago, has written extensively on the fundamental importance of early education and intervention with children.[21] He notes that education and skills help drive economic prosperity, that the demand for higher skills is growing, and that remediation (teaching skills to the unskilled) is costly and not very effective.

Heckman marshals strong evidence to support his position. The return on education dollars is much higher for preschool programs than for interventions with older children or adults.[22] An example is the Perry preschool program, where a program costing $12,148 per child returned $54,170 by decreasing later education costs, welfare payments, costs to the criminal justice system, and losses to crime victims. Such a program increases the number of people gainfully employed and paying taxes.[23]

Using Heckman's logic, but replacing education with nutrition and physical activity, the case for early intervention may be equally compelling. The importance of health and vitality to economic prosperity is obvious—a sick nation cannot create, work hard, and compete. The costs of remediation (weight loss) are high, and programs have limited effectiveness. And, hidden behind the cold numbers on costs, benefits, and the economy, are real people. Being unhealthy, lethargic, stigmatized, left out, and the victim of discrimination hurts a child and the adult that child becomes.

Ignoring the problem carries enormous costs. If people concerned with health cannot win the hearts of America's children, others will. Others have.

Looking Away in the Face of Crisis

Until very recently, obesity has been ignored as a serious issue, much less as a national crisis. Biology and drugs, not the environment and prevention, have been emphasized. There are countless signs of this disregard. To name a few:

- Obesity has been a raging problem for many years, yet the first report issued by the Surgeon General on obesity did not come until 2001.[24]
- Government funding for research on obesity is a small fraction of what one would expect given its high prevalence and medical consequences.

- In 1995, the Institute of Medicine released an insightful report saying that the environment, and not genetics, was responsible for increasing obesity.[25] Yet government funding for biological research and treatment still dwarfs that for environmental contributors and prevention.

Beyond Belated: Explaining the Slow Response to Crisis

Describing this national oversight does not explain it. Why have obesity and its prevention been ignored so long?

Weight bias, stigma, and discrimination are major reasons.[26] Any problem resulting from perceived misbehavior by a disrespected group is likely to be overlooked until escalating disease rates simply cannot be ignored. Parallels with AIDS are clear. Victims of that disease belonged to stigmatized groups. Many in society felt those with AIDS got what they deserved and deserved what they got, hence efforts at prevention began far later than necessary.

Obesity has been considered a consequence of weak discipline, laziness, psychological dysfunction, and other personal failings, explaining widespread discrimination in areas such as education, employment, and medical care.[27] It is widely believed that obese people are responsible for their condition and that they—not physicians, insurance companies, or the nation—should be responsible for its remedy. Empathy, caring, and kindness, much less federal dollars for research, do not flow freely to people who are disliked.

Another distraction has been the focus on biology and genetics in the research community. A great many advances have been made and more will come, but biology has not delivered a cure and obesity remains very resistant to treatment. The field has all but ignored prevention.

In addition, obesity has been low on the national agenda because the food industry pressures legislators, attempts to influence national nutrition guidelines, and opposes measures such as food labeling that would help consumers understand what they are eating.[28] The industry is organized, well-funded, and expert at lobbying, and hence has friends in high places and formidable power.

In November of 2002, top White House and cabinet officials met with the Board of Directors of the Grocery Manufacturers of America

(GMA), the world's largest food industry lobbying group. Secretary of Health and Human Services Tommy Thompson urged food companies to be aggressive with their critics and heralded the industry for its fine job in promoting healthy eating.[29]

Sometimes defense of the status quo comes from surprising sources. The education lobby (school systems, superintendents, etc.) has been among the most vigorous opponents of efforts to rid schools of snack food and soft drinks. They value the health of children, but need the money.

Add together the powerful forces resisting change, and one sees that the food fight the nation must have is likely to be ferocious.

The Good Food Versus Bad Food Debate

Throughout this book we refer to "healthy" and "unhealthy" foods. This runs counter to the stance of the American Dietetic Association, which holds that no food is good or bad, that every food can be part of a good eating plan.

> "It is the position of the American Dietetic Association that all foods can fit into a healthful eating style."[30]
>
> —American Dietetic Association position statement

This approach has some utility when professionals deliver dietary counseling to individuals. It may help prevent expectations that eating a forbidden food will set off binges or that favorite foods are off limits. We adopt this philosophy ourselves when addressing nutrition in the clinical setting.[31]

The food industry evokes the "good/bad" gospel repeatedly when food is criticized, saying it is unfair to demonize any one food and inferring that no food should be targeted for change. All food, therefore, is blameless.

All foods and beverages can fit into a healthy diet. . . .
—NATIONAL SOFT DRINK ASSOCIATION[32]

Policies that declare foods 'good' or 'bad' are counterproductive. . . .
—GROCERY MANUFACTURERS OF AMERICA[33]

. . . no single food causes obesity or weight gain.
—CHOCOLATE MANUFACTURERS ASSOCIATION (WITH TECHNICAL
ASSISTANCE FROM THE AMERICAN DIETETIC ASSOCIATION)[34]

No single food is to blame.
—NATIONAL CONFECTIONERS ASSOCIATION[35]

We agree that no one food is to blame for obesity, but to be distracted by the "no bad foods" argument is a mistake. From a public health perspective, it is folly to not believe that some foods are better than others. The nation should consume less bacon and more broccoli, fewer hot dogs and more whole grains, less ice cream and more fruit. This does not imply that a person should never touch bacon, hot dogs, or ice cream, but rather that changing the balance of some foods relative to others is a means for improving America's health.

Before progress can be made on changing the American diet, there must be collective agreement that the population should be eating more of some foods and less of others, else we place equal value on bacon cheeseburgers and vegetables. Failing to assign value has a stifling influence, skirts key policy decisions that must be made, and helps defend the ruinous status quo.

Is a Braver New World Possible?

The nation's reticence to tackle the obesity problem has allowed an epidemic to flourish, our children to be victimized, and business to prevail over health, much like what occurred with tobacco. It leads the United States to illogical and bizarre places, where schools must sell soft drinks and snack foods to survive financially and where children are not protected from forces that can make them unhealthy.

The responsibility to protect children is deeply ingrained in American morality. Children need protection from a food and activity environment that is out of control.

Individuals can act, as can parents, families, schools, communities, states, businesses, the nation, and the world. But there must be a stimulus. That stimulus is now beginning to take shape. It is concern, even outrage, over the human suffering caused by this environment, especially in children. Suffering is least defensible when children are affected, and children are the most startling victims of the toxic environment.

Mobilizing both individuals and the nation requires as its centerpiece bold and decisive changes in public policy. Progress is possible, but only if the nation, from its individual citizens to the largest corporations, from the local school board to the President, takes several steps:

1. Acknowledge the massive nature of problems caused by poor diet, inactivity, and obesity, appreciate the resulting human suffering, and recognize the costs to the nation.
2. Resist the seductive argument that people are doing this to themselves, thus justifying inaction.
3. Appreciate that there are victims—our children deserve more from us.
4. Understand that prevention must take priority and that children are the logical initial focus.
5. Stand up to the food companies to prevent undue influence on nutrition policy and obesity initiatives.
6. Hold the food industry accountable for targeting children.
7. Provide parents and children skills to deal with the toxic environment.
8. Develop creative ways for institutions such as schools to help solve the national problem.
9. Do everything possible to allow and encourage the population to be more physically active.

10. Change the basic economics of food so that it is easier and less expensive to eat a healthy diet.

The environment should produce healthy and happy citizens. It must help parents raise healthy children, provide schools with alert and vigorous pupils, offer businesses healthy employees, and create conditions in which the nation's people can thrive. Profound change is necessary.

DIETARY MAYHEM:
What We Eat, Why We Eat,
and the Impact

[W]e've changed the environment that we live in in an incredibly short time—one generation or perhaps two generations at most, and this has challenged our ancient metabolism, which for thousands of generations has been geared to fighting famine.

—RESEARCHER ANDREW PRENTICE[1]

Here we are in the 21st Century, surrounded by more cheap and plentiful food than has been available since the Garden of Eden, and Americans are still struggling to learn how to eat.

—SALLY SQUIRES[2]

Eating in American culture is like swimming in a tsunami. The best of intentions get pulled under by massive forces.

What we eat is easier to explain than why we eat. The tapestry that is modern eating is woven with influences from biology, psychology, and the food environment, influences that vary greatly from country to country and person to person.

There has long been debate pitting genetics versus environment in the genesis of obesity. Both have obvious importance, but controversy arises when considering which prevails over the other and which should be the focus of efforts to reverse the epidemic.

Is the Environment Causing the Obesity Epidemic?

There are several ways to tackle this question. One is to track changes within countries over time. The World Health Organization (WHO), for example, shows increasing obesity in nation after nation. Such rapid increases cannot be ascribed to shifting biology or changes in the world's gene pool. The WHO agrees with scientists who study this process that the changing environment is responsible.[3]

There are many examples of countries in transition.[4] Studies show time and again that weight increases as lifestyles become more modern and westernized. Tracking such changes within countries is instructive; however, it does not prove that the environment is responsible. A helpful means of separating environment and biology is to study related individuals who live in different environments. One group of scientists obtained weights for 247 individuals who had migrated to West London from the Punjab in India.[5] They were compared to 117 of their siblings who remained in Punjab. Those in West London had 19 percent higher body weights (in addition to higher blood pressure, cholesterol, and fasting blood glucose).

A striking case occurs in America. The Pima Indians, living primarily in Arizona, migrated to the United States from Mexico, where most were subsistence farmers. Eric Ravussin and colleagues have compared Arizona Pimas to a group with Pima ancestry living in a remote and mountainous part of northern Mexico. The Arizona Pimas eat nearly twice the calories from fat and weigh much more (44 pounds for the average woman). The American Pimas have extremely high rates of childhood obesity and have the highest rate of diabetes in the world.[6]

A fascinating discovery was made by German researchers who found that lifespan is affected by the month in which a person is born.[7] People in Austria and Denmark born in October–December live longer than those born in the spring, presumably because such babies undergo key *in utero* development in months when their mothers had access to a healthier diet, particularly fresh fruits and vegetables, and may also have been more active.

These scientists then did two clever things. First, they looked at longevity data in Australia, where the seasons are the reverse of those in the Northern Hemisphere. The data were shifted by a half-year; those people born April–June lived longest. Second, they studied British immigrants to Australia. Their lifespan was similar to those seen in the Austrian and Danish groups. The early food environment is quite important.

As the environment modernizes, diet and physical activity deteriorate, weight increases, and disease follows. In modern conditions, biology is important but the environment steals the show.

Balancing Genes and the Environment

The genetics of obesity has been studied for decades. The agriculture industry knows how to breed cows, pigs, and other animals to optimize body fat. Human studies began when Albert Stunkard from the University of Pennsylvania, working with scientists in Denmark, found that adults who had been adopted early in life had weights more closely resembling those of their biological than their adoptive parents. Stunkard then found that twins reared apart have similar weights to those reared together, again showing genes to be important.[8]

Much research has now been done on human genes and obesity.[9] Sophisticated techniques are being used to identify genes that predispose people to weight gain and to diseases like diabetes. In scientific parlance, 25 percent to 40 percent of the variability in population body weight can be explained by genes (as the weight of the population changes, 25 percent to 40 percent of the fluctuation is attributable to genetics). Given that obesity is usually blamed on personal failing, these numbers underscore the importance of biology, but still, 60 percent or more of the influence can be attributed to the environment.

Biology can act on body weight by affecting food preferences, hunger, fullness after eating, metabolic rate, conversion of excess calories to body fat, whether weight loss is easy or hard, and much more. As an example, Barry Levin showed that laboratory animals genetically programmed to be obese have multiple brain abnormalities that prime them to gain weight when high-calorie food is available. These abnormalities largely disappear when an animal reaches a steady obese weight. New neural circuits can then develop that make the obesity hard to change, and these circuits can then be passed along to subsequent generations.[10]

Without a "willing" biology, a person simply will not become obese. If a person is capable of gaining weight, how much is gained will be heavily influenced by genes. Sadly, biology is "willing" in the majority of people and is easily activated by the obesifying environment. Biology, therefore, allows obesity to occur, but the environment causes it to occur.

> In summarizing vast amounts of research on body weight, well-known obesity expert George Bray said, "Genes load the gun, the environment pulls the trigger."[11]

What Drives Eating?

Eating is governed by an exquisite network of biological, environmental, and psychological factors. The balance of these factors is different from meal to meal and varies from person to person. To attack a problem such as obesity, it is important to understand which factors are most important overall and which are the most logical leverage points for making change.

Genes Overwhelmed by a Modern World

A number of experts suggest that biology has evolved to withstand threats of starvation from an unpredictable food supply. Over many thousands of years and across countless generations, humans who adapted to scarcity were able to survive and reproduce. Darwinian natural selection took place, leaving a human race with finely tuned abilities to eat large amounts when food is available, seek out a variety of foods, and selectively focus on foods high in energy density (calories).

Several fascinating accounts of this process explain how humans have evolved:

> [B]ecause of the scarcity and unpredictability of food in nature, humans and other animals have evolved to eat to their physiological limits when food is readily available, so that excess energy can be stored in the body as a buffer against future food shortages.[12]

The theory that evolution has set the stage for today's obesity cannot truly be tested. We cannot go back in time to observe evolution and cannot exert enough experimental control over free-living humans to test the theory today. However, we can examine whether various species behave in ways consistent with the theory. Here the science gets extremely interesting. One way to look at the environment while holding biology constant is to study animals.

An Important Study. Michael Tordoff at the Monell Chemical Senses Center in Philadelphia used lab rats to test the widely accepted concept that animals have "nutritional wisdom" (under normal conditions they will eat a healthy mix of foods).[13] When given separate containers of fat, protein, and carbohydrate, animals usually balance their intake of nutrients and maintain good health. Tordoff speculated, however, that this regulatory system might break down if animals had access to larger amounts of energy-dense foods. He gave animals single cups of fat, protein, and carbohydrate, similar to what had been done previously. But in addition, some rats received three additional cups of either protein, carbohydrate, or fat.

Tordoff stopped the study after only eight days. Four of the seven animals given extra carbohydrate and three of seven given extra fat ate so little protein that they failed to thrive. All eight animals given extra protein and seven of eight given only one cup of each nutrient grew as expected. Carbohydrate and fat had equally life-threatening effects by creating protein malnutrition. Nutritional wisdom vanished as the environment grew toxic.

Tordoff then examined this phenomenon using liquid calories from sucrose (sugar) solutions. Animals were given either one bottle of water, five bottles of water and one bottle of sucrose solution (sugar water), or one bottle of water and five sucrose bottles.

The animals with one sucrose bottle gained more weight than those getting water only, but the big effect occurred in animals with five sucrose bottles. They drank more sucrose and took in more calories than the animals given one sucrose bottle. Significant increases in body fat were seen after only eight days. At the end of the experiment, the five-sucrose-bottle group had 33 percent more body fat than the animals getting one sucrose bottle and 85 percent more body fat than the animals getting just water. The five-sucrose-bottle animals dropped their food intake somewhat to compensate for the influx of liquid calories, but not nearly enough to maintain healthy body weight. Other researchers have shown that normal weight animals often become obese when given access to sucrose solutions.[14]

Tordoff's rats were betrayed by their own bodies, simply by transforming their environment into a rat "convenience store."

Yet More Evidence

The Tordoff study with rats was preceded by other research, some using different species, showing that animals given access to a diet high in fat, carbohydrate, and calories will ignore nutritious foods, overeat, gain weight, and become unhealthy. Anthony Sclafani, a scientist at Brooklyn College, was among the first to show that a "supermarket" diet consisting of foods like Oreo cookies, Hershey bars, marshmallows, cheese curls, salami, and other human favorites produces marked obesity.

Sclafani and colleagues also examined the effect of variety in the diet and found that animals will eat more and gain more weight when given a varied diet as opposed to having a single food repeatedly. Sclafani proposes that variety increases food intake by allowing animals to express individual nutrient preferences (some prefer fat and others carbohydrate) and by thwarting the monotony and reduced intake that comes with eating a single food,[15] a phenomenon called "sensory specific satiety" studied extensively by Barbara Rolls at Pennsylvania State University.[16]

Another key factor studied by Rolls and colleagues is the energy (calorie) density of foods; food intake is greatest when foods are dense with calories (accomplished by maximizing fat and carbohydrate). The positive side is that people moderate their intake more effectively when water is added to foods, thus decreasing energy density and helping people feel full with less food.[17]

The Ultimate Explanation for the Epidemic

Putting together animal and human research, we see significant danger in modern conditions. Animals and humans are drawn naturally to an energy-dense diet and therefore seek out sugar and fat, variety, and flavors associated with fat and carbohydrate. The conditions that make animals and humans overeat in the laboratory are precisely what people face in everyday life. Genes cannot adapt quickly enough, and while we wait for evolution to take its course, humans are locked into a biology that responds poorly to the modern environment.

These animal studies would predict high sugar intake when children are offered soft-drink machines at school and that overeating will occur when people are offered cheeseburgers, fries, and pizza.

It is clear in our minds that the environment has caused the obesity epidemic. Others have come to the same conclusion. Scientists James Hill and John Peters say in the journal *Science*:

The current epidemic of obesity is caused largely by an environment that promotes excessive food intake and discourages physical activity.[18]

Similarly, an Institute of Medicine report on obesity highlighted that:

[T]here has been no real change in the gene pool during this period of increasing obesity. The root of the problem, therefore, must lie in the powerful social and cultural forces that promote an energy-rich diet and a sedentary lifestyle. (p. 152)[19]

Herein is the impetus for this book. The environment must change.

What People Eat

It is surprisingly hard to know what people eat because of the crude
technology available to study food intake. Scientists can do no better
than ask people what they eat. There are different ways of doing this,
some more sophisticated than others, but when the day is done, scientists rely on what people tell them.

Self-reports of food intake are prone to several distortions. Some
people may be unwilling to report all they eat or may recall things inac-
curately because of self-consciousness. For example, a person whose diet
for a day consists of two Egg McMuffins and hash browns for breakfast, a Whopper and fries for lunch, pizza for dinner, and root beer,
chips, and cookies in between, may hesitate to confess. It is also hard to
recall how much is eaten after the fact. Recalling the amount of cereal
poured into a bowl or the number of potato chips pulled from a bag is
difficult, particularly because serving sizes have grown so large.

There is plenty to suggest that dietary data are inaccurate.[20] In 1996,
for instance, the average person reported consuming about 2,000 calories per day. Were this true, the population should not weigh so much.
People report eating less fat now than in the 1970s, but fat in the food
supply has increased by 25 percent.

Marion Nestle points out several clear changes in food consumption.[21] Calorie intake has increased, even by self-report data. Such
research shows a 200-calorie-per-day increase from the 1970s to 1996.
Larger increases are suggested by studies tracking calories in the U.S.
food supply, which have risen from 3,300 per person in 1970 to 3,800
in the late 1990s.

Intake in all major food groups has increased. Accompanying the
positive increase in fruit and vegetable intake are increased consump-
tions of meat and dairy products and of particular concern, foods high
in fat and sugar. Nestle notes:

. . . *we can conclude that the increased calories in American diets comes
from eating more food in general, but especially more of foods high in fat
(meat, dairy, fried foods, grain dishes with added fat), sugar (soft drinks,*

juice drinks, desserts), and salt (snack foods). It can hardly be a coincidence that these are just the foods that are most profitable to the food industry and that it most vigorously promotes.[22]

> In 2002, Frito-Lay launched its line of Go Snacks. Doritos, Cheetos, and Fritos can now be purchased in plastic containers the size and shape of a water bottle. Frito-Lay says this new packaging "fits the active, fast-paced lifestyles of today's consumers. Anytime, anywhere—even on the run—Go Snacks let Americans stay on the go without going hungry for their favorite snack foods."[23]

Driven to Sweetness

Sugar makes things taste good, is added to a vast array of foods, is the sole source of calories in many soft drinks, can have negative physical effects, and is pushed hard by the sugar and sweetener industries.[24] One authoritative review of sugar and health concluded that ". . . high sugar intake should be avoided. Sugar has no nutritional value other than to provide calories."[25] Yet according to the U.S. Department of Agriculture (USDA), the average American consumes 152 pounds of sugar each year. This is thirty pounds more than two decades ago.

Sugar comes naturally in foods, such as fructose in fruits and lactose in milk. The big problem is sugar added to products as they are produced. Soft drinks are a prime example. A twenty-ounce bottle of Pepsi or Coke has fifteen teaspoons of sugar. Other key sources of sugar are pastries, fruit drinks, candy, and other sweets.

Soft drink consumption in children ages eleven through seventeen has doubled in the past twenty years.[26] The consumption of added sugar (sugar beyond what occurs naturally in foods) is double what the USDA says it should be. A report from the National Academy of Sciences highlighted an additional concern: people with diets high in added sugars have lower intakes of key nutrients.[27] There is a detailed discussion of sugar in soft drinks in Chapter 7.

Even consumers who read food labels may not realize when sugar is added to products because it comes in forms like high-fructose corn syrup, dextrose, and maltose. Three years ago, the Center for Science in the Public Interest (CSPI) petitioned the FDA to require food manufacturers to clearly label the amount of added sugar, but no action has been taken. Michael Jacobson, director of CSPI, attributes the delay to lobbying by the powerful sugar and sweetener industries. The Sugar Association lobbied the USDA to change the wording of the current dietary guidelines on sugar, hence consumers are asked to use "moderation" rather than "limit" their sugar intake.[28]

Adding sugar is a cheap way to make foods taste good. In Skippy Super Chunk peanut butter, for example, roasted peanuts are the first ingredient and sugar is the second. High-fructose corn syrup is the third ingredient in Heinz Ketchup and the first in Kellogg's Strawberry Nutri-Grain yogurt bars. Sugar is the second ingredient in Nabisco Honey Maid Graham Crackers. Marion Nestle, nutrition expert at New York University, pointed to a survey in *Consumer Reports* magazine showing that consumers found sweetness just as important as peanut flavor in choosing their favorite peanut butter.

George Bray, a pioneer in studying obesity, made an important observation about increases in the consumption of high-fructose corn syrup, which is manufactured from corn starch and was introduced widely into the food supply in the 1970s.[29] Bray notes that fructose is sweeter than either sucrose (table sugar) or glucose and has different physical effects. It does not stimulate insulin secretion, which is related to people feeling full, but does stimulate the formation of fat cells. Bray found that the rise in use of corn syrup paralleled almost exactly declining intake of milk and rising prevalence of obesity.

Ore-Ida, owned by Heinz, is marketing Funky Fries—French fries "available in five funky varieties." Among them are fries coated with cinnamon and sugar and others coated with chocolate. Perhaps unaware of the irony, Heinz says, "Simply put, they're not what a potato is supposed to be."[30]

Dietary Fat and Obesity

There is raging controversy over the role of fat in the diet. Studies of large populations do not show consistent relationships between reported fat consumption and obesity. More carefully controlled studies tracking individuals over time *do* suggest a link. For instance, investigators at the University of Minnesota followed 826 women and 218 men over a three-year period.[31] During this time, there was a clear relationship of dietary fat with weight gain. Another study of more than 2,500 employees at thirty-two work sites found weight gain associated with the intake of both high-sugar and high-fat foods (sweets, French fries, meat, etc.).[32]

A recent study in Finland addressed the fat issue in a clever way.[33] Researchers studied identical twins where one twin was obese and the other not. Because the twins have the same genes, differences in weight must be caused by behavior and the environment. The obese twin reported a preference for fatty foods three times more often than the nonobese co-twin. The authors concluded that acquired preferences for foods high in fat are related to risk for obesity.

High consumption of fat is what one would predict from the animal studies mentioned earlier. One group of scientists, after reviewing all studies on fat and weight change, concluded that reducing dietary fat helps prevent weight gain in normal weight individuals and produces weight loss in those who are overweight.[34] James Hill and colleagues at the University of Colorado Medical Center note that:

. . . it is clear that consumption of a high-fat diet increases the likelihood of obesity and that the risk of obesity is low in individuals consuming low fat diets.[35]

Furor over Fat and Carbohydrate

On July 7, 2002, the *New York Times Magazine* published an article by Gary Taubes on what people eat and why they gain weight. Entitled "What If It's All Been a Big Fat Lie?," the article made the magazine cover, which showed a steak with butter melting over the top. Taubes had lost weight himself on the Atkins low-carbohydrate diet. The lead paragraph said:

If the members of the American medical establishment were to have a collective find-yourself-standing-naked-in-Times-Square-type nightmare, this might be it. They spend 30 years ridiculing Robert Atkins, author of the phenomenally-best-selling Dr. Atkins' Diet Revolution *and* Dr. Atkins' New Diet Revolution, *accusing the Manhattan doctor of quackery and fraud, only to discover that the unrepentant Atkins was right all along. Or maybe it's this: they find that their very own dietary recommendations—eat less fat and more carbohydrates—are the cause of the rampaging epidemic of obesity in America.*[36]

The article caused immediate furor, and struck a resonant chord because it transformed the complex obesity story into a simple one of a villain (carbs) and an unlikely hero (fat). Tell people they can eat all the fat they want and you've got a winning story, just like Atkins wrote a winning diet book.

The article challenged the doctrine that fat is the main reason the population is overweight, brought needed attention to carbohydrates, and rightfully noted that segments of the industry peddling foods high in sugar cannot be exempt from criticism. It also had problems and was later criticized roundly by the very experts Taubes quoted.[37]

The major problem is that Taubes, similar to Atkins, minimized fat as a contributor to obesity. Common sense suggests otherwise. Fat contains twice the calories per gram of either protein or carbohydrate and is widely present in the food supply. The number of fast food restaurants has exploded; their universal food is French fries. Onions are fried, zucchini is fried, cheese is fried, and ice cream is fried.

Let's say hypothetically that fat and carbohydrate each explain 50 percent of increased food consumption and weight gain in the population. Fat intake then declines, but increasing carbohydrate consumption more than compensates, leading to an overall increase in calorie intake and rising levels of obesity. Fat may now be 40 percent of the problem and carbohydrate 60 percent, but it would be illogical to dismiss the 40 percent contribution.

There is a lively debate on fat in the scientific literature,[38] and one can build a case on either side of the issue. Taubes criticizes scientists who emphasize fat and ignore carbohydrates, but he and Atkins made the same mistake, just reversing the nutrients. The greatest risk of this debate is that it diverts people from the big picture—the nation eats too much of just about everything (except healthy food). Forcing scientists or the public into the juror's box to decide whether fat or carbohydrate contributes more to obesity is like debating whether tornadoes are worse than hurricanes.

People consume too many calories, which is the key to the obesity problem. Sugar may be more the problem with some and fat with others—not everyone has the same food preferences. Most people probably have trouble with both. An analysis of patterns of women in the Framingham Heart Study, a large study of heart disease in Massachusetts, found that overall diet was a stronger predictor of a woman's likelihood of becoming overweight than was intake of any nutrient.[39]

Is Food Addictive?

This question has enormous implications. Among the more important are what foods schools might be allowed to serve, what foods should be permitted to be advertised to children, whether warning labels might be justified, and whether food companies are vulnerable to lawsuits claiming health damages.

There has been a lively debate on food addiction for years, with most attention focused on carbohydrate (sugar). Early studies by Judith and Richard Wurtman at MIT suggested that people who stop eating carbohydrates will experience strong cravings, something akin to cravings for cigarettes, alcohol, or drugs. Based on these findings, Judith Wurtman wrote a popular book called the *Carbohydrate Craver's Diet*.[40] Other scientists took issue with the Wurtmans' findings and doubted whether carbohydrate craving exists at all.[41]

More recently, Bartley Hoebel, Carlo Colantuoni, and their colleagues at Princeton University did careful testing of rats to examine whether an addiction for sugar might occur. They knew that palatable foods stimulate neural systems in the brain that are considered important in drug dependence. They wanted to test whether changes in the brain produced by sugar reflect physical addiction. The results are striking.[42]

In the first study, these researchers allowed rats access to a sugar solution (25 percent glucose) and their standard, healthy laboratory diet. They were then deprived of food for twelve hours and then given free access to the sugar solution and the lab diet for twelve more hours. This cycle then repeated. The animals voluntarily doubled their sugar intake within ten days and developed a pattern of eating large amounts in the first hour when given access to food. After thirty days, the scientists found that the excessive, intermittent sugar intake had sensitized receptors in the brain in a way similar to some drugs of abuse.

The second study involved a similar procedure, but the animals' sugar intake was stopped at the end of the experiment to test for signs of withdrawal. Stopping addictive drugs produces characteristic effects on both the behavior and brain chemistry of animals. The researchers found just these signs in the animals that consumed sugar and stopped. The changes in the behavior and brains of these animals were like those seen with highly addictive drugs, such as morphine, leading the scientists to suggest that the rats had become sugar-dependent.

> "Laboratory rats given a high-sugar diet and then withdrawn from sugar experience changes in both behavior and brain chemistry similar to those seen during withdrawal from morphine or nicotine."[43]
> —Princeton University scientists

These are startling findings but coincide with what little is known from work with humans. People who struggle with eating often state emphatically that they are addicted to sugar, sweets, or food in general, although psychological factors could be at work.

Adam Drewnowski from the University of Washington did research on food craving in the 1980s using the drug naloxone.[44] This drug blocks opioid receptors in the brain. Opioids are chemicals related to pleasure that can be activated by addictive drugs. Blocking opioid action with naloxone reduces cravings in drug addicts. In Drewnowski's work, naloxone reduced the pleasure people reported from snack foods and suppressed consumption of high-sugar and high-fat foods. Drewnowski points out that most foods people crave contain both fat and sugar (such as chocolate, ice cream, and cake) so if addiction is occurring, either or both could be implicated.[45]

More studies must be done with both animals and humans to determine whether sugar is addictive, but if it is, practices such as heavy advertising of high-sugar products to children, adding sugar to foods, and systematically increasing portion sizes may take on new legal and public policy meaning. Research on sugar addiction must be a priority.

Lifestyle Factors That Promote Obesity

The simple story is that biology seeks out an energy-dense diet, the environment provides it, and we have runaway obesity. The way the environment acts on eating and activity, however, is a puzzle with many pieces. Only hubris would lead us to say we have all the pieces and can fit them into place. Much, much more work must be done before all the responsible factors can be identified and we understand how they interact with each other. For instance, the economics of food, exercise, and obesity is a key area where work has just begun (see Chapter 9).[46] For now, we can point to several aspects of lifestyle that likely contribute to obesity, knowing that the list is incomplete.

Television, Video Games, Computers, and Obesity
Starting more than fifteen years ago with William Dietz and Steven Gortmaker leading the way, scientists began investigating whether the amount of time a person watches TV is associated with risk for obesity.[47] The early studies suggested a strong relationship between TV watching and obesity.

About forty studies have now been done, one after another showing that TV time is coupled with both obesity and poor food consumption in children and adults, males and females, and people across countries, including the United States, Spain, Australia, and Mexico.[48] Another by-product of watching television is risk factors for cardiovascular disease such as worsening triglycerides, LDL cholesterol, HDL cholesterol, and blood sugar control.[49] Several leading figures in the field, including William Dietz from the Centers for Disease Control and Prevention and Thomas Robinson from Stanford University, have emphasized reduced TV watching as a national policy priority.[50]

Television viewing occupies a startling proportion of people's lives, even with infants and very young children.[51] The well-known statistic is that children graduating from high school have accumulated more hours before the TV than in school, and this must be added to the hours people spend with video games and computers. Studies have now shown links between obesity and having a TV in a child's bedroom and that children who watch TV during meals watch more TV overall.[52] Researchers in both Boston and New York have found that children in families where watching TV occurs during meals watch more TV in total, eat fewer fruits and vegetables, and consume more pizza, snack foods, and soft drinks.[53] One study found that metabolic rate declines in children while watching TV.[54]

Eating Away from Home

The National Restaurant Association says the nation now has 858,000 restaurants. The average household spends $2,116 per year ($846 per person) on food away from home. Fifty-four billion meals are eaten per year at restaurants or at school or work cafeterias.[55]

Eating out often means eating a lot and eating poorly, for both adults and children.[56] The frequency of eating out is associated with higher calorie and fat intake and increased body weight, while eating meals at home is associated with better calorie intake. One study of more than 16,000 children found that the more days a week children ate dinner at home with the family, the more likely they were to have healthful eating patterns (more fruits and vegetables, less fried food and soft drinks, less fat, a lower glycemic [sugar] load, and more fiber).[57]

> More than 40 percent of adults eat at a restaurant on a typical day.[58]

It is not surprising that calorie intake increases in children who eat out. Marlene Schwartz at Yale led a nutrition analysis of children's menus at the nation's five leading fast-food restaurants (McDonald's, Burger King, Kentucky Fried Chicken, Wendy's, and Taco Bell) and the five leading family restaurants (Pizza Hut, Applebee's, Denny's, Red Lobster, and Outback Steakhouse).[59] The meals exceeded dietary recommendations in fat and calories and were lower in fiber. The problem was especially severe in the family restaurants because of larger portions. The most common entrée for children was chicken pieces breaded and fried (nuggets, tenders, strips), and, of course, French fries were nearly universal.

> Researchers at the University of Minnesota found that the frequency of visits to fast-food restaurants by children was related to:
> - increased intake of soft drinks, cheeseburgers, French fries, pizza, total fat, and calories
> - decreased intake of fruit, vegetables, and milk[60]

People like to eat away from home because good-tasting food is enticing. Time-constrained, stressful lifestyles make it difficult to prepare meals at home. Children seeking toys and foods they see on TV pressure parents for trips to restaurants. In the case of fast food, eating out takes little time, the kids may have a play area, and as with all restaurants, someone else does the preparation, serving, and cleaning.

> The Olive Garden restaurant chain, wanting its customers to order less water and more of other beverages, worked with Coca-Cola to develop the H_2NO program. Crew education kits trained Olive Garden staff on "beverage suggestive selling techniques," and both sales managers and servers were given beverage sales goals. Participating restaurants showed significant increases in beverage sales along with "reduced tap-water incidence."[61]

Snacking

Snack food is a huge business. The industry's main organization, the Snack Food Association (SFA), represents more than 800 companies that manufacture "potato chips, tortilla chips, cereal snacks, pretzels, popcorn, cheese snacks, snack crackers, meat snacks, pork rinds, snack nuts, party mix, corn snacks, pellet snacks, fruit snacks, snack bars, granola, snack cakes, cookies and various other snacks." The SFA states that Americans buy more than $32 billion of snack foods every year.[62]

Foods eaten between meals comprise a growing portion of the nation's calorie intake. One study with children and another with young adults compared snacking patterns from the 1970s to the 1990s.[63] Snacking increased in all age groups. In the young adults, the number of snacks per day increased by 14 percent and the calories consumed per snack increased by 26 percent. In children, the amount eaten per snack stayed about the same, but the number of snacks increased.

Snacking is linked to obesity,[64] and convenience makes snacking easy. Food companies do heavy promotion of snack foods, convenience stores and vending machines make the foods accessible, and television provides both the time and inducement to snack.

A survey in England found that "For every healthy product targeted specifically at children, there are more than 10 products which are 'nutritional disasters,' with high levels of saturated fat, sugar or salt. . . ."[65] This is probably an underestimate, as the survey did not include candy, soft drinks, or snack chips.

The Glorification of Overeating

Overeating is glorified, to the point it is a spectator sport. It is common to see people eating large amounts in food advertisements, asking for large sizes, or making light of eating too much. ("I can't believe I ate the whole thing.") Recipes for "sinful" desserts are in magazines juxtaposed with articles on how to lose weight.

Pie-eating contests at county fairs have given way to televised championships where the best gorgers become minor celebrities. The hot dog–eating contest held by Nathan's in New York gets national coverage. The Fox TV network broadcast "The Glutton Bowl," which featured a series of eating events with a "world champion" being crowned. Contestants ate massive amounts of mayonnaise, beef tongue, butter, and in the last event, animal brains. The announcers used language like "the world's greatest athlete" to describe the victor.

And yes, there is the International Federation of Competitive Eating (IFOCE). This group seeks "to achieve objectives consistent with the public interest—namely, creating an environment in which fans may enjoy the display of competitive eating skill." This group, which sanctioned the Glutton Bowl, has a list of IFOCE records on its website. Among them are four 32-ounce bowls of mayonnaise in eight minutes by Oleg Zhornitskiy, one gallon and nine ounces of ice cream in twelve minutes by Ed "Cookie" Jarvis, fifty-seven cow brains (17.7 pounds) in fifteen minutes by Takeru Kobayashi, and 137 chicken wings in thirty minutes by Bill "El Wingador" Simmons.[66]

While Mayor John Street of Philadelphia spearheaded a major fight against obesity, Philadelphians flocked to the Wing Bowl hosted by a local sports radio station. This chicken-wing contest outgrew a local hotel and then the Spectrum sports complex when crowds exceeded 12,000. It finally landed in the First Union Center where the 76ers and Flyers play.

Bad enough that adults do this, but it is especially dispiriting to see eating contests for children, sometimes sponsored by institutions such as schools and museums.

- The Rye Playland in Rye, New York, holds hot dog–eating contests for both adults and children on July 4.
- The Seagate Beach Club in Brooklyn holds a "children's division" competition of their pie-eating contest.

- Troy, Ohio, holds a pie-eating contest for contestants age six and up.
- The highlight each year at the annual Children's Day at Missouri Town outside Blue Springs, Missouri, is the pie-eating contest.
- The Children's Museum of the Sierra in Oakhurst, California, along with the Girl Scouts of Oakhurst host the Children's Play Center, which includes a costume contest, Halloween parade, ice cream–eating contest, and chocolate pie–eating contest.

Poor Access to Healthy Food

There has been growing concern that certain segments of the population are prone to poor diet because they do not have access to healthy foods. Maya Rockeymoore from the National Urban League, for instance, said, "In some neighborhoods, it's easier to get an artery-clogging piece of fried chicken than it is to get a fresh apple. Many urban community dwellers would love to have better eating habits, but if there's no grocery store nearby, you're talking about getting on public transportation with a grocery cart."[67]

We discuss this issue of being poor in Chapter 9, but several facts are clear. Access to healthy foods is limited in impoverished areas. One can argue demand—that food establishments provide what people want (fast foods, snack foods, and soft drinks) and that poor people want these foods. Studies suggest otherwise. When healthy food is made available to poor populations, diet improves.

The Consequences of an Obesity Epidemic

Obesity is a major-league problem. It increases risk for many serious diseases, can be disabling, and has a very negative impact on the quality of a person's life. It also comes bundled with the behaviors that cause it, namely poor diet and physical inactivity. These affect health, irrespective of their impact on weight.

Is Epidemic *an Overstatement?*

Epidemic is used time and time again by the press to describe the spread of obesity. The press harvested the word from experts, who interpret data from studies but also see the human tragedy the numbers represent. *Epidemic* has been used by the Centers for Disease Control and Prevention to describe conditions in the United States and by the World Health Organization to describe the global picture.[68]

> Almost two-thirds—64.5 percent—of Americans (127 million people) are overweight or obese.

The World Health Organization sets the definition of *overweight* at a body mass index (BMI) of 25 kg/m^2 and obesity at a BMI of 30 kg/m^2. These numbers correspond to about 20 percent and 40 percent above ideal body weight, respectively. You can obtain your own BMI using one of many tables and programs for doing so.[69]

The most recent national statistics on obesity were collected during a nationwide study completed over two years, 1999–2000.[70] During the period 1988–1994, 55.9 percent of Americans were overweight and 22.9 percent were obese. Now 64.5 percent are overweight and 30.5 percent are obese. The number of people with very high body weights where disease risk is extreme (BMI $\geq$ 40) has tripled in the last decade. Prevalence is rising so fast that increases can be detected year by year. Because of the worsening environment, we expect the numbers will rise still higher. Simply stopping the rising tide would be a major victory.

Special Problems in Minority Groups

Shiriki Kumanyika at the University of Pennsylvania is a leader in studying health issues in minority populations.[71] She shows that compared to whites, the prevalence of obesity is higher in males from every single racial group yet studied (including African Americans, Cuban

Americans, American Indians, and Alaskan Natives, among others). With a few exceptions, the picture is the same for minority women. Children from minority groups also suffer a disproportionate burden of obesity.[72]

The high prevalence of obesity in minority populations is especially troubling when one considers their vulnerability to disease. African Americans have greater increases in blood pressure when they gain weight, and the years of potential life lost from diabetes is extremely high in African American, Hispanic, and Native American populations. Asian groups begin to show increased disease risk at weights considered healthy in other groups.

Kumanyika notes that a variety of economic, cultural, and biological factors may explain increased obesity in minority individuals. These include:

- **Risk from the physical environment:** targeted marketing by food companies, poor foods in neighborhood stores, lack of supermarkets, distance to fitness facilities, neighborhood crimes, and so on
- **Risk from the sociocultural environment:** high-calorie traditional cuisines, insecurities about having enough food, cultural attitudes about physical activity, and so on
- **Risk from the economic environment:** family income and cash-flow problems, cost of exercise equipment, limited government investment in park and recreation facilities in inner cities, and so on[73]

How Bad Is Obesity?

We use strong words like *epidemic* and *crisis* to describe the current situation with obesity. We believe they are fully justified. The picture is so bad that a group from the University of Minnesota published an article entitled "Can anyone successfully control their weight?"[74] They tracked the weights of 854 people from the community during a three-year period. Only one in twenty (4.6 percent) lost weight and kept it off, and only one in four (24.5 percent) avoided weight gain during the three years. More than half (53.7 percent) gained weight in the first twelve months. Let's examine the health consequences of statistics such as these.

> American children may be the first generation in modern history to live shorter lives than their parents did.

Obesity and Physical Disease

Research has shown links between obesity and more than thirty medical conditions.

Medical Conditions Associated with Obesity

Osteoarthritis	Heart disorders
Rheumatoid arthritis	Hypertension
Birth defects	Impaired immune response
Breast cancer	Impaired respiratory
Cancer of esophagus and	function
gastric cardia	Infections following wounds
Colorectal cancer	Infertility
Renal cell cancer	Liver disease
Cardiovascular disease	Low back pain
Carpal tunnel syndrome	Obstetric and gynecologic
Chronic venous insufficiency	complications
Daytime sleepiness	Pain
Deep vein thrombosis	Pancreatitis
Diabetes (Type 2)	Sleep apnea
End stage renal disease	Stroke
Gallbladder disease	Surgical complications
Gout	Urinary stress incontinence[75]

Risk for disease increases the more weight goes up, hence additional weight gain in a person already overweight will elevate risk further. As a person goes from normal weight to very obese, the risk of coronary heart disease increases nearly 60 percent in men and 179 percent in women. Diabetes increases fivefold for men and eightfold for women.

Obesity also increases risk of premature death. It does this primarily through its associations with cardiovascular disease, Type 2 diabetes (90 percent of people with Type 2 diabetes are overweight), and some cancers.[76] When a person reaches criteria for obesity (BMI of 30), risk of death is elevated by 30 percent. When BMI reaches 40, risk of death is 100 percent higher than for a person at normal weight.[77] To place these BMI numbers in perspective, a 5'5" woman weighing 180 pounds would have a BMI of 30; her BMI would be 40 if she weighed 240 pounds. A 6' man weighing 220 pounds would have a BMI of 30, and at 295 pounds would have a BMI of 40.

As science marches ahead and methods for studying disease become more sophisticated, the news about weight and health grows even worse. Recent studies, for example, have shown that obesity increases risk for heart failure, that excess weight may trigger inflammation that causes heart attacks, that obesity combined with cigarette smoking leads to substantially increased risk for heart disease, and that obese women who are pregnant risk developing gestational diabetes, having very high blood pressure, and having babies with serious health problems.[78]

Medical problems caused by obesity often cluster together. One such cluster, called the Metabolic Syndrome, occurs when people have at least three of the following five conditions: (1) waist measurement more than forty inches in men or thirty-five inches in women; (2) triglycerides of 150 or greater; (3) HDL, or "good" cholesterol, less than 40 in men or less than 50 in women; (4) blood pressure of 130/85 or more; and (5) fasting blood sugar of 100 or more.

Having the metabolic syndrome is quite common, and it is linked with particularly increased risk for developing diabetes and cardiovascular disease and for dying prematurely.[79] The number of people with the syndrome ranges from 7 percent of people in their twenties to about 43 percent of people in their sixties. Rates are especially high in African American and Mexican American women.

Quality of Life

Diseases caused by obesity, such as heart disease and diabetes, can seriously impair a person's life. Going blind, losing limbs to amputation, and being homebound are examples, but there are many more. The list of diseases mentioned earlier begins to tell the story, but even in people without these specific diseases, obesity brings high risk for physical limitations, psychological problems, and economic and social disadvantage.[80]

The physical burden of excess weight can affect even the most routine activities. Climbing stairs, maneuvering into an automobile, finding comfortable chairs, and walking any distance can be difficult. Physical tasks one does many times a day become sources of pain and embarrassment.

Because obesity is a stigmatized condition, overweight people, especially children, are teased, reminded repeatedly of their bodies, and victimized by discrimination. The discrimination itself would make most people anxious, depressed, and hypervigilant, but the diminished education and employment opportunities it causes can have a real impact on income and security.

Overweight people often internalize negative social messages and come to feel badly about themselves. Diminished self-esteem, poor self-confidence in social situations, and other psychological fallout are common. This is hardly a surprise—negative messages about overweight people, unfair as they may be, are relentless. Even people who are resilient have trouble defending themselves against the barrage. Children can be especially hard hit by this social bias.

Health Care Costs

Obesity costs lots of money. The costs are incurred by individuals, insurers, businesses, the country, and the world. Costs will only increase if prevalence rises.

Health care costs associated with obesity are $70–$99 billion per year in the United States.[81] Overweight individuals have 36 percent higher inpatient and outpatient costs and 77 percent higher medication costs.

Adding in lost productivity, time away from work, and other costs not included in these figures, the total cost to the nation is hard to comprehend. Countries such as Canada, France, and Japan are just a few of those also concerned with rising costs.

> Around 7 percent of all U.S. health care expenditures can be attributed to obesity.

Roland Sturm, an economist with the Rand Corporation, has produced what may be the most startling numbers of all. He found that obesity now surpasses smoking in its negative effects on health and health costs and bestows on the individual the same risk as aging two decades.[82]

Children

Obesity in children is a problem of major significance.[83] Rates are growing around the world; the medical, psychological, and social consequences are harsh; and the primary causes, poor diet and declining activity, are themselves growing worse.

Obesity in children has increased two- to threefold in the United States in the last twenty-five years. The increase in minority groups is double that in white children. The prevalence of overweight children during the period 1988–1994 was 10.5 percent for ages twelve through nineteen, 11.3 percent for ages six through eleven, and 7.2 percent for ages two through five. The numbers now are 15.5 percent, 15.3 percent, and 10.4 percent, respectively. The increase in child obesity has been nearly 3-fold in England; 3.5-fold in Brazil and Haiti; and nearly 4-fold in Ghana, Australia, and Egypt.[84]

Consequences

Early concern about childhood obesity centered on its role in predicting adult obesity and hence adult diseases. Seventy percent of obese children become obese adults; obesity in children is related to risk for disease as much as fifty years later.[85] The epidemic of childhood obesity we see now will have major consequences for years to come.[86]

Childhood obesity also has immediate health effects, some devastating. Excess weight gain in children can cause lipid problems, high blood pressure, blood clotting abnormalities, asthma, and other serious disturbances. One of the most serious is the clustering of risk factors for heart disease known as insulin resistance syndrome, now identified in children as young as five years old.

> Overweight children who develop Type 2 diabetes may have heart attacks and need coronary bypass surgery before they reach age thirty.

Problems with glucose tolerance and insulin resistance place severely overweight children at risk for Type 2 diabetes, a disease once seen only in adults.[87] These children risk having diabetic complications, including heart disease, stroke, blindness, limb amputation, and kidney failure, before they reach age thirty.

Researchers in France found that early signs of heart disease were much more common in obese than in thin children. Obese children had stiffer carotid arteries and unhealthy changes in the artery lining. Canadian researchers tracked children who developed Type 2 diabetes before age seventeen for fifteen years after they were diagnosed. As young adults, they were experiencing blindness, amputation, kidney failure requiring dialysis, pregnancy loss, and death.[88]

Also noteworthy are the psychological and social consequences of being an overweight child. Social exclusion, teasing, and antifat media messages are common, and there is discrimination in education. As a result, poor self-esteem and other problems are very real issues for these children.[89]

As with adults, health care costs for obese children are escalating rapidly. A study comparing hospital discharge records in children ages six through seventeen from around 1980 to those from the late 1990s found that discharges for diabetes doubled, obesity and gallbladder disease tripled, and sleep apnea increased fivefold. The amount of total hospital costs attributed to obesity in children quadrupled.[90]

It is sad to witness the humiliation, shame, and pain suffered by overweight children and heartbreaking to think of heart attacks in young people barely out of college. The toxic environment is powerful and acts early. Children need our help.

A large percentage of young adults ages seventeen through twenty, from whom military recruits are drawn, do not meet U.S. military weight standards. Weights are particularly high among minority youth, who form a disproportionate percentage of those in military service.[91]

Personal Responsibility

Our stance on the causes of obesity is admittedly deterministic—with the right biology and a bad enough environment, the average person will become overweight. But how does this square with personal responsibility? Do people have any control over the way they eat and how much they exercise? What about old-fashioned willpower?

Scientists cannot yet dissect a person's weight into the separate contributions of biology, environment, and failures of personal responsibility. Balancing these factors thus becomes a matter for speculation, and opinions vary widely. Some people believe that obesity comes from lack of personal responsibility, so measures aimed at changing the environment are considered unfair and only interfere with personal choice. They draw on the long history in our country of emphasizing personal responsibility. Beginning with the Puritan work ethic and the "pull yourself up by the bootstraps" philosophy, people are expected to show discipline and are assigned blame when things are not right.

Without saying so explicitly, the nation has tried the personal responsibility approach to solve the nation's weight problem. People are blamed for being overweight and are under extreme pressure to lose the extra pounds. But as the pressure to be responsible (and thin) has grown, the prevalence of obesity has risen. We cannot say the pressure caused obesity to increase, but arguing that even more pressure would help is not defensible. Advocates of personal responsibility typically fall silent when asked what more could be done based on their philosophy.

Parental Responsibility

Personal and parental responsibilities are complex issues in the case of children. Young children do not have the maturity to make healthy choices and respond most often to immediate gratification. They do not control their environment, and even if they did, they do not possess the psychological resources to structure a healthy environment. They are easy prey for the food companies, and the companies begin their work early.

> A company called Munchkin Bottling arranged to have soft drink logos like Mountain Dew and Pepsi placed on baby bottles. Babies are four times more likely to consume soft drinks from these as from standard bottles.[92]

Certainly parents play a role and could be major allies in the fight against obesity. One problem is that their own diets have deteriorated

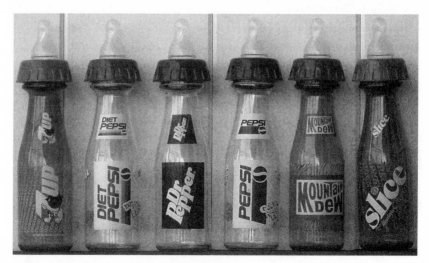

Figure 2.1 Baby Bottles with Logos (Photo courtesy of Matt Brownell.)

and their activity has declined. Research shows that parents' diet and exercise patterns predict a child's likelihood of being overweight, giving rise to the term "obesigenic families."[93] Parents need help to change their own lifestyles and to raise healthy children.

Parents must compete with television, movies, candy fund-raisers, schools filled with soft drinks, snack foods, and fast foods, and peer pressure to eat. They go toe-to-toe with creative people on Madison Avenue whose job is to win the hearts of their children. Children see ten advertisements *per hour* when they watch TV, most of them for unhealthy foods. Even the most motivated parents find themselves overpowered.

Yes, parents can forbid their children to watch TV and can keep unhealthy foods out of the house. But it is harder to shield children from food ads on billboards, cartoon and movie characters associated with food, and, of course, all the food the children encounter at school and from peers. Being a parent is hard enough without having to fight these forces.

Of Course Personal Responsibility Is Important

Calling on people to make better decisions and providing them with the skills to do so should always be the first step, always the default. This is consistent with our country's character and also with psychological principles; people who change through their own efforts have enhanced self-esteem and maintain the changes longer.

But personal responsibility is sometimes not enough. The country waited many years hoping for smokers to stop and for parents to protect their children from the tobacco companies. It was a good try, but insufficient, so local and national leaders stepped in with decisive action. High taxes have been levied on cigarettes, smoking has been prohibited in public places, and strong sanctions have been imposed for the marketing and sales of cigarettes to minors.

Our country has had a long history of intervening with regulation and legislation when personal responsibility falls short. People are required to wear helmets on motorcycles, wear seatbelts, buckle their children in car seats, obey speed limits, not pollute the environment, and so forth.

George Bray draws an interesting parallel between the prevention of dental caries (cavities) and the prevention of obesity.[94] Preventing cavities has a personal responsibility solution. If people brushed their teeth frequently, flossed as recommended, and did not eat sweets, cavities would be reduced greatly. But people are not perfect; hence, the nation does not rely solely on personal efforts to minimize tooth decay. So fluoride is introduced into the water to make it easy for people to protect their teeth.

People deserve an environment that promotes good health; it is fundamental to the country's vitality, productivity, and security. But they get the opposite—a finely crafted set of conditions that make it very difficult to eat reasonably and be active. If parents are to raise healthy children, if schools are to produce vital minds and bodies, and if future generations of Americans are to be healthy and happy, the environment must change.

Conclusion

The world is undergoing an immense transition in diet and patterns of physical activity. Millions upon millions of people are affected adversely by these changes, with the numbers growing by the day. The list of diseases caused by poor diet, physical inactivity, and obesity is long and disheartening. Beyond disheartening is the suffering caused by the combination of these diseases and the psychological and social consequences of being overweight.

Obesity is a major issue because (1) vast numbers of people are affected; (2) the prevalence is growing; (3) rates are increasing in children; (4) the medical, psychological, and social effects are severe; (5) the behaviors that cause it (poor diet and inactivity) are themselves major contributors to ill health; and (6) treatment is expensive, rarely effective, and impractical to use on a large scale.

Biology and environment conspire to promote obesity. Biology is an enabling factor, but the obesity epidemic, and the consequent human tragedy, is a function of the worsening food and physical activity environment. Governments and societies have come to this conclusion very late. There is much catching up to do.

SPREADING THE AMERICAN GOSPEL: On the Way to an Obese World

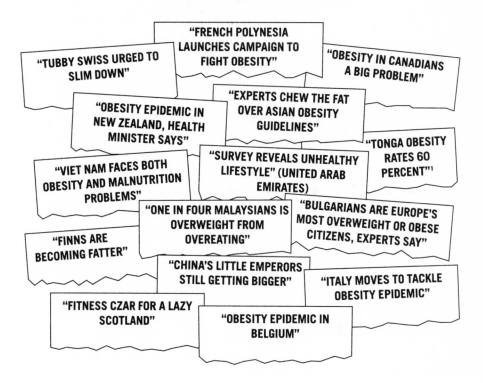

"FRENCH POLYNESIA LAUNCHES CAMPAIGN TO FIGHT OBESITY"

"TUBBY SWISS URGED TO SLIM DOWN"

"OBESITY IN CANADIANS A BIG PROBLEM"

"EXPERTS CHEW THE FAT OVER ASIAN OBESITY GUIDELINES"

"OBESITY EPIDEMIC IN NEW ZEALAND, HEALTH MINISTER SAYS"

"TONGA OBESITY RATES 60 PERCENT"[1]

"SURVEY REVEALS UNHEALTHY LIFESTYLE" (UNITED ARAB EMIRATES)

"VIET NAM FACES BOTH OBESITY AND MALNUTRITION PROBLEMS"

"BULGARIANS ARE EUROPE'S MOST OVERWEIGHT OR OBESE CITIZENS, EXPERTS SAY"

"ONE IN FOUR MALAYSIANS IS OVERWEIGHT FROM OVEREATING"

"FINNS ARE BECOMING FATTER"

"CHINA'S LITTLE EMPERORS STILL GETTING BIGGER"

"ITALY MOVES TO TACKLE OBESITY EPIDEMIC"

"FITNESS CZAR FOR A LAZY SCOTLAND"

"OBESITY EPIDEMIC IN BELGIUM"

And so the list goes—on and on and on.[1]

Much of the interest in obesity by the world press is prompted by surveys done by health ministries in various countries showing increased prevalence.[2] Escalating problems are clear in China, Canada, and Cameroon; Samoa, Spain, and the Seychelles; Poland, Paraguay, and Palau, just to begin.

Dr. Stephan Roessner, a scientist from Sweden and President of the International Association for the Study of Obesity, said, "There is no country in the world where obesity is not increasing. Even in [developing] countries we thought were immune [such as Zimbabwe and Gambia], the epidemic is coming on very fast. The frightening thing is that so far nobody has succeeded to stop it."[3] The World Health Organization (WHO) has declared obesity a global epidemic.[4]

The first major WHO obesity report, which declared the global epidemic, was in 1998. Only four years later, the WHO presented a picture even more dire.[5] More than 25 percent of Egyptian children are obese; the numbers are similar for Chile, Peru, Germany, and Mexico. Fifteen percent to 20 percent of four-year-olds are obese in Zambia and Morocco.

> In some areas of Africa, overweight children outnumber malnourished children three to one.

Obesity is increasing across all segments of society, adults and children, young and old, rich and poor, males and females. Rates are rising in Alaskan Eskimos, the Evenki (reindeer herders in Siberia), and the Walpiri (Australian Aborigines).[6] Few pockets in the world are left untouched.

Why the Global Crisis?

The simple answer is that people are eating more and exercising less. Why this occurs is more complex.

"Because they can" is a glib but probably correct answer. Economic factors, globalization, increasing urbanization, advances in energy-saving devices, and the glamorization of high-calorie, high-profit foods by the food industry, to name a few of the likely explanations, interact with biology to make overeating and sedentary behaviors very likely (see Chapter 2).

Physical inactivity joins eating as a central explanation for rising obesity. An article in the *Wall Street Journal* noted that:

- Swedish lumberjacks who may have burned 7,000 calories per day in heavy physical labor are being replaced by machines.
- Highway construction in Malaysia is being done with heavy machinery rather than picks and shovels.
- Bicycle sales in areas of China are declining and more people are buying motor scooters.[7]

Nutrition Transition

Barry Popkin from the University of North Carolina has coined the term "nutrition transition" to explain global changes in diet.[8] He has done the most thorough global examination of nutrition and activity changes, and defines five nutrition patterns that characterize different countries at different times:

- **Pattern 1: Collecting Food.** Food comes from hunting and gathering. The diet is high in carbohydrates and fiber and low in fat. Activity levels are high and there is little obesity.
- **Pattern 2: Famine.** Diet is less varied, scarcity occurs, and malnutrition is common. Obesity is rare.
- **Pattern 3: Receding Famine.** Consumption of fruit, vegetables, and animal protein increases as do inactivity and leisure time.
- **Pattern 4: Nutrition–Related Noncommunicable Disease.** The diet is high in fat, cholesterol, sugar, and other refined carbohydrates, and low in polyunsaturated fat and fiber. Sedentary behavior increases. Obesity increases as does chronic disease.
- **Pattern 5: Behavioral Change.** The desire to prevent disease leads to changes in diet and physical activity, sometimes self-driven by consumers and other times stimulated by government action.

Many countries are in pattern 3 or 4. In particular, many developing nations are making a rapid transition from receding famine to energy-dense diets and declining physical activity.

A good example is Popkin's analysis of China, an important case study both because the population is so large and because the Chinese experience may portend what occurs in other countries. The percentage of calories from fat in the Chinese diet was 10 percent in the 1970s, but now one-third of families eat a diet with more than 30 percent of calories from fat. The number of televisions has risen dramatically, and the number of jobs requiring physical labor is decreasing. Popkin points out that as countries like China have advanced from food shortages to a healthier diet, the line is quickly crossed where eating too much and weight gain become key concerns:

Changes in diet and activity patterns are fueling the obesity epidemic. These rapid changes in the levels and composition of dietary and activity/inactivity patterns in transitional societies are related to a number of socioeconomic and demographic changes.[9]

Following the U.S. Lead

Nation after nation is experiencing the same social, economic, and technological forces that have crafted America into an obese nation. High-calorie food is becoming more available around the globe. Technology's steady march forward is removing physical activity in most countries. Diseases caused by poor diet and inactivity follow on the heels of the changing environments.

Many cultural changes can increase eating and diminish activity. For instance, the growth of urban centers increases distance between masses of people and those who grow food, exposes people to more prepared and fast foods, and makes physical labor less likely. As another example, more women entering the workplace means less time (and economic incentive) for meals to be prepared at home.

Many factors contribute to obesity in a nation. Some are probably not yet recognized. The balance of factors varies from culture to culture, so the entire blame cannot be placed at the feet of any one cause, any one food, any one company, any one institution, or any one national policy. To say, however, that all foods, companies, institutions, and policies bear no blame is also shortsighted.[10]

The World's Food Supply in Transition

It would be convenient but wrong to blame the global epidemic only on the spread of American food. Other factors (like declining physical activity) are influential, but it is also the case that eating outside the home is rare in countries like India and China and that food patterns are determined much more by local factors than by outside influences.

The American experience *is* instructive to the extent that factors damaging diet and activity in the United States are occurring around the world. American food and lifestyles entering other countries may signal problems in the making.

Perhaps more than any American export, our food has powerful symbolic importance to the world's inhabitants. Both revered and hated, our food represents affluence and innovation. People in China, Australia, Spain, or the Bahamas may buy a Big Mac or have Kentucky Fried Chicken not only because the food tastes good, but also because it represents the perception of a good life. They buy a dream.

> When the first McDonald's in Kuwait opened in Kuwait City in 1994, 15,000 customers lined up for opening day.[11]

American food also represents the bloated U.S. lifestyle and American domination of the world. It may portend, in the eyes of non-Americans, obesity, poor health, and disability, along with takeover of local culture and further enrichment of America. Fair or not, our food generates strong feelings.

The spread of American food involves many companies. Coca-Cola, for instance, is in 200 countries selling 230 brands.[12] Frito-Lay, now part of PepsiCo, sells its snack foods around the globe. Mars Incorporated, makers of M&M's, Twix, Milky Way, Snickers, Starburst, Skittles, and more, has an M&M's website with messages in Danish, Spanish, Portuguese, and other languages.[13] The most controversial piece of the food picture, however, is fast food. Being the leading purveyor, McDonald's draws both admiration and ire, and it does so around the world.

> A McDonald's in Moscow's Pushkin Square serves 40,000 people every day.[14]

Over half of McDonald's sales come from outside the United States; Asian-Pacific sales alone accounted for almost 18 percent of that total in 2000.[15] With its 30,000 restaurants in 118 countries, McDonald's has a key global impact.[16] McDonald's opens a new restaurant every 17 hours[17] and is the world's largest user of beef.[18] KFC has more restaurants outside than within the United States.[19]

> **Which does not belong?** McDonald's sells each of the following overseas except:
> - Kiwi Burger
> - McHuevo
> - McNifica
> - McAfrika
> - McKoala
> - McLaks
> - Samurai Pork Burgers
> - Maharaja Mac
>
> **Answer:** McKoala

McDonald's modifies its selections to suit local needs, of course. Monthly, 3.2 million customers in India avoid taboo products such as beef and pork (Muslims are not to eat pork, and the Hindu religion holds cows sacred) and have a mutton burger called the Maharaja Mac. Respecting the many vegetarians in India, McDonald's separates vegetable and meat products during cooking.[20] McDonald's and its partners are planning to invest about $75 million dollars in the Indian market to more than triple the number of restaurants.[21]

In China, McDonald's has 350 restaurants and a workforce of 38,000. Workers make less than U.S. wages, but are paid more than many other employees in China, causing college graduates to line up for job opportunities.[22] Japan has more than 3,000 McDonald's franchises serving rice dishes and a fried chicken sandwich with soy sauce and ginger. Thai customers order Samurai Pork Burgers, a teriyaki-spiced sandwich that may have contributed to the chain's 10 to 15 percent increase in expansion in 1999 alone. Hong Kong has 158 franchises, which is one restaurant for every 42,000 residents, not far from the U.S. number, which approaches one restaurant for every 30,000 Americans.[23]

McDonald's is not the only fast-food company with a strong foreign presence. In New Delhi, India, seventeen McDonald's are joined by twenty Domino's Pizzas, eleven Pizza Huts, and nine Wimpy's franchises.[24] In 1989, Kentucky Fried Chicken was the first foreign fast-food franchise allowed to enter China. It has 490 outlets and a twenty-year goal of 5,000 franchises. A Nielsen poll ranked KFC the most recognized foreign brand in China, over Coke, Nestle, and Mickey Mouse. Chinese outlets have the most per-store sales worldwide.[25]

Pizza, considered by some the most representative of American fast foods, is a big seller abroad, creating fierce competition among chains such as Pizza Hut and Domino's. The top seller for Domino's in Japan is a pizza with mayonnaise, potatoes, and ham or bacon, while those in Hong Kong want Cajun spices and satay, according to Pizza Hut. The Thai request lemongrass and lime on their pizzas; people in England want tuna and sweet corn. Domino's has 2,094 chains in sixty-one countries, while Pizza Hut maintains 4,000 outlets in ninety countries.

Foreign fast-food companies competing in their own countries against American chains have learned American tactics. Bangkok restaurants have begun delivery service, following in the footsteps of KFC. Almost half of KFC's orders there are filled by delivery.[26]

> Dunkin' Donuts opened its 1,000th international shop in Thailand in 1995. Its 5,000th shop worldwide opened in Bali, Indonesia, in 2000. Dunkin' Donuts sells 6.4 million donuts per day (enough to circle the earth twice), totaling 2.3 billion donuts per year.[27]

What makes McDonald's, KFC, Coca-Cola, Pizza Hut, and Dunkin' Donuts thrive overseas? Certainly they are "pushed" into countries by American business interests, but there is pull as well. The foods taste good for the biological reasons discussed in Chapter 2. Technology inspires the economy, hence more people have more money and eating out is a treat. More demanding work makes convenience and "fast" food more attractive. Whether or not American food survives abroad, its presence reflects changing conditions.

Culture Shock, Backlash, and Bricks

Fierce debates occur over the place of fast food in foreign cultures. On one side are arguments that the companies simply respond to demand, so by definition their presence is accepted, even wanted. They provide local jobs, may purchase local supplies, and in some cases are owned by local businesspeople (who can cut their way through extensive red tape). One-quarter of McDonald's foreign outlets are owned by local individuals.[28] Some locals welcome the introduction of standards for cleanliness, foods they feel are safe, and even clean toilets.

Fast-food franchises are special in some cultures because of novelty and well-known advertising icons and because all things American are held in awe. Local people are known to save money to expose their children to "American culture" at fast-food chains, buying less expensive food for themselves later.

At the same time, there are worries that fast-food franchises threaten local customs and values and represent the worst of American influence. Complaints of homogenization of culture and standardization of cuisine are common, along with disapproval of local money going to U.S. companies.[29]

There have been protests in more than fifty countries at McDonald's restaurants alone.[30] Regular protests by anarchists occur in Paris and London.[31] Restaurants in Prague and Cape Town have endured attacks such as bricks hurled through windows.[32] Hindu activists have demanded that the Prime Minister shutter all McDonald's in India, which they consider an affront to the culture (especially after revelations that McDonald's used beef products to make its French fries).[33] Protests in New Delhi caused police to increase security and surveillance around all fast-food outlets. During the American bombing of Afghanistan from Pakistani airspace, Pakistan's Kentucky Fried Chicken outlets became targets for stoning and riots by virtue of their association with American culture.[34] Mexico's most famous living artist, Francisco Toledo, led a campaign to prevent the opening of a McDonald's restaurant in the main square of Oaxaca, a colonial city famous for its food.[35]

KFC entering India has become a celebrated case study in resistance to globalization.[36] The first KFC in India opened in 1995. Tens of thousands of people protested. Many stories emerged, including one in which local officials accused KFC of selling carcinogenic foods to farmers who protested anticipated changes in local agriculture. Farmers joined with antiglobalization demonstrators to pressure KFC in places such as Bangalore, and KFC has since abandoned business in India.

In *Fast Food Nation*, Schlosser notes: "The overseas critics of fast food are more diverse than America's old Soviet bloc adversaries. Farmers, leftists, anarchists, nationalists, environmentalists, consumer advocates, educators, health officials, labor unions, and defenders of animal rights have found common ground in a campaign against the perceived Americanization of the world. Fast food has become a target because it is so ubiquitous and because it threatens a fundamental aspect of national identity: how, where, and what people choose to eat."[37]

The Unique International Opportunity

History provides foreign nations with an opportunity no longer available to the United States. America has grown wise to the negative effects of poor diet and obesity, but poor foods and the companies selling them are cemented into both the U.S. economy and the American psyche. The horse has left the barn.

Most countries are not this far down the road. If alert to early signs of change, early response may be possible. Among the signs are:

- diminishing activity as a part of work
- diminishing activity in day-to-day life (transportation)
- more time devoted to sedentary activities (television, etc.)
- more opportunities for eating (food in schools, vending machines, restaurants, etc.)
- more eating out and snacking and increasing portion sizes
- increasing availability and promotion of energy-dense foods
- economic forces that encourage unhealthy eating (less time to prepare meals, etc.)

The United States can change only by retrofitting an entrenched and toxic environment. Other countries may be able to create a better fit between modernization and healthy lifestyles. Preserving native cultures may be one leverage point, but preventing the ravages of poor diet and inactivity is sensible on economic and humanitarian grounds. Countries can seize this special opportunity by shaping policies to their needs. Regulating food advertising may be possible in some countries, as may keeping poor foods from schools, helping children walk or bike to school, instituting food labeling regulations, and so on. Regional or even worldwide efforts might be especially powerful.

Success Stories

A number of countries in the world are alert to the obesity crisis and are beginning to take action.[38] Creative approaches are being tried, some with good results, but most programs are in the early stages of being evaluated. There is much countries can learn from one another.

Major Dietary Change in Mauritius

In Mauritius, a small, developing nation in the Indian Ocean, people had very high levels of cardiovascular risk factors and diabetes. One problem was a universally used cooking oil called ration oil that is high in palm oil (high in saturated fat). A five-year program began in which the government reduced palm oil in cooking oil and launched a program that encouraged lifestyle changes. This effort produced impressive changes in diet and cholesterol.[39]

Lessons from Finland

One of the earliest and most extensive lifestyle change programs occurred in Finland, centered originally in the district of North Karelia. In the early 1970s, Finnish men had the highest rates of heart disease in the world. To improve diet and other lifestyle factors, an ambitious program was launched that included education, TV announcements, and work with food and catering companies.

Over a period of twenty years, striking changes were made. The number of people using butter on bread went from 60 percent to 5 percent. Similarly, the number of people drinking fatty milk declined from about 40 percent to about 6 percent. Use of vegetable oil for cooking went from 2 percent of the population to 34 percent. These are only a few of the positive developments. From 1971 to 1995, the rate of ischemic heart disease dropped by 73 percent in North Karelia and 65 percent in all of Finland.[40]

Initial Efforts in Brazil and China

Brazil has undertaken a variety of programs to improve diet. Labeling is now required for packaged foods, legislation has been enacted to improve school food programs, work sites have been targeted for educational programs, and major efforts have been used to educate the public about healthy eating. Results are not yet available, but the Brazilian effort has shown that consensus requiring the input of multiple parties (health professionals, government, businesses, schools, etc.) can be reached and that creative programs can be implemented.[41]

A National Plan for Nutrition in China, along with programs for smoking and physical activity, has been implemented in recent years. With pork and fat intakes increasing and soy intake decreasing, efforts are being aimed at increasing vegetable consumption in northern China by using price adjustments and subsidies and increasing the conception and production of soybean products. Limited results have been reported thus far, but China is one of the few places where policy changes such as altering the price of food have been tried.[42]

Taking Action

Many countries are following the regrettable path taken by the United States. Diets grow worse, physical activity declines, and obesity increases. The U.S. experience has shown the extraordinary cost of waiting too long to act.

Nations at the early stages of the problem are in an ideal position to anticipate what looms ahead and to inoculate their citizens. We suggest that nations be aware of the warning signs mentioned above, but in addition they need to:

- Be aware that programs to feed hungry nations can overshoot the mark. Providing calories at low cost is a priority when shortages are the issue, but when availability of poor foods becomes extreme, overnutrition can supersede malnutrition as the top priority.
- Track the prevalence of obesity in both children and adults. Increasing prevalence in children in particular should be considered an ominous warning.
- Resist the temptation to blame individuals for the problem and to rely solely on calls for personal responsibility. The environment will overwhelm any such efforts.

- Recognize the need to intervene early and to address the problem of prevention in children. Treatment is difficult, costly, and not very effective, so prevention is an obvious focus.
- Do not permit the negative influences of food companies to flourish without challenge. Brand loyalties and preferences for certain foods can be difficult to reverse once established. Regulation of advertising may be a necessary step. Children need to be protected from inducements to eat unhealthy food.
- Enlist institutions designed to protect children, such as schools, to avoid contributing to poor diet and inactivity. They should be engaged as agents for positive change.
- Develop and test strategies for intervening in local environments. Encouraging local creativity is likely to generate many new approaches that may be adapted for use elsewhere. An example is a system for setting local priorities developed by Boyd Swinburn and colleagues in New Zealand that is sensitive to local customs and takes advantage of local resources.[43]
- Establish a culture in which promoting unhealthy food is unpopular, much as the United States has done with tobacco. Public pressure on celebrities to endorse only healthy products and popular publications refusing to advertise some products are examples of changing a culture. Each such move helps mobilize public opinion.

Conclusion

Obesity, poor diet, and physical inactivity are problems around the world. Many factors are responsible, but some common economic, social, and cultural themes are clear. There are opportunities for the world to learn from America's history, its mistakes, and its innovations. Many countries may have the opportunity to intervene before the environment grows so bad it can no longer be subdued.

PART 2

THE TOXIC ENVIRONMENT

EXERCISE MAYHEM:
Unendangering
Physical Activity

*Imagine a future like this: every community in America enjoys the benefits
of a seamless network linking trails, sidewalks, on-road bicycling facilities,
and mass transit. Such a network would connect homes, schools, shops,
families, and friends. It would provide residents—young, old, and in-
between—the choice of mobility without the automobile. Such a vision is
not anticar. In fact, it would benefit drivers by getting people off the road
that now have no other transportation choice. A national commitment to
creating communities conducive to walking and biking would do wonders for
improving the health of our people and the places where they live.*

—Congressional Testimony of Keith Laughlin, President
of the Rails-to-Trails Conservancy[1]

In this time of controversy on how to respond to raging obesity, all
parties agree on one thing: physical activity is a key player. It is central to health, well-being, and weight control and must increase if there
is hope of reversing the obesity epidemic.

The environment, much as it encourages overeating, makes sedentary behavior almost inevitable. As with food, one can take the individual responsibility approach, educate or implore people to be more
active, and then hope for the best. This may be helpful for some people
in some settings, but broader change is necessary. Scientist Steven Blair
of the Cooper Institute and colleagues say just this:

Clinical interventions and mass appeals to be more physically active are limited in effectiveness against the background of increasingly sedentary lifestyles. Exercise scientists and public health officials need to turn attention to public policy and legislative initiatives to restructure physical and social environments to encourage more activity and discourage sedentary habits.[2]

People were once paid to exercise—jobs required physical work. Today the most physically demanding feature of many jobs might be swiveling in a desk chair. Most streets are not safe for walking, biking, or playing. Stairs in many buildings are inaccessible, dark, and unattractive. Few children walk or bike to school, and once they arrive, inactivity is the norm. Energy-saving devices make nearly every physical action require less effort.

This environment of inactivity is a blueprint for banking rather than burning calories. As the population eats more, substantial increases in exercise would be needed just to keep weight stable. But activity has declined and declined a lot. This is bad news because exercise can help prevent weight gain and reduces risk for many of the leading causes of death.

One study found that 14 percent of all deaths could be attributed to the combination of diet and physical inactivity. Another estimated that 23 percent of all deaths from major chronic diseases could be attributed to sedentary lifestyle.[3]

A Primer on Exercise and Health

The study of physical activity and life span began with the 1873 book *University Oars* by John Edward Morgan.[4] He followed men who had rowed in the famous (and strenuous) Oxford–Cambridge crew race in England. The rowers lived longer than their more sedentary peers.

Sophisticated research on the topic started with the pioneering work in the 1960s by Jeremy Morris in London and Ralph Paffenbarger in

California, but even before, some experts believed that exercise was necessary for good health. Cardiologist Paul Dudley White, personal physician to President Eisenhower, defied prevailing wisdom when Eisenhower had a heart attack by suggesting that the heart needed exercise to be strong, not rest to be preserved.

Jeremy Morris compared the health of London bus drivers to that of conductors who made repeated trips up and down the stairs of double-decker buses collecting tickets. The conductors had better health. Morris found similar results comparing letter carriers to postal employees with desk jobs. In the United States, Ralph Paffenbarger studied people with physically demanding jobs, such as longshoremen. He found what has now been cemented into scientific truth—more physical activity leads to better health, longer life, and better quality of life.

Then came a generation of top-rate scientists who specified the effects of exercise on health, among them Blair, Russell Pate, Jack Wilmore, William Haskell, Peter Wood, and Michael Pollock. Two landmark events were the 1996 publication of the Surgeon General's Report on Physical Activity and Health (edited by Blair) and the broad changes in exercise recommendations issued jointly in 1995 by the Centers for Disease Control and the American College of Sports Medicine (Pate and Blair were key figures).[5]

The universal agreement about the importance of physical activity has moved it to the top of the priority list for national agencies, helped along by scientists who believe it is an easier problem to tackle than food and by a food industry that would like nothing better than to focus attention on activity rather than eating. Changing eating habits requires battling with powerful combatants, while no groups are organized to fight physical activity. This is an area, therefore, where considerable innovation and consensus are possible.

A Population Good at Being Still

Health experts recommend at least thirty minutes of physical activity per day, but few people accomplish this.[6] Twenty-seven percent of American adults engage in no physical activity at all, and 28 percent more are not regularly active. More than two-thirds of Americans are trying to lose weight or maintain their current weight, but only 20 percent of this group exercises more than 150 minutes per week. Low as these numbers are, they might overstate activity; sedentary adults tend to overestimate the intensity of their physical activity.[7] Women, older people, non-Hispanic African Americans, and Mexican Americans are most likely to be inactive.

Most discouraging is inactivity in children.[8] Almost half of all children do not participate in *any* regular physical activity. Fifty-five-year-old adults are more likely to get regular exercise than are twelve- to seventeen-year-old children. In addition, activity declines during adolescence; by ages sixteen to seventeen, 56 percent of black girls and 31 percent of white girls have no leisure-time activity at all.

> Only 13 percent of all trips to school are made by walking or bicycling. Fewer than 10 percent of children walk or bike to school regularly, down from 66 percent thirty years ago.[9]

Study after study shows that the absence of physical activity is related to poor health. The reverse is also true—people who get regular exercise have less disease, engage less in other unhealthy behaviors, and live longer.[10] Being active is linked to lower rates of heart disease, diabetes, high blood pressure, stroke, and colon cancer, among other diseases. A study of 73,000 postmenopausal women found impressive reductions in risk of cardiovascular events (heart attacks, stroke, etc.) with either regular walking or more vigorous exercise.[11]

Being inactive also hurts children.[12] Indicators of heart disease can be found in childhood. Inactive children have higher blood pressure and lower levels of HDL (good) cholesterol. Lack of exercise combines with poor diet to produce obesity in children, which can lead to Type 2 diabetes.[13]

Studies have shown considerable benefit of regular physical activity on mental health and well-being.[14] Some studies, for instance, have found that exercise is as effective for depression as both medication and a widely used form of psychotherapy. Other psychological issues such as anxiety also tend to improve as people become more active.

It is interesting to ask whether inactivity causes obesity or the reverse. Overweight people are more inactive than their thinner peers,[15] and the prevalence of obesity has risen while physical activity has declined. But gaining weight makes exercise less likely, so it is possible that obesity causes inactivity and not the reverse.

Following a cohort of people over time (longitudinal research) is better for defining cause and effect. Two such studies in Denmark found that physical activity did not predict later obesity, but obesity predicted drops in activity.[16] Balanced against this are studies showing that low levels of physical activity predict weight gain.[17] While the science is not yet perfectly clear, it appears that people with low levels of activity are prone to weight gain and that people who increase activity derive considerable benefit.

There is no doubt that exercise helps people lose weight, but more importantly, helps with maintenance of weight loss.[18] The central role of exercise in weight maintenance is shown with the National Weight Control Registry, a group of more than 3,000 successful maintainers assembled by James Hill at the University of Colorado and Rena Wing at Brown University.[19] The average person in the registry has lost sixty-six pounds and kept it off for six years. Being physically active is the factor most consistently related to weight maintenance.

Fat and Fit?

Groundbreaking work on fitness and weight has been done by Blair and colleagues at the Cooper Institute.[20] They have shown that the advantages of being fit are striking and that people can be fit even if they are fat. Blair and others had a big impact by showing that physical (cardiorespiratory) fitness is related to longer life and that even moderate levels of activity greatly reduce risk for major killers such as heart disease. Even activities like regular walking are now considered beneficial.

But most striking is the discovery regarding fitness in overweight individuals. People who are overweight *can* be physically fit and thus have lowered risk of disease. A remarkable finding is that heavy people who are fit have lower risk than thin people who are unfit. This information offers considerable hope; overweight people can improve their health even if weight loss is difficult to achieve.

Blair's group in Dallas followed with more discoveries. Among them were that: (1) for men, being lean is associated with good health only in those who are fit; (2) low fitness in men with Type 2 diabetes carries very high risk; (3) the lowest risk for the metabolic syndrome occurs in those most fit; and (4) fitness provides protection against cardiovascular disease in men who already have one major risk factor (hypertension).

While one can be fat and fit, it is important to remember that there is a strong tendency for obesity to be coupled with inactivity. Most overweight people are inactive for reasons of embarrassment, low self-confidence with sports and exercise, lack of programs designed for their needs, and, of course, the physical burden of the excess weight.

Why All the Inactivity?

Many factors converge to make the population inactive. As with the food environment in transition, the nation was late to respond to the troubling changes in physical activity until a crisis existed.

Advances in Technology

It is widely agreed that technology, while it fuels economies and aids humankind, also promotes obesity by reducing the need for physical activity.[21] Let's chronicle a day in the life of Mr. America, not the pumped-up specimen who wins muscle contests, but the average person.

Mr. America rises in the morning, uses an electric toothbrush and coffeemaker, and then has a meal in a can (such as Slim-Fast) or visits a drive-in window. Buttons open his car and garage doors. In his car he uses power steering and brakes, a switch rather than a crank to open the window, and a button rather than a dial to tune the radio. Adjusting the outside mirrors no longer requires a reach. At work he uses an elevator rather than stairs, a computer rather than a typewriter, E-mail rather than walking to speak with a colleague, and a hard disk rather than a file cabinet to store information.

Back home after work, the TV remote lets him change channels dozens of times without moving from the chair and a microwave helps him prepare dinner. He can slice meat with an electric knife, chop vegetables with a food processor, and make drinks with a blender. Dishes will be cleaned with a dishwasher and trash compacted by a machine. There is about a fifty-fifty chance he would have avoided even this little effort by going out to dinner. Playing golf could be done with a cart, cutting the grass with a self-powered mower, and shopping with the Internet. Separately, each convenience may not seem important, but the cumulative effect, added over days, weeks, months, and years is enormous.

> The tiny bit of exercise required to buy food while pumping gas (walking to and from the convenience store) may soon disappear. Computer touch screens on gas pumps are being tested that will allow you to select items in the market. The Fritos, Coke, and Twinkies will be charged to your credit card and hand-delivered to your car.

Technology has made us lazy and has stifled the creativity needed to structure environments that encourage activity. Few buildings have convenient, centrally located, and attractive staircases. Unsafe, busy streets and the absence of bike paths make people reluctant to walk or bike to work or school. Only a minority of communities have paths designated for walking and biking.

An Auto-Centric Country

If you happen to be a car, truck, or bus in the United States, you're in the right place. Trillions of dollars have been spent helping you get around and insuring that the population uses you as much as possible.

You don't have much competition, because most streets and highways are not suitable for people who wish to move about by foot or bicycle.

Suburban sprawl is part of the reason; as things spread out, people must use cars. Neighborhood schools and downtown stores have given way to schools away from the population and strip malls on busy streets.[22] Jeffrey Koplan and William Dietz from the Centers for Disease Control and Prevention (CDC) cite U.S. Department of Transportation figures estimating that one-fourth of all trips are less than one mile in distance but 75 percent are made by car.[23]

A report entitled "Mean Streets" by the Surface Transportation Policy project notes that streets are dangerous, so people avoid walking or biking. The most dangerous of all are in:

[P]laces where sprawling development has often left pedestrians stranded. Wide roads have been built without sidewalks or frequent crosswalks, and high-speed traffic makes those roadways particularly deadly. In many areas, intersections with crosswalks may be as much as a half-mile apart, leaving pedestrians with no safe way to cross the street.[24]

The same report noted that the number of trips taken on foot has dropped by 42 percent in the last twenty years.

> A study done across eight provinces in China found that people who lived in a household with motorized transportation had an 80 percent increased chance of being obese. Men who acquired a motorized form of transportation were 100 percent more likely to become obese than those who did not.[25]

In old neighborhoods, where there are sidewalks, safer streets, and opportunities to walk to schools and stores, people get more activity.[26]

Television, Computers, Video Games

Of all aspects of technology, television watching has probably been the most often studied by obesity researchers. As mentioned in Chapter 2, there is a robust connection between the amount of television people watch and both their likelihood of becoming obese and of having elevated risk factors. TV may affect obesity by increasing the desire to eat, but also keeps people sedentary.

A number of studies have examined whether people who watch TV are more likely to be sedentary, with some studies showing this to be the case and others not.[27] We suspect that competing sedentary activities, such as time on the computer, may dilute the relationship that is seen between TV and physical activity. For instance, two people may be highly sedentary, but one watches television and the other uses the computer. A study including these two people would not show an association of television watching with inactivity because the two people would cancel each other out.

Children are engaged with the computer. Surfing the Internet, playing games, and connecting with friends occupy children for hours at a time, in some cases making television itself passé. To be a child no longer requires a trip to the library, the park, or a friend's house. An ad for Dell Computer shows children at home around a computer with the caption "Stay in and Play."

Schools

In many schools, being physically active every day is a distant memory. Some require no physical education at all; others require little. When children are in PE classes, much of the time they are not moving. As of 2000, Illinois was the only state to require daily physical education in all schools.

It is hard to blame school administrators. The same financial realities that make soft drink money appealing, as explained in Chapter 7, necessitate spending cutbacks. The pressure to improve achievement scores motivates administrators to protect a school's educational core, so classes thought not to contribute to performance on standardized tests disappear. As an example, Georgia's school overhaul bill eliminated mandatory PE in grades six through eight, mandating PE only for grades kindergarten through five. The change occurred when thirty additional minutes of academic courses were added to the curriculum. As a result, PE was cut in order to protect programs such as band and chorus.[28]

Schools and activity are not the same partners they used to be.[29] Thirty-five percent of students in high school do not engage in regular vigorous physical activity, and almost half do not play on sports teams. Only 29 percent participate in physical activity classes, a decrease from 42 percent in 1991, and of course few children walk or bike to school. In fact, bicycle sales have decreased from the 1970s. One study found that children spend only twelve to thirteen minutes daily engaged in vigorous physical activity, compared to ten hours in sedentary activities. Two hours weekly of sport or physical activity is the national goal in Britain, but only 25 percent of children currently meet this goal.[30]

If children do not engage in structured activity through classes, they will not be active elsewhere in school. A study in San Diego found that only 2 percent of girls and 6 percent of boys chose to be active during unstructured time.[31]

The Chrysler Fund Amateur Athletic Union tested youth fitness and found that among 9.7 million six- to seventeen-year-olds, children are getting weaker overall and slower on endurance runs. There has been a 10 percent decrease in distance run scores and an 11 percent decrease in "satisfactory" ratings on the entire test.[32] The Shape of the Nation Report stated that most high school students participate in only one year of physical education between ninth and twelfth grades.[33] Even those who do get formal physical education may not actually exercise. In many cases, the PE instruction does not conform to exercise recommendations: in 1997, only 70 percent of high school students enrolled in PE reported being physically active, compared to 81 percent in 1991.[34]

In an average gym class, a child is aerobically active for only 3.5 minutes.[35]

Whether or not a school requires PE, facilities make a difference. James Sallis and colleagues in San Diego studied 25 public middle schools and found that children were four to five times more likely to be active in schools with good physical facilities and adult supervision.

The researchers concluded, "The main findings of this study can be summarized by paraphrasing a line from the movie *Field of Dreams*: If we build it, they will come—and be active."[36]

Creative Means of Increasing Physical Activity

A number of experts have called for public health approaches to increasing activity, focusing on community interventions, removing barriers to exercise, and changing the environment.[37] Some creative programs have been developed to encourage people to move more.[38] These programs represent only local victories thus far, but if supported, might have an impact nationwide.

Colorado on the Move

An ambitious and innovative program, Colorado on the Move (COM), has been launched by James Hill and colleagues at the University of Colorado Health Sciences Center.[39] The innovation is in finding an inexpensive means of increasing physical activity (people get step counters and information on activity) and in connecting with people through many channels (schools, work sites, churches, walking clubs, physicians, etc.). The ambition comes from Hill and colleagues wanting to increase activity in Coloradoans first and then go nationwide.

The objective is to prevent weight gain in the population by increasing physical activity. Hill figures that the exercise message (get more steps) is simpler to convey than complex messages about nutrition, that the step counter is an inexpensive means for achieving this objective, and, as we mentioned earlier, there are no enemies. COM funding, in fact, comes from insurance, pharmaceutical, and other health-related companies, but also from Kraft, General Mills, Kellogg, McDonald's, Coke, Pepsi, and the National Cattlemen's Beef Association.

There is some consensus that 10,000 steps per day is a level helpful for both health and weight control. The Colorado on the Move group found that only about 15 percent of children and even fewer adults in

Colorado meet this level. The goal of COM is for people to make a 2,000-step per day increase in their activity, on the way to the final goal of at least 10,000 per day.

People can buy step counters from the COM website for $19, can be put in touch with community organizations and other resources, and have access to information on physical activity, weight, and health. Work sites, schools, churches, and other institutions are encouraged to start activity programs and are given ideas on implementation (e.g., teachers are given suggestions for integrating small bouts of activity into classroom instruction).

The Colorado on the Move program is now being evaluated, but the initial signs are positive. The program has generated a wide base of financial support; has been very visible in the state; has been embraced by business, education, church, and government leaders; and has generated considerable interest from the public.

Health Partners 10,000 Steps

Health Partners, a Health Maintenance Organization in the Minneapolis area, has also made innovative use of step counters.[40] Members of the organization are provided with step counters and encouraged to increase steps, with an ultimate goal of 10,000 steps per day. Information on physical activity is made available on the Web, but in addition, participants receive a personal action planner, a tracking log for steps, seven motivational mailings over eight months, and prize drawings as an incentive for participation.

The program is very popular, and data from the first ninety-two participants showed good results. There was a 69 percent increase in the number of steps in the first eight weeks, with 31 percent of the participants reaching the 10,000-step goal. At the eight-month mark, more than 90 percent felt they were meeting health recommendations for physical activity and 65 percent were still using the step counter.

Encouraging Use of Stairs

Using stairs is one opportunity to increase activity in daily life. Using stairs burns more calories per minute than most other physical activities, can be done in small or large amounts, and is available to most people at home, at work, and in other settings. Elevators, escalators, and moving stairs move double the population of the United States and Canada combined *each day* (210 billion passengers each year in the United States).[41] Ross Andersen of Johns Hopkins University estimates this saves 34 million pounds worth of calories each year in excess weight.

Over a period of about twenty-five years, a number of scientists have tested whether signs posted at the base of stairs would increase the number of people choosing stairs over escalators and elevators. Every study has worked!

A first study in Philadelphia was done by one of us (KB) along with Albert Stunkard and Jan Albaum in 1980. More than 45,000 people were observed using stairs versus escalators in a center city shopping mall, commuter train station, and bus terminal. After finding that only 5 percent of people used the stairs, we placed a sign between the stairs and escalators. Produced by Tony Auth, Pulitzer Prize–winning political cartoonist from the *Philadelphia Inquirer*, the sign said "Your Heart Needs Exercise, Here's Your Chance." Stair use nearly tripled, increasing significantly in both thin and heavy people.[42]

In 1995 researchers in Scotland used a sign saying, "Stay Healthy, Save Time, Use the Stairs" where stairs and escalators were adjacent in a city center underground (subway) station. Twenty-two thousand people were studied and stair use increased from 8 percent to about 16 percent.[43]

In two studies researchers from Johns Hopkins University tested signs that encouraged stair use for either heart health or weight control. Both led to significantly increased use of stairs.[44] Finding that the signs had a greater impact on white than black individuals, the scientists designed a second study to increase stair use specifically in African Americans. They showed a picture of an African American woman in a sign that said, "No time for exercise? Try the stairs." While more whites than blacks used the stairs, the sign worked as intended and had a large impact on African American individuals.

Researchers at the University of Minnesota tested the impact of using signs and having artwork and music in stairwells of office buildings. The sign alone did not increase stair use, but there were significant increases when artwork and music were used together.[45]

A team from the University of Texas at El Paso used a sign with a family message ("Do It! For the Life of Your Family") that had the words in both Spanish and English. They tested the effects of the sign in an airport, bank, office building, and university. Overall, stair use increased from 3 percent to 9 percent. While this may not seem like a big increase, the number of people potentially affected is very large and the cost of the sign is very low.[46]

These studies show that an inexpensive approach can increase use of stairs significantly. The most successful studies did not get stair use much above 15 percent to 20 percent, so there is much room for improvement, but even at this level the impact could be substantial because so many millions of people would be affected.

Schools on the Move

Many schools have implemented plans to increase physical activity, some in quite creative ways. Even if schools have required physical education, the way it is implemented will make a big difference. Increasing time in PE classes where children mostly stand around is not likely to have a health impact nor to teach children a love of activity that carries on in later years.

The issue of activity in schools is not specific to the United States. An Irish study found that less than 40 percent of primary school children exercised vigorously, while 75 percent spent more than two hours each day with the TV or computer.[47] One elementary school in Thailand launched a fitness and diet program after learning that it had one of the highest obesity rates in the country; almost 900 of the 4,000 elementary school students were classified as overweight. The program led 400 of the 900 children to lose weight.[48]

A district in the United Kingdom proposed an auto-free zone for a quarter-mile area around the school to reduce traffic and encourage children to be more active.[49] This was necessary because the number of children getting regular PE in the UK had fallen dramatically. The Kids for Life program in the UK aims to counteract that trend, scheduling forty-five-minute activity sessions designed to reach all primary school children, athletic or not. The program was introduced to 1,000 primary schools in June 2000.[50] Seventy-five schools in Nova Scotia have begun using step counters to help children be more active.[51]

CATCH and SPARK Programs. As creative as they are, most programs in schools have not been tested, so it is not possible to know whether they work or are worth the cost. A striking exception has been a series of programs undertaken in San Diego by James Sallis, Philip Nader, Thomas MacKenzie, and their associates. These researchers have shown that physical activity can be made fun, can be integrated into the school curriculum, and can truly increase physical activity.

The two most notable projects sound like alphabet soup, but are quite innovative. They are CATCH (Child and Adolescent Trial for Cardiovascular Health) and SPARK (Sports, Play, and Recreation for Kids).[52] These programs have been implemented to incorporate activity into the school routine, to increase movement in PE classes and in school in general, and to encourage children to be active outside of school. The results have shown improvements in children's physical activity, diet, and medical outlook, and in some cases have shown enduring effects that last for some years beyond the end of the program.

There are good, tested programs available as communities and schools enhance their focus on physical activity.

Does Exercise Time Interfere with Academics? Physical education is often curtailed in schools because academic classes are considered more important; time in PE is thought to interfere with learning because other classes get pushed aside. This was put to a test in a two-year study in San Diego by examining standardized test scores. Having a physical education course did not interfere with academic performance; in fact, students receiving physical education outperformed those who did not on several subjects. A British study also found no damage to academic performance.[53]

At a conference on "Learning and the Brain," researchers lamented PE cuts in schools, noting that exercise may improve brain function, elevate mood, and promote learning. Exercise improves blood flow to the brain and spurs cell growth, leading some to compare the brain to muscle, which performs best when exercised. Research by Chuck Hillman and colleagues at the University of Illinois showed that physical fitness is related to increased decision speed on a response test.[54]

There are a number of reasons why physical activity would be linked with better academic performance. Exercise can decrease stress and anxiety and increase self-esteem in adolescents. Active children are less likely to smoke or use drugs and are more likely to behave well and stay in school. Research with adolescents shows that low physical activity is associated with lower fruit and vegetable consumption; higher cigarette, alcohol, and marijuana use; more time watching TV; less use of seat belts; and perception of low academic performance.[55]

Activity Programs Sponsored by the Food Industry

The food industry has been active in creating or supporting programs designed to increase physical activity. Some programs are quite good.

Launched in 2002, the Kidnetic program (www.kidnetic.com) is an engaging, colorful, and appealing program dealing with both diet and activity, aimed at children ages nine through twelve. It was developed by the International Food Information Council (IFIC). IFIC's description of its aim and backing is "to communicate science-based information on food safety and nutrition to health and nutrition professionals, educators, journalists, government officials and others providing information to consumers. IFIC is supported primarily by the broad-based food, beverage and agricultural industries."[56]

The Kidnetic program has excellent content and was designed with the input of a number of professional organizations (American College of Sports Medicine, American Academy of Family Physicians, and National Recreation and Park Association, as examples). It has helpful information, cute characters, a way for children to discuss important issues, and more.

Also launched in 2002, Coca-Cola has a Step With It! program that encourages children to be more physically active. It was developed with the National Association for Sport and Physical Education. The Step With It! program encourages children to be more active, giving children step counters and encouraging them to have a minimum of 10,000 steps per day.

The Upsides and Downsides to Industry Programs. Industry has the money to develop state-of the-art materials, websites, and means for dissemination. Organizations of health professionals do not have such resources, nor do state health departments, parent groups, or others who wish to promote exercise.

Two key questions must be addressed. The first is whether these programs work. They might have been tested for appeal, and the number of hits to websites may indicate interest and visibility. But this is different than showing that people truly use the programs. Do the programs in fact lead to lasting (or even temporary) changes in physical activity?

The second question pertains to the broader context in which these programs exist. We must understand the total impact on children before proceeding. The nation must know whether: (1) sponsorships by food and beverage companies divert attention from the food and drinks they sell; (2) companies like Coca-Cola have implicit or explicit expectations of what schools will do in return when a program is offered; (3) sponsorship affects children's image of a company and the likelihood of consuming its products; and (4) the overall impact is positive or negative, adding together the impact on activity, food intake, emotional attachments to specific food companies, and so on.

Community Programs

Community approaches shift the focus from the individual (a medical/clinical model) to a public health approach that emphasizes changes in the physical environment and in social networks and structures.[57] These have considerable potential.

The KidsWalk-to-School Program, a program supported by the U.S. Department of Public Health, the Centers for Disease Control and Prevention, the National Center for Chronic Disease Prevention and Health Promotion, and the Division of Nutrition and Physical Activity, is designed to encourage children to walk or bike to school in groups accompanied by adults. The program has a website that provides information on physical activity in general and on getting to school in particular, as does a similar program in England.[58]

Chatelaine, a Canadian media group, and The Canadian Association for the Advancement of Women and Sport and Physical Activity (CAAWS) have created On-the-Move Walking Clubs to inspire women to enjoy exercise with their friends. Chatelaine maintains a "virtual fitness talk forum" to help women connect with other walkers.[59]

The Bikes Belong Coalition maintains a website devoted to seeking funding for bicycle facilities.[60] In California, the organization supports the LA River Bikeway Project, which will provide a path for an expected 5,000 bicycle commuters and 2,500 recreational cyclers daily.[61] California communities, in conjunction with local governmental agencies, have organized conferences on using community design to promote exercise.[62] The London Cycle Network, planned for completion in 2008, will provide 1,800 miles of new bicycle tracks.[63]

The National Trails System Act of 1968 led to the Rails-to-Trails Conservancy, which has been successful in converting abandoned railroad tracks to trails for bicycles and pedestrians. Another federal program, the Intermodal Surface Transportation Efficiency Act, implemented in 1991, calls for federal transportation funds to be directed to states for bicycle and walking projects.[64]

The Rails-to-Trails group has had an important impact. It focuses not only on helping local communities plan and build trails, but on national policy to make funds available for building more trails. There is support for their efforts in scientific studies; trails in communities get used and increase physical activity.[65]

In testimony before the U.S. House of Representatives Subcommittee on Highways and Transit, Keith Laughlin, President of the Rails-to-Trails Conservancy, noted several examples where community and federal funds have been used to build trails:

- The Pinellas Trail, forty-seven miles long, runs from St. Petersburg to Tarpon Springs, Florida. It now has 90,000 users per month. Approximately 67 percent of trips are for commuting or with a destination in mind, rather than simply recreation.
- The Monon Trail is a thirteen-mile corridor between Indianapolis and Carmel, Indiana. This trail connects many local

destinations, including parks, libraries, museums, cafes, bike shops, workplaces, schools, and a farmer's market. This former railroad right-of-way is once again becoming a transportation corridor.

• The Burke-Gilman Trail is eighteen miles long, running between Seattle and Bothell, Washington. This beautiful trail is now used by 2,500 bicycle commuters each day, connecting to many destinations in Seattle.[66]

The Centers for Disease Control and Prevention has undertaken a number of initiatives regarding physical activity. One has been to collect and disseminate information on programs proven to help increase activity. A major emphasis has been on community programs that have the potential to affect large segments of the population.[67]

Some very clever programs have been developed, implemented, and, in a few cases, tested. These provide a place to begin when thinking of creative ways to make the nation more active.

Is Activity Sufficient by Itself?

A key question in the overall effort to prevent obesity is whether the battle can be won by focusing on food or physical activity alone. Ideally, activity alone would be sufficient. People like to eat, food tastes good, and fighting the food industry is daunting. However, we believe that changes in both areas are necessary, for the following reasons:

1. Poor diet increases disease risk even in people who are active and are not overweight. Similarly, being sedentary increases risk even in people who eat well and are thin. Maximum health benefit will occur if the population changes both eating and activity.
2. Studies have shown that combining diet and exercise is more effective than using either alone in helping people maintain weight loss.

3. It is not clear whether simply making exercise available will compel enough people to increase activity to lower the prevalence of obesity.
4. Some people will probably respond more positively to changing exercise, others to changing food intake, and yet others to both. Attacking the problem on all fronts probably offers the greatest hope.

Success Stories
Biking to School in Oxfordshire, England
Less than 1 percent of children in England bike to school, but about 50 percent do at Watchfield primary school in Oxfordshire. Each morning a "train" of children on bicycles led by an adult winds through the village, picking up children along the way. Parent guards at the middle and end of the train keep the group in tight formation. Response by parents, teachers, and children has been very positive, with teachers saying the children are more alert and perform better at school.[68]

Travel to School in Marin County
Activists in Marin County, California, urged parents to walk the routes their children take to school and make a list of hazards (intersections without crosswalks, uneven sidewalks, etc.). The parents then lobbied local government officials to change things. This was part of a two-year campaign to make safer bike paths and bike lanes. The number of students who used the routes doubled.[69]

National Cycle Network in Britain
In England, 2 percent of trips are made by bicycle compared to up to 20 percent on the European continent. To improve things, 6,500 miles of cycling trails, expected to increase to 10,000 miles by 2005, have been created in England, using car-free paths and traffic-calmed roads. The routes are very popular and in some areas, communities have been creative in publicizing use of the trails and of making them appealing

(e.g., adding sculptures). The network is promoted in part by Sustrans, an organization devoted to sustainable transportation.[70]

Wheeling Walks

Researchers at West Virginia University, supported by the Robert Wood Johnson Foundation, initiated a program in the city of Wheeling using television, radio, and newspaper ads to increase walking. One ad, for example, shows a happy couple giving up a television show so they can walk together. The program was associated with a 32 percent increase in the number of people who walked at least thirty minutes daily five times a week, compared to 18 percent in a control community where the ads were not shown.[71]

Indy in Motion (in Indianapolis)

Initiated through the national group Partnership to Promote Healthy Eating and Active Living, Indy in Motion has brought together numerous groups and organizations in Indianapolis to promote healthy lifestyles. One program, "A Walk in the Park," supports walking and other activity programs in nine city parks.[72]

Project Active in Dallas

Researchers at the Cooper Institute developed an innovative program that can be used to counsel individuals or small groups about being physically active. The two-year program, which emphasizes integrating activity into day-to-day routines, improves physical activity, fitness, and disease risk factors.[73]

Increasing Activity at Xerox

A four-year study found that Xerox employees who participated in the company's wellness plan designed to encourage healthier lifestyles had fewer worker's compensation claims and lower costs for on-site injuries. Xerox reported a return of five to one on their investment for this program.[74]

Sisters Together: Move More, Eat Better

Developed through the Weight-control Information Network of the National Institutes of Health, this program is "designed to encourage Black women 18 and older to maintain a healthy weight by becoming more physically active and eating healthier foods."[75] The program began in Boston and is expanding. It includes work with radio and TV stations, written materials, and a creative means of community organizing.

Planet Health

This Boston program, developed by Steven Gortmaker, Karen Peterson, and colleagues at Harvard, is "an interdisciplinary curriculum focused on improving the health and well-being of sixth- through eighth-grade students while building and reinforcing skills in language arts, math, science, social studies, and physical education."[76] This is a creative program woven through the school curriculum. In a study of 1,295 students, the Planet Health program

- decreased TV time for both boys and girls
- increased fruit and vegetable consumption in girls
- reduced the prevalence of obesity in girls
- reduced increases in calorie intake in girls
- improved the remission of obesity in girls

Taking Action

Increasing the nation's activity can improve health and well-being, but another beneficiary may be the environment. The distance people travel by car has increased dramatically, while travel by bus, bicycle, and foot has declined. Rising pollution and traffic congestion are two of the consequences. Encouraging transportation by foot and bicycle could be considered a pollution-control strategy and a means of conserving fossil fuels.[77]

In 2000, President Clinton asked the Secretary of Health and Human Services and the Secretary of Education to propose strategies for increasing activity in the nation's youth.[78] Clinton issued a report entitled "Promoting Health for Young People Through Physical Activity and Sports" in November of 2000 outlining ten strategies for encouraging exercise and sports for children. Daily physical education classes for children in grades kindergarten through twelve was a major focus of the report, which also suggested creating community recreation facilities, involving the family, and encouraging after-school programs.[79]

In 2002, President Bush declared "If you're interested in improving America, you can do so by taking care of your own body" and that "people ought to work out every day, one way or another."[80]

It is clear that there is national concern over declining physical activity. Having national leaders inspire people to be more active is good, but much, much more needs to be done. Increased funding for the Centers for Disease Controls and Prevention to address issues of diet and physical activity is a good beginning, but the necessary change in our culture is so fundamental that more funding, more innovation, and more community programming will be needed to have an impact. We propose the following as measures to consider.

Develop a National Strategic Plan to Increase Physical Activity

Many approaches to increasing physical activity have been tried and tested. Increasing activity is possible, in both children and adults, with programs having been tested in schools, work sites, clinics, doctors' offices, and communities. What is needed is a national strategic plan to place all these approaches in a public health context and to devise a plan for the nation. A number of leading scientists have written on such public health priorities.[81]

A national plan would establish priorities among approaches, identify the most critical target populations, balance the likelihood of success against cost, and, most of all, establish a blueprint that brings together research, community organizing, and the efforts of health professionals into a coordinated effort. The Centers for Disease Control and Prevention is the logical organization to coordinate the development and implementation of a national plan.

Earmark Transportation Funding to Increase Activity

Transportation funding is enormous. Much of the funding is grouped into a single appropriations bill, the Transportation Equity Act for the 21st Century (TEA-21). TEA-21, up for reauthorization in 2003, is currently funded at $217 billion over six years. The funding can be used for multiple purposes, but almost all goes for roads, bridges, and, to some extent, public transportation.

Only a few programs anywhere in the country are funded by this bill to deal with walking or cycling. The Surface Transportation Policy Project (STPP) estimates that the amount spent on highways and bridges is $72 per person, compared to 55 cents per person for pedestrian projects. This group notes that facilities for cars crowd out opportunities for cycling and walking, being a pedestrian is dangerous, more people are overweight in places where people walk less, and fewer people are walking to work, down even from 1990.[82]

The STPP, along with a broad coalition of health, government, and business groups called the Alliance for a New Transportation Charter, proposes that a percentage of the next TEA-21 bill be allocated for pedestrian and cycling projects. This begins with recognizing that transportation funding can affect health. Once funding is available, programs can be undertaken to design neighborhoods for walking and cycling, retrofit existing streets to promote "traffic calming," equip transit buses with bike racks, and so on.

We believe that such action is one of the most rapid and powerful means of making progress on physical activity. Contacting your members of Congress and becoming more informed on these issues (www.transact.org) is an excellent way to be involved.

Design Activity-Friendly Communities

Planning new communities can be done to make physical activity more likely. Building sidewalks, bike lanes, trails, and parks, and insuring that children can get to school by walking or cycling is essential in modern-day America. Existing communities can be modified when possible to help stimulate activity. Such an effort requires the commitment of local, state, and national leaders and agencies. School boards and PTA groups, state education and transportation agencies, and housing groups are all relevant parties.

Build Facilities Knowing They Will Be Used

There is scientific evidence that people will use exercise facilities if constructed. This has been shown with bike/walking paths and trails and with facilities in schools. However, barriers to use must also be considered. If children can bike to school but parents have concerns with safety, if a community builds a path but the location does not promote biking to work, and if hills and busy intersections inhibit use, participation will be hampered. People must also be educated on the benefits of being active, which in turn helps create support for building sidewalks, bike paths and lanes, better crosswalks, and recreational facilities.[83]

Promote Walking and Biking to School

The CDC's KidsWalk-to-School and other similar programs are an excellent start and will help raise public awareness of travel to and from school as a means to improve health. For the seed to grow into a national increase in activity, city planning, transportation policy, and education must all intersect with physical activity as a priority. Walking and biking to school can be an ideal way to program activity into daily life. Public relations campaigns will be necessary to sensitize children, parents, and teachers to the importance of this issue.

Increase Physical Activity in Schools

Schools are an ideal site to improve activity.[84] Even in places where PE is required, it is not always delivered. Middle school gym is required by the state in Maryland, but some counties consider it an elective. In counties with fewer elective slots, exercise is more likely to be sidestepped.[85] Likewise, New York mandates PE for kindergarten through third grade, but 40 percent of local schools fail to comply.[86] Following existing regulations would be a good start.

Gym classes can involve much time standing around, listening to instructions, or waiting in line. Innovative programs have been developed to correct this problem. These should be used more systematically.

Making these changes could have a real impact, and guidelines exist for how to implement programs.[87] The group P.E.4Life has very helpful information for activity programming in schools.[88] A study in North Carolina found that PE could be changed in a way that leads to more true activity and that such classes produce beneficial effects on body fat and blood pressure.[89]

Decrease Sedentary Behavior

One way to increase activity is to decrease what competes with it. In working with overweight children, Leonard Epstein and colleagues have had good success with teaching children to decrease time spent watching television, playing video games, and using the computer.[90]

William Dietz of the CDC and Thomas Robinson of Stanford have been leading proponents of decreasing sedentary behavior (particularly watching TV) as a means for helping overweight children.[91] Robinson did an important study with third- and fourth-grade students. He studied two elementary schools, one having no change in the curriculum and the other receiving a six-month, eighteen-lesson classroom curriculum to reduce the use of TV, videotapes, and video games. When the program ended, children receiving the special curriculum weighed significantly less than the children in the other school.

There is an interesting question here—whether people who decrease particular forms of inactivity will use the time to be more active. Research with children is promising. Ultimately science should help identify people for whom increasing activity or decreasing sedentary behavior will be more effective.

Offer Incentives for Physical Activity

The British National Health Service helps subsidize exercise costs. This occurs to a small extent in the United States, but mainly for exercise rehabilitation programs after someone has had a heart attack. The British system helps people pay for exercise as a means of prevention.

Whether through the government or insurance companies, providing more systematic incentives to be physically active might be a cost-effective means of reducing disease.

Promote Work Site Activity Programs

There is a long history of physical activity and other health promotion programs being used in work sites.[92] There is still debate over whether they are cost-effective, but such programs can be considered a benefit by employees, improve health, and have a positive impact on work-related factors (time off from work, productivity, etc.). Some, but not nearly all, companies support these programs.

One barrier is that many people work in small businesses with too few employees to justify developing a program. Government incentives for businesses to have such programs might stimulate wider development and might lead to creative approaches, such as small businesses in a community forming partnerships to pay for programs and facilities.

Help Physicians Encourage Physical Activity

Thinking that primary care physicians could be a major means of motivating people to be physically active, researchers in San Diego have been using a program called PACE (Patient-Centered Assessment and Counseling for Exercise). The program provides physicians with motivational and counseling skills that can be used in brief office visits to encourage their patients to be more active. The program has reported positive results, as have others, including the Activity Counseling Trial.[93] While only a minority of people may be affected by this approach, a small number multiplied across thousands of physician practices, especially considering the low cost, can be significant.

Conclusion

Increasing physical activity is central to addressing the obesity crisis. Many factors in our culture are barriers to activity. These social and economic factors, such as suburban sprawl and more widespread use of energy-saving devices, are a mounting presence even in developing countries. Encouraging the population by exhortation is likely to help to some extent but must be combined with innovation in changing the environment. It must be easy for people to act in a healthy manner, so times, places, and incentives for people to be physically active must be engineered into daily life.

5

TELEVISION, MOVIES, CELEBRITIES, AND THE SEDUCTION OF CHILDREN

The commercial exploitation of children . . . is particularly egregious. Recognizing that children are not fully mature with regard to making informed decisions, we control the promotion of alcohol, firearms, and tobacco. Yet we assume that young children can rationally decide about food choices that have important health consequences, and we expose them to intense marketing of products that are largely devoid of nutritional value but replete with calories.

—WALTER WILLETT, HARVARD NUTRITION RESEARCHER[1]

Test Your Advertising IQ

Your brain sorts through thousands of images and sensations each minute. Memory discards most of this input but stores what gets through the filters.

Advertisers must compete with all else going on (what they refer to as clutter) just to get your attention, much less have their jingle or slogan stored away so you don't forget. Let's see how well the food companies do.

Take a moment to jot down which food is associated with the slogans listed below.

(a) Melts in your mouth, not in your hand
(b) Break me off a piece of that _____ bar
(c) It's the real thing
(d) They're magically delicious
(e) No one can eat just one
(f) The best part of waking up is _____ in your cup
(g) Silly rabbit, _____ are for kids
(h) He likes it! Hey, Mikey!
(i) We love to see you smile
(j) Have it your way
(k) M'm, M'm good
(l) They're Grrrreat!
(m) I go cuckoo for _____
(n) Taste the rainbow
(o) Do the Dew
(p) Finger lickin' good
(q) Obey your thirst
(r) Snap! Crackle! Pop!
(s) The other white meat
(t) Billions & billions served

Answers[2]

Advertising Age magazine listed the top 100 ad campaigns, jingles, slogans, and icons of the century. Coke, McDonald's, and Pepsi were in the top fifteen campaigns of all time.[3] Among the top ten jingles of the century were:

1. You deserve a break today (McDonald's)
3. Pepsi Cola Hits the Spot (Pepsi)
4. M'm, M'm good (Campbell's)
6. I wish I were an Oscar Meyer Wiener (Oscar Meyer)
9. It's the real thing (Coca-Cola)

Food captured seven of the ten top advertising icons:

2. Ronald McDonald
3. The Green Giant

4. Betty Crocker
6. The Pillsbury Doughboy
7. Aunt Jemima
9. Tony the Tiger
10. Elsie

In 1998, 89 percent of children under age eight visited McDonald's at least once a month. Their vice president of marketing said that McDonald's goal for the following year was 100 percent. A study of nearly 10,000 children showed that 100 percent of those in the United States recognized Ronald McDonald; the figures were 98 percent in Japan and 93 percent in the United Kingdom.[4]

The Key Question

Both the food industry and its critics can agree that massive money is spent on food advertising and that food slogans, jingles, and advertisements have become fixtures in American culture. But here the agreement stops.

Industry claims that advertising is only effective at moving people toward brands of products they will use anyway: a child might be tugged by General Mills to eat Count Chocula or by Kellogg to want Disney Buzz Blasts, by Pepsi to want Gatorade or by Coke to want Powerade. Such advertising, so the industry says, does not compel children to want sugared cereal or soft drinks more than they would otherwise.

On the other side are those who believe that images of unhealthy food are implanted in the American brain and that it defies common sense (and now research) to say that food advertising does not increase consumption.

The resolution of this argument is important. If the nation's consumption of sugared cereals, soft drinks, and fast food is unaffected by advertising, getting stirred up about food advertising makes no sense. Who cares if a child eats Count Chocula rather than Lucky Charms? If the assumption is wrong, however, reining in food advertising becomes logical, with special protection afforded to those least capable of protecting themselves (children). About one-third of the $30 billion spent each year on food advertising is targeted at children.

About $10 billion per year is spent on advertising food to children. A study of Australian children ages nine to ten indicated that more than half believe that Ronald McDonald knows best what children should eat.[5]

How Much Advertising Is There?

Television is the leading means of persuasion for the food industry. The average American watches 1,567 hours per year, or 3–4 hours per day.[6] America's children spend more time watching television than doing anything but sleeping. At least 96 percent of American homes have one TV; 65 percent of eight- to eighteen-year-olds and 32 percent of two- to seven-year-olds have a TV in their bedroom. By age seventy, the average person has spent seven to ten years watching TV.

The Better Business Bureau noted that children watch the equivalent of a fifty-day "marathon" of television each year, most of which occurs on weekday afternoons and Saturday mornings, when parents may not be supervising.[7] The *Boston Globe* reported that African American households watch 10.5 hours of TV daily (76 hours/week) versus 54 hours a week in other households. The National Assessment of Education Progress found that 34 percent of people with poor reading skills watched six hours or more of TV daily, compared to 6 percent of the best readers. And most of the children watching six hours or more were African American.[8] One study found that 17 percent of children eleven months old or younger, 48 percent of those ages twelve to twenty-three months, and 41 percent of those ages twenty-four to thirty-five months watch more TV than recommended by the American Academy of Pediatrics. These early viewing habits persist into later childhood.[9]

Major networks show between 8.5 and 10.3 minutes of commercials per hour of programming, many for food.[10] In 1997, food advertisers spent $1.4 billion to promote food on network television and $1.2 billion to promote restaurants and drive-ins. On syndicated television, food advertisers spent $369 million on ads for snacks and soft drinks, followed by $144 million on restaurants and drive-ins. Restaurants and drive-ins were the largest advertisers on local TV, spending $1.3 billion. Food stores and supermarkets ranked fifth, spending $336 million for local advertising.[11]

Some parts of the food industry are especially aggressive with advertising. The advertising budget for soft drinks in 1998 was $115.5 million, for popular candy bars it was $10–$50 million, and for McDonald's the budget was more than $1 billion. Compare that with the National Cancer Institute's $1 million budget for its 5 A Day campaign or the $1.5 million for the National Cholesterol Education Campaign of the National Heart, Lung, and Blood Institute.[12] A UK-based magazine ranked McDonald's the most prolific advertiser in the world in 1997.[13]

TV advertising is convincing. Forty-nine percent of American adults view television as the most authoritative advertising medium, followed by 24 percent for newspapers. Almost three-fourths vote television as the most exciting medium. Sixty-six percent find it the most persuasive, and 78 percent believe it to be the most influential.[14]

Critics of regulating food advertising say that parents can turn off the TV, but TV only begins the onslaught. Ads on billboards; product placements in movies; food logos in schools; splashy signs on vending machines; and ads on buses, taxis, and even police cars contribute to the blitz. Every child is exposed.

Children as Market Objects

Children were identified as a separate market for advertisers in the 1960s.[15] The concept developed quickly, and now there are conferences, books, and ad agencies all focused on children as consumers. Marketing handbooks encourage businesses to target children and provide strategies to "unlock the secrets to children's hearts."[16] As a result, marketing to children has doubled since 1992.[17]

Targeting children is partly to develop the next generation of adult customers, but what children spend right here, right now is remarkable. American children ages five to fourteen spend $20 billion each year and influence the spending of about $200–$500 billion annually.[18] Children ages four through twelve had access to $31.3 billion in 1999 from allowances, jobs, and gifts, and they spent 92 percent of it.[19]

> "It isn't enough to just advertise on television. . . . You've got to reach kids throughout their day—in school, as they're shopping at the mall . . . or at the movies. You've got to become part of the fabric of their lives."[20]
>
> —Carol Herman, Senior Vice President, Grey Advertising

Content of Television Directed at Children

The average American child sees 10,000 food advertisements each year, just on television. Children watching Saturday morning cartoons see a food commercial every five minutes. The vast majority are for sugared cereals, fast foods, soft drinks, sugary and salty snacks, and candy; few promote foods children should eat more frequently such as fruits and vegetables.[21] Between 1976 and 1987, the ratio of high- to low-sugar ads increased from 5:1 to 12.5:1.

Researchers complained about advertisements for unhealthy food as early as 1973,[22] but the situation has worsened. One study found only ten nutrition-related pubic service announcements versus 564 food advertisements during 52.5 hours of Saturday morning TV.[23]

Companies offer meals with toys and characters to entice children. In one holiday season, three fast-food companies competed for children with major promotions. Burger King featured the Rugrats, McDonald's had *A Bug's Life*, and Taco Bell used the Taco Bell Chihuahua. When asked who would win, an analyst stated, "Maybe in the end, they all win. . . . I can easily see kids wanting stuff from all three promotions—and especially around the holidays, if the kids want it, it's hard for parents to say no."[24]

> Forty percent of McDonald's advertising directly targets children. In 1998, Coca-Cola paid the Boys and Girls Clubs of America $60 million for exclusive marketing in more than 2,000 clubs.[26]

Keebler used aggressive marketing to make their Chips Deluxe brand the company's top-rated cookie in 1997. Promotions included a Chips Deluxe "Create Your Own Cookie Contest" and the introduction of "Dude," an animated character in Chips Deluxe ads to make the brand relevant to children. Revenues increased by 25 percent.[25]

Does Food Advertising Work?

Given the $30 billion per year spent on food advertising, we must assume it works and that people buy more of the advertised food. The core question, though, is whether advertising changes the overall diet, especially in children.

Children view television with less skepticism than adults and therefore are particularly vulnerable to advertising.[27] Research with fifth- and sixth-graders showed that more than half believed every commercial they viewed in the study. Children have difficulty distinguishing between advertising and programming and before age eight do not understand that the intent of commercials is to sell a product.[28]

A study of children ages six through eight found that 70 percent believed that fast foods were healthier than food from the home.[29]

Awareness

Advertisers employ many methods to get attention, but chief among them is the use of easily recognizable characters and cartoon figures. The hope is that children will transfer the emotional attachment they feel about a character to a product. A study of 229 preschoolers showed that even very young children recognize and remember brand logos.

In a study of children ages nine through eleven, 94 percent knew that Tony the Tiger sells cereal and 81 percent knew that frogs sell beer. Slogans were also well recognized; 80 percent knew the "What's up Doc?" Bugs Bunny slogan, 73 percent recognized the "Bud-weis-er" frogs' slogan, and 57 percent the Tony the Tiger "They're Grrrreat"

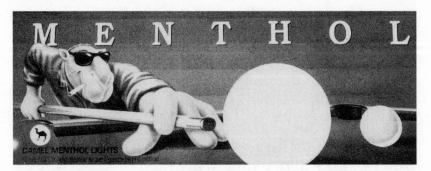

Figure 5.1 Banned

slogan.[30] Thirty percent of three-year-olds and 91.3 percent of six-year-olds were able to match Joe Camel to a cigarette.[31] An experiment with eight-year-olds asked, "Who would you like to take you out for a treat?" Tony the Tiger and Ronald McDonald were more popular choices than the children's parents.[32]

Attitudes and Behavior

Ads also change attitudes. In children ages two through ten, a single exposure to an advertisement produces more favorable attitudes toward the product.[33] Ten- to thirteen-year-olds who are aware of beer commercials hold more favorable beliefs about drinking, have greater knowledge of beer brands and slogans, and show increased intent to drink as adults.[34] TV watching has been linked to unhealthy nutrition perceptions in fourth and fifth graders.[35]

Awareness and attitude changes notwithstanding, the ultimate test is whether advertising affects behavior. Poor eating practices are correlated clearly with the amount of TV a child watches. A study with three- to five-year-olds found that TV time is linked to the purchase-influencing attempts of the children at the grocery store. Cereal and candy are two of the most requested items and two of the most advertised foods.[36] First graders watching ads for high-sugar foods choose more sugary foods, both advertised and nonadvertised.[37]

As discussed in Chapter 2, watching TV is linked to increased snacking and caloric intake and decreased nutrient quality among children.

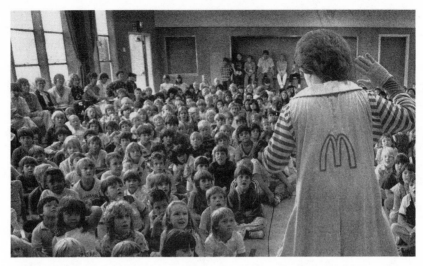

Figure 5.2 Embraced (Permission granted by the photographer, Evan Johnson.)

The number of hours of TV viewed each week is correlated with what children ask their parents to buy, what parents do buy, and calorie intake.[38] Children whose families watch TV during mealtimes have poorer diets than those who do not.[39] Although one study of tenth to twelfth graders found no association between viewing commercials and snacking,[40] other studies continue to find a relationship.

> "Although advertisers insist that their intent is to promote brand selection, an unacknowledged consequence is increased product consumption."
> —American Academy of Pediatrics[42]

While generally consistent, these studies can only take us so far in understanding how food advertisements affect diet. There is only circumstantial evidence that the ads cause poor eating. It is possible that some third factor, say level of education or parents' nutrition knowledge, drives both the amount of TV seen and the diet of a child. One could also argue that something about watching TV other than the food ads leads to weight problems, with physical inactivity the logical candidate. An interesting way to address these issues would be to compare children who watch commercial TV to those who spend the same amount of time watching videos or public TV. This would control for the effect of activity and would help isolate the effect of food ads. Some experts, however, believe the question has been answered—TV promotes increased consumption.[41]

We can conclude that more TV means more food ads, and with more ads comes deteriorating diet. It is hard to imagine that the barrage of ads children see from their earliest years does not create desire for the foods they see. Children should not be fair game for the food companies.

> The risk of obesity in a preschool child increases by 6 percent for every hour of television he or she watches per day. If there is a TV in the child's bedroom, the risk of being obese is increased by 31 percent.[43]

The Mating of Giants: TV and Movie Companies Consorting with Food

Partnerships have evolved between the food industry and companies involved in the fantasy and play world of children. Movie figures have been in fast-food children's meals for many years, but the phenomenon is spreading far beyond. There are now dozens of food products associated with the most popular children's television and movie characters.

> "Mary Clark of Noblesville [Indiana] gave her husband, Buddy, a list of all the places he has to eat lunch for the next two weeks. Buddy Clark will have to eat at Burger King, where he can get one of four Teletubbies characters with a child's meal. Star Wars premiums are available at Taco Bell, Kentucky Fried Chicken, and Pizza Hut; Friday, McDonald's begins offering its third set of Teeny Beanie Babies free with Happy Meals. Buddy Clark can enjoy the food; the toys are saved for the grandchildren."[44]

A colleague told us of her four-year-old daughter at the supermarket seeing Betty Crocker's Disney Princess Fruit Snacks with Cinderella, Snow White, and the Little Mermaid on the box.

Daughter: "I want that."
Mother: "What is it?"
Daughter: "I don't know."

Such anecdotes underscore the obvious—that for these partnerships to be so pervasive, foods must help promote TV shows and movies, and the characters help sell food. The four-year-old child probably had faith that whatever was in the box would taste good (would be high in sugar, fat, or both).

Infiltrating the Aisles

In order to get a snapshot of the TV/movie and food pairings, one of us (KB) made a field trip to the nearest supermarket with two expert observers (a boy age eight and girl age fourteen).[45] We examined all food items and made note of each instance of a character/food pairing (see Figure 5.3).

The table does not include food products associated with sports stars and organizations (NASCAR paired with pudding, Kobe Bryant paired with Nutella), movie actors (Scorpion King characters paired with Reese's Bars), bands (O-Town paired with Frosted Cheerios), or one food paired with others (Nestle Crunch in Yoplait yogurt, M&M's in ice cream sandwiches).

Most items we found would not be on lists of foods children should be encouraged to eat. After finding these 59 products in a single store, it seems clear that selling unhealthy foods with TV and movie characters is common practice and that using them to sell healthy foods is rare.

Nickelodeon and Disney Lead the Plundering Herd

Many companies (thirteen in our local tally) negotiate the rights for their characters to the food industry, but Nickelodeon and Disney appear to lead the way. Each owns characters immensely popular among children.

Company	Character	Food
Nickelodeon	Blue's Clues	Nabisco Fruit Treats, Mott's Berry Flavor Applesauce
	Bob the Builder	Brach's Fruit Snacks
	Jimmy Neutron	Quaker Chewy Granola Bars, Quaker Life Cereal, Quaker Cap'n Crunch Cereal, Quaker Cap'n Crunch Peanut Butter Cereal
	Rocket Power	Nabisco Cheese Nips
	Rugrats	Nabisco Fruit Treats, Kraft Macaroni and Cheese, Mott's Fruit Punch Applesauce, Popsicle Cookie Sandwich
	Sponge Bob	Nabisco Fruit Treats, Nabisco Cheese Nips, Saputo String Cheese
	Waldo	Franco American Pasta with Meat Balls
Disney	Beauty and the Beast	Kellogg's Corn Flakes
	Buzz Lightyear	Betty Crocker Fruit Snacks
	Country Bears	Act II Microwave Popcorn
	Disney Princesses	Betty Crocker Fruit Snacks
	Mickey Mouse	Betty Crocker Fruit Snacks
	Mickey Mouse	Disney/Minute Maid 10 percent juice
	Monsters Inc.	Orville Redenbacher's Microwave Popcorn
	Tigger	Disney/Minute Maid 20 percent juice
	Winnie the Pooh	Disney/Minute Maid 100 percent juice
	Winnie the Pooh	Betty Crocker Fruit Snacks, Keebler's Rumbly Grahams

Figure 5.3 Television and Movie Characters Used to Promote Food

Company	Character	Food
Cartoon Network	Dexter's Laboratory	Kellogg's Pop-Tarts, Kellogg's Apple Jacks
	Johnny Bravo	Keebler Munch'ems, Kellogg's Apple Jacks
	Powerpuff Girls	Keebler Powerpuff Girls Sandwich Cookies, Hunt's Pudding Snack Pack, Edy's Grand Ice Cream
Hanna Barbera	Scooby Doo	Oscar Meyer Lunchables, Betty Crocker Fruit Snacks, Hunt's Pudding Snack Pack, Kraft Macaroni and Cheese, Edy's Grand Ice Cream
Sesame Street Workshop	Bert and Ernie	Apple & Eve 100 percent juice
	Big Bird	Sesame Street Animal Crackers
	Elmo	Sesame Street Cheddar Snack Crackers, Sesame Street 100 percent juice, Apple & Eve 100 percent juice
Miramax	Spy Kids	Frito-Lay Funyons, Frito-Lay Doritos, Frito-Lay Snack Mix, Tony's Pizza
Public Broadcasting System	Arthur	Juicy Juice 100 percent juice
	Clifford the Dog	Brach's Fruit Snacks, General Mills Kix Cereal
Marvel Characters	Spider-Man	Kellogg's Pop-Tarts, Kellogg's Corn Pops
Universal Studios	Scorpion King	Reese's Bars
	The Mummy	Reese's Bars
Houghton Mifflin	Curious George	Stop & Shop Fruit Snacks
Warner Brothers	Looney Toons	Hunts Snack Pack Pudding
Nintendo	Pokémon	Betty Crocker Fruit Rolls
20th Century Fox	Homer Simpson	Kellogg's Corn Pops

In a job announcement for a position with the "Promotion Marketing" team at General Mills, a key responsibility is to "Negotiate promotional tie-ins with third parties such as Disney, Microsoft, and Mattel." A promotion planner named Sarah is quoted in the "Our Careers" website of General Mills, as saying, "We work with tie-in partners to ensure successful promotions that greatly impact higher volume levels."[46]

Disney has a long history of helping sell fast foods, sugared cereals, and more. Its clout, reach, reputation, and creativity are what make parents believe Disney can be trusted. You can take young children to Disney movies and count on them seeing reasonable content. This trust might be threatened as the public objects to food alliances.

Children's meals at McDonald's or Burger King often include Disney characters as toys, and characters are used to sell pudding, snack chips, fruit snacks, ice cream, and more. Disney has established a relationship with Kellogg's in which prominent Disney characters become icons used to sell cereals. The cereal boxes have "Kellogg's—Disney-Pixar" in bold letters across the top of the box, with the Tinkerbell character flying above. The Kellogg-Disney portfolio includes Buzz Blasts (with Buzz Lightyear the icon), Hunny Bs (Winnie the Pooh and other Pooh characters), and Magix (Mickey Mouse), all highly sweetened cereals. The Kellogg-Disney partnership is important to both companies:

"We're excited about the possibilities with this alliance," said Kellogg spokesman Neil Nyberg. Kellogg's co-branded goods will be served at Disney's theme parks and resorts as well as promoted through its entertainment properties, which include radio stations, film production companies, and television stations.

For Disney, it is an opportunity to partner with a company that connects with children and parents, said Andy Mooney, president of Disney Consumer Products, which licenses the Burbank, Calif.-based company's characters.

"Clearly in the case of cereal, Kellogg is a global leader in their category the same way Coca-Cola is a leader in carbonated beverages," Mooney said.

Mooney said his goal is to put Disney products in front of consumers on a daily basis.[47]

The mating of Disney characters with food happens in a carefully choreographed way. For instance, the Buzz Lightyear character (from *Toy Story*) was in McDonald's Happy Meals. Then the movie was released and Kellogg's—Disney-Pixar placed Buzz Blasts cereal on supermarket shelves. McDonald's helps promote the movie and its spin-off products like pajamas, toys, lunchboxes, and bedding, and Buzz draws kids to McDonald's. Kellogg's then gets a boost from both Disney and McDonald's. Everyone wins.

A three-way partnership was established between Disney Interactive, General Mills, and EarthLink (an Internet provider).[48] Netactive created a CD game to help Disney promote *Toy Story 2*. The CD provided three hours of free play and was packaged in five million boxes of Frosted Cheerios and Cinnamon Toast Crunch cereals. Consumers playing the game could then buy the software online for $9.99 or receive it free if signing on with EarthLink. General Mills had growth as high as 63 percent during this period, which was more than double the growth of *Toy Story* cereal without the premium. General Mills, through its subsidiary Betty Crocker, also pairs with Disney in selling fruit snacks.

Disney and Frito-Lay announced a multiyear agreement in which Frito-Lay products will be featured at restaurants and food kiosks in Disney's theme parks, but in addition Frito-Lay will sponsor park attractions, including California Screamin' presented by Lay's in Disney's California Adventure and Disney's Typhoon Lagoon Water Park presented by Cheetos at the Walt Disney World Resort. Frito-Lay also will receive naming rights to the baseball stadium at Disney's Wide World of Sports Complex, currently home to the Atlanta Braves spring training and double-A Orlando Rays, which will be renamed Cracker Jack Stadium.[49]

Product Placement in Movies and Television

It is common practice for companies to pay for their products to appear in movies and on television. Products sometimes appear by happenstance, but in many cases, money changes hands and products get featured. This practice began many years ago, but is now so common that there are more than 100 product placement agencies and even a professional organization to represent them, the Entertainment Resources Marketing Association (ERMA). ERMA notes:

The greatest home run in product placement since E.T. scarfed up a pack of Reese's Pieces came with BMW's launch of its Z3 roadster last fall. When the car became James Bond's preferred ride in the 007 flick Goldeneye, *the hype and glitter surrounding this placement became an event unto itself, generating hundreds of millions of dollars worth of exposure worldwide. The deal won BMW and its marketing partners a Super Reggie as the top promotion of the year. Beyond the accolades and the press clips, though, the placement helped drive BMW's business as discounts for the Z3 vanished and waiting lists stretched out for months.*[50]

One leading firm, Feature This!, with offices in six countries, notes how powerful placement can be, especially when celebrity endorsements are implied: "The cost of celebrity endorsements is usually exorbitant and many celebrities refrain from such activities. However, product exposures act as implied celebrity endorsements."[51]

The tobacco companies were early adopters of product placement. In 1980 Rogers & Cowan, a Beverly Hills public relations company representing RJR Tobacco Company, sent this memo to RJR:

The Cannonball Run—*To be released by 20th Century Fox. Through special arrangements with producer Al Ruddy, we have arranged important visibility for several R.J. Reynolds products in the film. This comedy stars Burt Reynolds, Farrah Fawcett, Roger Moore, Dean Martin, Sammy Davis, Jr., Dom DeLuise, Bert Convey, Terry Bradshaw, Bianca Jagger, Mel Tillis, and others. In the film, there will be numerous scenes showing cigarette smoking in a most favorable light and in some of these scenes we will actually see one or more of our brands. Additionally, Burt Reynolds plays scenes wearing a Winston jacket and Winston racing cap.*[52]

Similarly, food is featured prominently in movies and TV, perhaps by accident, but perhaps not. A few examples, featuring just one food company:

- *Sleeper* (1973). Woody Allen awakens from an operation to be 100 years in the future. Allen walks in front of McDonald's.
- *Bye, Bye Love* (1995). Three divorced men struggle with custody and raising children. The movie begins with mother and father exchanging children at a neutral location, McDonald's. McDonald's is shown many times in the movie as parents exchange children.
- *George of the Jungle* (1997). George is transported from the jungle to San Francisco. He lands on top of a taxi with a McDonald's placard and goes to a McDonald's drive-thru. A McDonald's representative was on location for the shooting to attend to the company's interests.[53]
- *The Flintstones* (1994). The movie shows a prehistoric shopping center with a "Roc Donald's."

This just begins the list. An anti-drug soldier comes across a Quarter Pounder wrapper from McDonald's in *Clear and Present Danger* with Harrison Ford, and Macaulay Culkin in *Richie Rich* has a McDonald's in his house.

The latest advance is virtual placement. An article in *Los Angeles Magazine* explains how this happens.[54] Products are inserted into program reruns as if they were there originally. For instance, Jerry Seinfeld might be eating cereal in an original episode but have a Cap'n Crunch box inserted electronically into the rerun. The food company is charged what a thirty-second commercial would cost.

You may also notice virtual advertisements on televised sporting events. A computer inserts what looks like a billboard on a stadium wall, scoreboard, and so on. While a pitcher peers at the catcher's signal in the World Series, there to the left of the catcher and umpire is a prominent product sign created by the computer.

The Industry of Marketing to Children

Marketing products to children is big business, with many people profiting. Most obvious is the food industry, but there are others including ad agencies and public relations firms who help promote the foods, the media who sell advertising space, consultants who establish deals between food companies and other enterprises (movies, schools, etc.), and, of course, all the places that sell food (supermarkets, convenience stores, drugstores, gas stations, schools, etc.). Add these together and you have powerful financial interests opposing change.

A number of organizations, publications, meetings, and marketing businesses exist to help companies sell products to children.

- *Kidscreen* magazine, in addition to covering children's marketing in its articles, convenes conferences such as one in New York City on "Advertising and Promoting to Kids."[55]
- Golden Marble Awards are given each year for the most effective advertising campaigns directed at children. Winners have included ads for Hostess snack cakes, Mountain Dew, Gatorade, Burger King, and McDonald's.
- A group called Kid Power Xchange is "the ultimate knowledge resource for youth marketers."[56] It holds the Kid Power Food & Beverage Marketing Conference. Workshops have included "Excitement in the Beverage Aisle—Taking Disney's Magic to the Grocery Store," "From Supermarkets to Soccer Fields: Kids' Wants, Moms' Behavior," and "Targeting Soft Drinks to Kids."
- *Selling to Kids* magazine publishes articles such as "The Best In-School Marketing Campaign" and "The 3 P's of Food and Beverage: Promotions, Premiums, and Partnerships," saying things like "With kids spending about a third of every dollar on

things they can put in their mouths, your product's image and sales can benefit from associations with brands in this segment."[57]

That these groups and activities exist is a sign that the business world, government leaders, and the general public believe that it is legitimate enterprise to sell products to children.

> A restaurant industry publication, *Restaurant Hospitality*, reported that "if there was one mantra that emerged from *Restaurant Hospitality*'s recent Kids Marketing Conference it was this: Kids are very important customers who can make a big difference to your bottom line."[58]

Take the Golden Marble Awards. On occasion these are given to companies who use marketing for good causes. For instance, a 2001 award was given to Campbell Mithun for an antismoking campaign. What is more common, though, is for a company such as Leo Burnett to win for a McDonald's ad using Britney Spears. Leo Burnett then lists its Golden Marble Awards among its accomplishments in order to sell itself to potential clients and employees.[59]

> "We always, always have kid-related programs."
> —1997 quote from Mary Miller, Vice President of McDonald's[60]

The Ethics of Advertising to Children

Some people and organizations believe that children's advertising is harmful and should not be permitted at all. In a position statement, the American Academy of Pediatrics declares that "Advertising directed toward children is inherently deceptive and exploits children under eight years of age."[61]

Stop Commercial Exploitation of Children (SCEC), a coalition of many child advocacy organizations, believes that marketing to children is exploitive and harmful to the nation's youth.[62] SCEC notes that the United States regulates advertising to children less than most other democratic nations.

The Center for Media Education (CME, formerly Action for Children's Television, ACT) was founded in 1991 as a national nonprofit organization to bring about federal change in children's television. The organization has been active in testifying to the Federal Communications Commission (FCC) and in creating the 1992 Campaign for Kids' TV that involved parent, education, and advocacy groups in the cause. In 1996, the CME was instrumental in persuading the FCC to require a minimum of three hours each week of educational children's programming.[63] The CME takes the approach that the media can be used for constructive causes and that political leaders should be urged to protect children from negative influences and harness the media to have positive impact.

The Center for Science in the Public Interest (CSPI) started an organization called "Kids Against Junk Foods" to raise health awareness among children. The CSPI has targeted major corporations in the fight to protect children. An example is the "Save Harry" campaign to protest Coke's exclusive global marketing rights to the Harry Potter movie.[64]

When the country's main pediatrics association, a broad coalition of organizations concerned with child welfare, an organization for media and children, a leading nutrition watchdog group, and a top medical journal[65] conclude that advertising practices are deceptive, exploitative, and harmful to the health and well-being of our children, there is reason for the nation to take notice. Our nation takes strong offense at the exploitation and harm of children, but only recently has the nation begun to view food advertising in this way. The food industry is concerned and is fighting back.

The Industry's Response

In the 1970s, the food industry was threatened by the possibility that the Federal Trade Commission (FTC) would regulate children's advertising. It fought off this threat in part by establishing its own self-policing group, the Children's Advertising Review Unit (CARU). Founded in 1974, CARU reviews advertising directed at children less than twelve years of age, but it has no legal recourse and seeks change only through voluntary cooperation with advertisers when claims are found to be misleading, inaccurate, or inconsistent with CARU guidelines. CARU supporters, including M&M Mars, Inc., Nabisco Foods, Hershey Foods, General Mills, and Frito-Lay, Inc., pay a fee to belong to the organization.[66]

Whether CARU is having an impact is difficult to assess. Children are bombarded more than ever by advertisements to eat unhealthy food, so from this perspective CARU either is not working or has minimal effects. One could argue, we suppose, that the situation would be worse if CARU guidelines were not in place. One thing is certain—what is being done currently is insufficient.

Power Versus the Common Good

Balancing the right of companies to market their products with the need to protect the public has always been tricky, but in some cases the government has taken decisive action—with tobacco, for example. This has not occurred with food. Two case studies illustrate this point.

Case Study 1. A physicians group in Australia, the Australian Divisions of General Practice, met with food manufacturers and asked for a ban on junk-food ads during afternoon television programming. Prior to the meeting, Robert Koltai, speaking for the Australian Association of National Advertisers, promised that his group and others would be aggressive in countering the perception that advertising contributes to poor diet.

What's alarming about this sort of challenge to advertising is that it proceeds on the basis that no one has control any more over their own behavior. It's nannyism, which says that as individuals or families we have no responsibility for what happens to us.[67]

Instead of working with medical authorities, the industry fights, using the familiar call for personal responsibility. Time will tell whether

Australia enacts such a regulation, but denying and fighting, a failed strategy for the tobacco industry, is a clear approach being taken by some segments of the food industry.

Case Study 2. In 2002, Coke and Pepsi distributors met with Governor Angus King of Maine about a state-sponsored media campaign initiated a month earlier by the Bureau of Health.[68] The "Enough Is Enough" campaign used radio and TV ads and letters to parents to warn young people about soft drinks.

The soft drink industry was represented by Dennis Bailey, owner of a Portland public relations firm and, conveniently, former press secretary to Gov. King. Also present at the meeting was Guy Johnson, from Johnson Nutrition Solutions in Kalamazoo, Michigan, who writes and testifies widely on behalf of the National Soft Drink Association.[69] Testifying before the New York State Assembly on soft drinks in schools, Johnson had said, "There is no nutritional reason why soft drinks, water, teas, sports drinks, and juices should not be made available to students and faculty."[70] Bailey said, "We object to being singled out. There is no scientific evidence that soda consumption causes obesity, and these ads draw that link."[71]

As Chapter 7 explains, there *is* scientific evidence linking soft drink consumption to childhood obesity. So, did Gov. King dismiss the self-serving lobbyists and use his influence for the state's children? Not exactly. The Governor's spokesperson announced that the "governor listens and understands" the soft drink lobbyists. The Bureau of Health reworked the campaign, with components scheduled to be used later (on increasing physical activity) being moved up.

Does the Government Offer Any Protection?

The FTC regulates advertising in America, focusing largely on false advertising and misleading statements (in representation or omission of facts deemed to be material).[72] The Food and Drug Administration (FDA) and the U.S. Department of Agriculture (USDA) share jurisdiction over claims made by food manufacturers. The FTC primarily regulates food advertising, while the FDA regulates labeling. The FTC may issue a temporary restraining order or preliminary injunction for suspected violation of its regulation. The penalty for violation of FTC provisions is a fine of up to $5,000 and/or a prison term of up to six months. Repeat offenders face a fine limit of $10,000 and imprisonment for up to one year.[73]

Current policies are inadequate. We agree with groups such as the American Academy of Pediatrics that children are being exploited by advertising and that change is necessary. The industry is not policing itself and the government falls short. The public health ramifications of poor diet are enormous, so it is time to declare current policies inadequate and take action to defend the nation's children.

Some Good News

One might expect that lessons learned from promoting unhealthy foods could be used to encourage consumption of better foods. If true, it would be wise to use this information to improve the nation's diet.

Research shows that children can be persuaded to eat healthy foods and can be taught to differentiate between persuasion and information in commercials.[74] One study found that children who watch public service announcements focusing on nutrition choose more vegetables, fruits, and other nutritious foods.[75] In another study, positive comments by an adult observer, along with pro-nutrition messages and ads for foods without added sugar, reduced three- to six-year-olds' selection of foods with added sugar.[76] A Canadian study found that children ages five through eight picked more candy than fruit following a candy commercial, but showing fruit commercials or public service announcements while eliminating candy commercials encouraged children to choose fruit.[77]

Simple reduction of time at the television can be effective as well. Thomas Robinson at Stanford used a school-based intervention to reduce TV, video, and video game use among children. Robinson found a significant reduction in weight among children in the intervention group compared to controls, along with decreased TV time and frequency of meals eaten while watching television.[78]

Parents have the power to shape children's TV viewing habits. One study showed that the most important factor related to a child's TV watching habits was the attitude of parents.[79] The American Academy of Pediatrics recommends limits on media exposure for children, skills to help children view TV critically, and discussion of media content with children.[80]

Studies have also shown that rules at home can modify physical activity and TV viewing. When television watching is made contingent on pedaling a stationary bicycle, for example, children exercise more and lose body fat.[81]

Success Stories

Smart-Mouth.org

Michael Jacobson, Margo Wootan, Bonnie Liebman, and others at the Center for Science in the Public Interest (CSPI) have devoted years to educating the public and policy makers about key nutrition issues, attending to issues such as labeling, packaging, and advertising of foods. CSPI publishes an excellent newsletter called the *Nutrition Action Healthletter* (www.cspitnet.org).

CSPI also has developed a nutrition site for children (www.Smart-Mouth.org).[82] Among its features is a character named Gus, whose Trust Gus quiz helps children learn about the food industry. For example, a child is asked whether the following statement is true or false: "Food companies encourage people to eat even if they're not hungry." The answer: "The more often you eat, the more money food companies make. Check out their ad slogans like 'don't just stand there, eat something,' 'crunch all you want, we'll make more,' or 'once you pop, you can't stop.' "

Swedish Government Action with the European Union

Sweden has been very active in lobbying within the European Union to ban television advertising to children. Making such an effort on a broad scale is a success by itself. If Sweden prevails and the European

Union develops a ban, it could lead the way for other countries to do the same.

Quebec's Consumer Protection Act

The Province of Quebec, Canada, enacted the Consumer Protection Act in 1978, which stated that "no person may make use of commercial advertising directed at persons under thirteen years of age." To determine whether advertisements are aimed at children, officials consider the nature and intended use of the advertised goods, the content of the advertisement, and the time and place it is shown.[83]

Pulled Support for Golden Marble Awards

A grassroots campaign in 2001 by Stop Commercial Exploitation of Children was mounted to encourage Scholastic, Inc. to withdraw its sponsorship of the Golden Marble Awards. Scholastic publishes the Harry Potter books and is the nation's leading educational publisher. Scholastic withdrew its support, with CEO Richard Robinson saying, "We wanted to let you know that Scholastic will not be a sponsor this year for the Kidscreen Conference. We appreciate your recognition that Scholastic has a long tradition of providing high quality products and services to teachers, children, and parents."[84]

Progressive Action in Other Countries

Greece bans toy ads until 10 P.M., while Belgium prohibits commercials five minutes before, during, and five minutes after children's programming. Norway and Sweden ban advertising directly to children under twelve.[85]

Taking Action

A number of steps are possible to protect children from commercial exploitation in general and food marketing in particular.

Stand Up to the Food Industry and Prohibit Children's Advertising

A Roper Poll found that 80 percent of adults believe that marketing and advertising exploit children by convincing them to buy things that are bad for them, and a marketing report found that 85 percent of adults believe that children's TV should be free of commercials.[86] Legislators, by yielding to pressure from the food industry, are out of step with public opinion. If a few courageous legislators can resist the pressure and start the nation thinking about banning children's advertising, public support could swell. It has been done elsewhere in the world.

At the Very Least, Level the Food Field

It is a national priority to reduce obesity in children, improve their diets, and encourage them to be active.[87] Standing in the way is the tremendous imbalance of promotion for unhealthy versus healthy food. Parents want their children to be healthy, educators want their children to be alert, and national leaders want the next generation of Americans to be vital, energetic, and fit. The unlevel playing field makes this unlikely.

If the food industry prevails in the political arena and the heavy promotion of unhealthy food continues, the nation must mount an effort to counter it. This would require considerable resources, because what must be countered are years of persuasion and trillions of dollars spent by the industry to change attitudes and eating behaviors.

Develop an Equal Time Mandate for Food Advertising

In the 1960s, the Fairness Doctrine from the FCC was interpreted in a way that mandated television stations to run antismoking spots if they ran commercials from tobacco companies. The antismoking ads worked. The tobacco industry decided it was not cost-effective to advertise on television any longer and voluntarily ceased TV advertising in implicit exchange for being permitted to advertise elsewhere.

The Fairness Doctrine has been repealed, but something similar applied to food advertising may be beneficial. Requiring advertisements for healthy foods or spots discouraging consumption of unhealthy foods may help counteract the effects of existing advertising. It would not make sense to confine the rule to advertising on television.

Create a Means for Supporting the Promotion of Healthy Foods

For pro-nutrition and physical activity messages to be powerful, compelling, engaging, and frequent enough to make a difference, funds will be necessary to generate and then disseminate material. Professional time might be available as pro bono work from advertising and public relations firms. Media outlets might also agree to use public service space for nutrition and activity programming. This may help, but would only be a start.

Generating funds to promote nutrition might be done in several ways. In Chapter 6 we recognize that schools may lose money if they cease the sales of snack foods and soft drinks. A way to replace this funding would be to enact a small state or national tax on soft drinks, snack foods, and fast foods, earmarking the money for schools. Revenue from such a tax might also create a "nutrition superfund" that would be used to support healthy eating campaigns for children.

Placing an assessment, fee, or tax on advertisements that occur for unhealthy foods would also be a way of supporting a nutrition superfund. Many states are using tobacco settlement money to establish antismoking campaigns, so there is a precedent for having an industry help counter the problems it creates. The food industry might be willing to pay now in hopes of avoiding paying a higher penalty later if held accountable for health damages.

The public has divided opinion on food taxes (see Chapter 9). More people support taxes if assured that the revenue will be used for a related, constructive purpose such as programs to promote healthy eating.[88] Support is likely to grow as the public becomes more aware of obesity as a national and world crisis and sees that so many people are affected.

Enforce Broadcasting Regulations

The Children's Television Act of 1990 mandated that broadcasters are required to have instructional programming/children's educational shows. Groups such as the American Academy of Pediatrics and the Center for Media Education note that the law's intent is violated routinely.[89] Among the problems are that monitoring is done only at the time of license renewal and that stations list public service announcements, short vignettes, and even cartoons as educational programming. Insuring that the educational environment on each station is consistent with the law's intent could be an important step forward.

Discourage Media Companies from Associating with Unhealthy Foods

One possible means of discouraging unhealthy eating would be to encourage media companies, such as Disney, Nickelodeon, the Cartoon Network, and Hanna Barbera, to cease connections with unhealthy foods. Using popular characters to promote healthy foods should be encouraged.

Disney does not associate its characters with cigarettes, probably because the damage to its reputation would be too great and questions arise on legal liability for promoting damaging behavior.

We cannot say that Buzz Blasts and Cinnamon Toast Crunch are the same as cigarettes. Cigarettes are illegal to sell to minors; the cereals are legal. Nicotine is an addictive drug, but whether foods can be addictive is not yet clear. Yet, a common principle might apply. If Disney helps increase sales of unhealthy foods, and children then increase consumption, can the case be made that Disney is harming the children? If parents begin to see things this way, Disney's reputation will suffer.

A company such as Disney might stage a public relations coup by announcing its products will only be used to promote healthy foods. The benefit could be considerable, and other companies might be forced to follow.

Work with Celebrities to Promote Healthy Eating and Activity

The food industry, being the powerful economic force it is, can afford even the highest paid celebrities to endorse its products. Michael Jordan for McDonald's, Shaquille O'Neal for Burger King, and Britney Spears for Pepsi are examples. Perhaps there is a way to harness their visibility and power in the service of improving diet.

Some Celebrities Endorsing Fast Foods and Soft Drinks

Michael Jordan	McDonald's
Kobe Bryant	McDonald's
Donald Trump	McDonald's
Cedric the Entertainer	McDonald's
Serena Williams	McDonald's
Venus Williams	McDonald's
Shaquille O'Neal	Burger King
BB King	Burger King
Jason Alexander	KFC
Halle Berry	Pepsi
Britney Spears	Pepsi
Barry Bostwick	Pepsi
Beyoncé Knowles	Pepsi
Mike Myers	Pepsi Twist
*NSYNC	Chili's
Michael Jordan	Ball Park Franks
Grant Hill	Sprite
Garth Brooks	Dr. Pepper

Both carrot and stick approaches may help. Celebrities would not endorse a product, no matter how great the reward, if public outrage were the consequence and future endorsements would be compromised. Hence, it is unlikely that Michael Jordan would promote Marlboro or that Britney Spears would promote Camel. If public sentiment turned against celebrities who endorse certain foods, the celebrities might take their endorsements elsewhere.

Some celebrities are civic-minded and embrace a wide array of social causes. Examples are soccer stars Mia Hamm and Kristine Lilly working with Safeway Supermarkets on the Eat Like a Champion program. If more such people take on healthy eating (or childhood obesity prevention) as their favored cause and then entice their celebrity peers to join in, tremendous change might be possible. These efforts would probably be seen quite favorably by the public, making such celebrities even more valuable in the endorsement marketplace.

Help Parents Help Their Children

The food industry claims that parents must take more responsibility if children are to develop healthier eating patterns. So fine, what would they suggest be done? Create massive education programs for parents? Design advertising campaigns to provide parents with the skills to work with their children? Devise penalties for parents who do not comply? Parental responsibility sounds good, but does not lead to helpful action.

Our nation has created an environment that makes it much too hard for parents to raise children who eat well and are active. Parents are subject to the toxic environment themselves, and even those who resist find it difficult to shield their children. Helping parents do their job is good policy.

Any means possible should be explored to assist parents. Websites, books, videotapes, and the like might be useful if they convey good information, can be distributed widely, get used, and affect the behavior of both parents and children. Creative programs through groups such as parent-teacher organizations might be helpful. Prenatal counseling for expectant mothers might work. There are many ideas to explore, most of them untested. They should be pursued, but we emphasize again that this can only be *part* of the solution.

Promote Media Literacy in the Schools

Some schools have media literacy programs designed to help children become educated consumers, identify themes used to sell products, and resist being exploited. Smoking prevention programs have used this approach for years to show children how tobacco companies glamorize smoking.

Food also is important to target in media literacy programs. How food is advertised, product placements in movies, and even how schools deal with foods (vending machines, fund-raising events, etc.) could all be subject to analysis. As long as children are exposed to food advertising, they deserve education that allows them to place what they hear in the context of good health.

Conclusion

Advertising aimed at children is powerful in presentation, overwhelming in amount, and pernicious in outcome. Many children do not recognize the purpose of advertising and cannot separate advertising from programming.[90] The Flintstones, for example, are TV and movie characters, but are also toys, vitamins, and cereals. Children find advertisements fantastically engaging because of fast-paced animation, clever story lines, and the use of captivating characters.

Groups with a strong interest in protecting children call for a ban on children's advertising. The food industry opposes any change. For the sake of public health, for the common good, and for the welfare of our children, which side deserves your support?[91]

6

JUNK FOOD 101:
Schools, Commercialism,
and Unhealthy Eating

When Susan Crockett walked Amy, her eight-year-old daughter, to her school bus stop last September, she was in for a surprise. The school bus that rolled up was covered with advertisements for Burger King, Wendy's, and other name-brand products. A few weeks later, Amy, a third grader, and Crockett's three older children arrived home toting free book covers and school planners covered with ads for Kellogg's Pop-Tarts and Fox TV personalities.

At Palmer High School [in Colorado Springs], students walk through hallways dotted with signs for national brands and local companies, eat in a snack bar sporting brand-new vending machines, use computers with ad-bearing mouse pads, and play basketball in a gym decorated with banners of corporate sponsors.[1]

Schools are an arena where our nation's relationship with food is acted out in remarkable ways. The play has villains and victims, unwitting players, social and economic issues as backdrops, and an unhappy ending (thus far).

The story's plot is straightforward:

- Schools are not funded sufficiently, and food and soft drink companies are there to "help."

- Schools depend on the companies and companies need new consumers. The marriage is consummated.
- Students love the foods, and there is little community resistance.
- Money flows year after year and becomes part of the operating budget, making it difficult to turn back.

The marketing of fast foods, snack foods, and soft drinks in schools occurs in many, many forms,[2] and has created a nutrition nightmare.

About a dozen teachers and administrators from the Fair Haven Middle School in New Haven, Connecticut, taking part in the McDonald's McEducation program, worked from 4:00 to 8:00 p.m. at the counters and drive-in windows to help the school raise money (20 percent of the profits). The walls of the restaurant were decorated with pictures the children had drawn of the golden arches, Ronald McDonald, and so on. Some parents and students helped out as well. One student explained how much fun he had behind the counter and wanted to help make the food. One teacher noted that it was nice for students to see their teachers outside the classroom.[3]

In testimony before the U.S. Senate, one of us (KB) said that schools are beginning to look like a 7-Eleven with books. This is an overstatement, of course, but when one adds together vending machines, school lunches, fund-raisers, food ads on school TV, arithmetic books where children count candy and snack food, and donut and pizza certificates as homework rewards, to name a few, one sees the many ways that food companies pursue children through the schools. The children have immense buying power already, and, of course, are tomorrow's adult consumers.

Schools may be the first battleground on which the war on obesity will be fought—and with good reason. There is opportunity for improving the health of the nation's children,[4] but only if parents, teachers, school officials, communities, and elected leaders agree there is a problem and become creative with solutions.

Eating Opportunities at School

The typical American school offers many opportunities to eat, the cafeteria being only one. Lunch programs often have a la carte foods beyond the core meal, which itself may not comply with federal nutrition guidelines. The a la carte foods may include some healthy choices, but more likely are snack foods, desserts, candy, and soft drinks. Most schools have vending machines, stocked overwhelmingly with foods and drinks high in sugar, fat, and calories. Some schools have snack bars; many have school stores. Fund-raisers have students selling candy. Students can bring food into school, student groups have bake sales, and, of course, many schools have convenience stores, donut shops, and fast-food chains located nearby.

A survey in Kentucky found that 44 percent of elementary schools have vending machines and 45 percent have school stores. The numbers for middle schools are 88 percent for machines and 30 percent for stores, and for high schools the numbers are 97 percent for machines and 80 percent for stores.[5]

The annual income per school from vending machines and school stores in Kentucky schools is significant.

	Vending Machines	School Stores
Elementary Schools	$3,146	$ 6,069
Middle Schools	$5,933	$13,223
High Schools	$9,736	$ 7,730

A statewide study of 610 secondary school principals in Minnesota found that 65 percent feel it is important to have a nutrition policy in school, but only 31 percent report that such a policy exists. Ninety-eight percent of the schools have soft drink machines and 77 percent have contracts with soft drink companies.[6]

It is important that parents, community leaders, and health professionals understand what children eat in school; the messages they receive about nutrition; how their school life affects overall eating; and how national, state, and local policies affect diet. Then it will become clear whether schools must change.

School Lunches

Watching children eat lunch at school is an amazing experience. Some bring; some buy. Many trade. Much gets thrown away. The school may have a fast-food company selling food or may make the same foods itself (chicken nuggets, cheeseburgers, pizza). Food served by schools may be ignored because lunch can be purchased from a machine or school store. Sometimes cafeteria lines are long and time is short, so machines and stores might be the only choice.

The National School Lunch Program

The National School Lunch Act, signed in 1946 by President Truman, is administered through the U.S. Department of Agriculture (USDA). The National School Lunch Program (NSLP) is a federally assisted meal program operating in more than 99,000 public and private schools and residential day-care institutions. Each school day, 25 million children receive low-cost or free lunches. Congress expanded the program in 1998 to include snacks served to children in after-school educational and enrichment programs.[7]

To participate, schools and school districts must meet federal lunch requirements and must offer free or subsidized lunches to eligible children. The schools then get cash subsidies and donated commodities from the USDA for each meal they serve. Lunches must contain no more than 30 percent of calories from fat (less than one-third of these calories from saturated fat) and one-third of the Recommended Daily Allowances for protein, vitamins A and C, iron, calcium, and calories. The program cost $6.4 billion in 2001.

The commodities part of the program is quite fascinating. Some healthy foods do indeed get provided to schools, but there are also major concerns. The Physicians Committee for Responsible Medicine concluded:

- The commodity system was designed with the dual purpose of providing food at low or zero cost to public schools while at the same time providing a guaranteed market for agricultural industry.

- There is a serious conflict of interest in the commodity system in that the USDA pledges to provide nutritious meals for our nation's youth and also to bolster the industries that produce foods that contribute to obesity, heart disease, and cancer. Many of the foods offered through this program are animal products that are rich in cholesterol and saturated fat—the same type of fat that the USDA recommends that schools reduce.
- Even when schools attempt to order the more nutritious items from commodity lists, they are often unable to do so due to low demand from other schools and, therefore, infrequent delivery of these items.
- Not only are commodities often unhealthy foods, they nearly always come from the wealthiest farmers. Huge agribusiness operations benefit far more from government subsidies than struggling small farmers. The General Accounting Office reports that between 1991 and 1999 the top 10 percent of recipient farmers received nearly 60 percent of total payments.[8]

The impetus for the NSLP was the desire to feed hungry children, whose learning was impeded by malnutrition. Obesity was not a concern. As years progressed, calorie overconsumption became a problem, leading to some beneficial changes, such as setting an upper limit on fat.

The NSLP potentially affects the diet of all children, not just those who receive its meals. Through requirements it can make of participating schools, the NSLP could eventually lead to sweeping changes in children's eating.

A la Carte Foods

Many foods in schools are sold a la carte (foods not part of the core school lunch or sold in vending machines). These might be served in the cafeteria as side items (French fries or bags of chips, for instance) or in school stores. The USDA defines any foods other than those served as part of the NSLP as "competitive" foods because children may use them to replace healthier foods served in the school lunch. The NSLP is regulated, but a la carte foods are not.

Since 1985 the federal government has attempted to regulate competitive foods. Congress is concerned still today. The House Appropriations Committee Report that accompanied the Agriculture Appropriations Act for fiscal year 2001 requested that the USDA prepare a report on competitive foods. Submitted to Congress in January of 2001, the report noted a wide discrepancy between dietary recommendations and what children eat overall. It also stated that competitive foods are "relatively low in nutrient density and are relatively high in fat, added sugars, and calories." The report concluded:

- Competitive foods have diet–related health risks.
- Competitive foods may stigmatize participation in school meal programs.
- Competitive foods may affect the viability of school meal programs.
- Competitive foods convey a mixed message.[9]

These conclusions are based on studies showing that the foods available as a la carte items are primarily snack foods, cakes, cookies, chips, crackers, candy, and soft drinks.[10] A la carte items are not healthy foods for the most part and are displacing healthier foods children might be eating. One study concluded:

. . . *the primarily high-fat snacks and calorie-dense beverages offered and sold to students via a la carte programs are displacing fruits and vegetables in the diets of young teens and contributing to total and saturated fat intakes that exceed recommended levels.*[11]

"Seconds after the buzzer sounds at 11:05 A.M., hundreds of pairs of Doc Martens, Skechers, and Air Jordans beat a path to the Nicolet High School cafeteria, where low-cost hot lunches are being snubbed for Taco Bell and Pizza Hut fast foods. 'Designer-label food' was added this school semester to the chow line to make Nicolet a 'warmer, friendlier place,' said Elliott Moeser, the School District's top administrator."[12] (Milwaukee, WI)

Food Woven Through the Curriculum

Children intersect with food in many ways in a typical school, some more obvious than others.

Channel One and Food Advertising

Television food ads have invaded the schools. Channel One shows ten minutes of news and two minutes of ads in its daily broadcast to school-children. In return, schools get "free" video equipment.[13] The broadcast reaches 12,000 schools, 400,000 educators, and eight million teenage viewers, and in return for access, each school receives $25,000 in equipment.[14] Ads cost about $175,000 for a thirty-second spot and are promoted as reaching 40 percent of American teens.[15]

Researchers studying the impact of Channel One found that 69 percent of commercials broadcast over a four-week period were for food products, which included fast food, candy, soft drinks, and snack chips. The study found that Channel One influenced the children's thoughts about the products advertised, enhanced their consumer orientations, increased their intent to purchase the products, and led to increased positive feelings about the products. The study did not, however, find that students at schools broadcasting Channel One were more likely than their peers to report buying the products.[16]

Some argue that children are exposed to marketing anyway, so schools may as well benefit. School officials have even argued that they have more control over the type of messages delivered when commercials are shown at school, thereby protecting children.

Some parents limit their childs's exposure to advertising, but Channel One, under the guise of education, has found a way under the radar. Channel One boasts of this, saying in one ad, "Channel One delivers the hardest to reach teen viewers. Channel One even penetrates the lightest viewers among teens."[17]

Advertising to children in school may undermine what children learn in health classes, uses time that could be devoted to education, adds to the already high level of advertising to which children are exposed, and may be seen as an endorsement of the advertised products by the school. Too little research exists on the impact of in-school advertising, but the negative impact can be imagined[18] or inferred from the amount food companies spend to advertise.

Channel One exposure sums to six hours of commercials per year and thirty-six total hours of time that could have been spent on instruction.[19] Participation may not be voluntary. Two Ohio teens who protested the programming by walking out were sent to the local juvenile detention center.[20]

Several states have begun to question the impact of Channel One and have ended contracts. Parents in several states have filed lawsuits against schools airing Channel One but refusing other activities.[21] Many of Alabama's public schools have distanced themselves from Channel One, spurred by the findings of Birmingham-based watchdog group Obligation, Inc., which provides information on the content and effects of the program.[22]

One report estimated that the number of school hours given to Channel One costs taxpayers $1.8 billion per year; the two minutes of commercials alone cost $300 million in lost school time.[23] Equipment rental would be cheaper. The study estimated an annual rental value of the equipment at $4,000 per school, but the value of the lost time at $158,000 per school. The study also reported that Channel One makes a $30 million annual profit.

If access to television news is important, schools could subscribe to services such as CNN Newsroom, which is commercial free and free of charge.

Infiltration of Educational Materials

Imagine the product exposure when young children learn their numbers by counting Tootsie Rolls, M&M's, and Skittles.[24] One company published a math textbook for elementary school students that included the following problems:

- Pop Secret popcorn claims that only 250 of every 500 kernels meet its high standards. Write a ratio comparing numbers of good kernels to the number examined in simplest form.

- Jerry and five friends bought a six-pack of Gatorade to drink after their baseball game. Each friend wants to pay for his share of the Gatorade. If the six-pack costs $2.49, how much does each friend owe to the nearest cent?
- What is your favorite color of M&M's? What fraction of that color do you think a package would contain?[25]

The company noted that it was not paid by the food companies, but this and other examples of the commercializing of education were criticized in the press.[26] The book was approved for use in fifteen states.

An article in an education newsletter cited more learn-by-counting-food books, including *Skittles Math Riddles, Reese's Pieces: Count by Fives*, and the *Hershey Milk Chocolate Bar Fractions Book*. Some bookstores, teachers, and even publishers have chosen to reject such books, and pediatricians and parents have spoken out against publicizing unhealthy food through academics.[27]

State laws that require textbook screening do not govern the use of corporate-sponsored "educational items." The Consumers Union evaluated corporate-sponsored materials and found that 80 percent favored the company's agenda and/or included biased or incomplete information.[28] Among the commercialized food-related materials they discovered:

Sponsor	Title
American Egg Board	*The Incredible Journey from Hen to Home*
Campbell Soup	*Prego Thickness Experiment*
Chef Boyardee	*Sharks Learning Activity Kit*
Domino's Pizza	*Encounter Math (Count on Domino's)*
Kellogg's	*Kids Get Going with Breakfast*
Mars, Inc.	*100 Percent Smart Energy to Go*
National Honey Board	*What's Buzzin'*
National Livestock and Meat Board	*Munchsters Talk About Food*
National Potato Board	*Count Your Chips*

Product placement in classroom material is orchestrated by savvy advertising companies who recognize the buying power of a captive student audience. Lifetime Learning Systems of Fairfield, Connecticut, advertised that companies can "take your message into the classroom, where the young people you want to reach are forming attitudes that will last a lifetime."[29] One cartoonlike ad showed kids rushing ahead with dollars in hand, the caption reading, "They're ready to spend, and we reach them."[30]

Food as an Academic Incentive

Incentive programs can support laudable goals like encouraging children to attend school, read, and do homework, but prizes tend to be things like donuts and pizza. The survey in Kentucky mentioned earlier found that the most common rewards for good academic performance, behavior, and attendance are pizza, candy, and soft drinks.

Several major food companies are involved. Pizza Hut's Book It! Program, in its seventeenth year, is a well-known example of an incentive program. Students are rewarded for meeting reading goals with free pizza, and now the program includes both elementary students and preschoolers. In a Detroit Elementary School, McDonald's constructed a Mini McDonald's where students could earn meals through reading, quizzes, and good school attendance. A mural of McDonald's characters was placed on the cafeteria wall.[31]

Dunkin' Donuts has a program called "Grade A Donuts: Honoring Homework Stars." Teachers can order a kit that includes an activity guide, "Homework Heroes" booklets for children, a classroom poster, and sets of coupons, each good for two free donuts. The program aims to "reward students and their homework helpers for good homework habits."[32]

Programs like these have both benefits and costs. We are not aware of whether these incentives improve school performance or whether food acts as a more powerful reward than alternative prizes like small toys. Drawbacks must be considered because such programs may influence food habits. Certainly other incentives could be used (movie passes, toys, etc.).

Selling Advertising Space in Schools

Placing advertisements or company logos in prominent locations has also become part of what schools sell to soft drink companies. Scoreboards with company logos are common, but other forms of advertising also occur. One university in Connecticut, where swim meets are held for children of all ages, has padded deck chairs around the pool with Coca-Cola in bright red letters against a white background. A Dallas high school near the Dallas–Fort Worth airport was paid to have the Dr. Pepper logo painted on its rooftop for advertising to arriving flights.[33]

Soft drink machines themselves are advertisements. The fronts of such machines are generally brightly colored and feature well-lit company logos, usually with pictures of the drinks. All students, no matter whether they buy the products, pass by the machines and are exposed to advertising.

School buses have become moving advertisements. Although the National Association of State Directors of Pupil Transportation and the National Conference on School Transportation have encouraged banning ads for safety reasons, buses continue to be covered. The New York City Board of Education hopes to raise $53 million annually by allowing ads on the district's buses.[34] Colorado school buses advertise 7 UP and Old Navy.[35]

Schools and food companies think of ever more clever ways to collaborate. Joining the age-old ads in school newspapers, yearbooks, and programs for theatrical, musical, and sporting events, there are reports of advertising and corporate logos on school-sponsored television stations, recognition on a school district's voice mail system, "spirit buses" with a school's logo along with the logo from Burger King, signs in hallways, and logos on posters, calendars, book covers, and mouse pads.[36]

Food as Fund-Raising

The National PTA held its 2002 convention in San Antonio. The *New York Times* published an article on the meeting, discussing not education but sugar.[37] The *Times* reported that the booths in the exhibit hall displayed software, books, testing materials, and candy. Mars, Nestle, and Hershey were among the "confectioners" who distributed free samples of candy and did their best to convince local PTAs to sell candy for fund-raisers.

Another exhibitor at the meeting was the Sugar Association. They distributed brochures saying that sugar does not cause obesity or tooth decay, and added, "If your child loves sweet treats, there's no need to worry." The association says that sugar used in moderation can be part of a balanced diet.

The National PTA and school administrators realize the inconsistency of selling candy to promote education. Many must have misgivings, but ultimately yield in an attempt to support the schools. The conflict between principle and practice is shown in the following two quotes:

National PTA supports policies that protect students from exploitation by prohibiting programs in schools that require students to view advertising.
—NATIONAL PTA POSITION STATEMENT ON
COMMERCIALIZATION IN SCHOOLS[38]

Shirley Igo, the National PTA President, said that when schools could not pay for their instructional programs, PTAs helped fill the gap, and that candy sales were only one way to do so.[39]

Two things might change the situation. Pressure and concern from both parents and teachers might make health salient enough to prevail over the need for revenue, and other ways could be developed to replace the money now generated from food sales.

In the End, What Do Children Eat in Schools?

With so many eating opportunities in schools, what parents see on a school lunch menu may bear little resemblance to what children actually eat. The school lunch itself might be a problem. The total fat and saturated fat content of meals in most schools is higher than that mandated by the NSLP.[40] Beyond the meal itself are the vending machines, a la carte items, school stores, and the like. Compared to schools with only the NSLP, children in schools with these additional eating opportunities eat fewer fruits and vegetables.[41]

The U.S. Department of Agriculture created a program called "Healthy School Nutrition Environments" in conjunction with several health organizations. Claiming that nutrition should be a priority in every school, the group pointed out that students "are flunking healthy eating."

- Only 2 percent of youth meet all the recommendations of the food guide pyramid; 16 percent do not meet any.
- Fewer than 15 percent to 20 percent of schoolchildren get adequate servings of fruits and vegetables.
- Only 16 percent of children meet the guidelines for saturated fat.
- Teenagers drink twice as much carbonated soda as milk; only 19 percent of girls get the recommended amount of calcium.
- Twelve percent of students report skipping breakfast, and only 11 percent have breakfasts with the recommended nutrients.[42]

This gloomy picture is reinforced by findings from the School Health Policies and Programs Study 2000. This national survey included information for all states and hundreds of school districts. Among the conclusions:

- Only eight of twenty-two food preparation practices recommended by dietitians to reduce fat, saturated fat, sodium, and added sugar are used in schools in any regular way.
- One-third of schools do not offer students a daily choice of two or more types of fruit or fruit juice, two or more entrées or main courses, or two or more vegetables.
- Nearly all high schools, most middle/junior high schools, and 25 percent of elementary schools have food and beverage machines.
- More than 40 percent of elementary schools allow students to buy food and beverages through vending machines, school stores, snack bars, or canteens, even though "young children may lack the maturity to make healthy and safe food choices."[43]

Overall, the report concluded that there is "a disturbing picture of the widespread availability of foods and beverages high in fat, sodium, and added sugar as a la carte choices, in vending machines, and in school stores."

The Physician's Committee for Responsible Medicine dispatched a team of dietitians to the nation's ten largest school districts to evaluate school lunches. The dietitians assembled information on a number of factors, including whether the lunch offered low-fat vegetable side dishes, whole or dried fruits as a side dish or dessert, and so on. The report card below shows the grades for each district.[44]

District	Grade
Broward County School District (Fort Lauderdale)	B
Dade County School District (Miami)	C
Fairfax County Public Schools (Virginia)	C
New York City Public Schools	C
Clark County School District (Las Vegas)	D
Dallas Independent School District	D
Los Angeles Unified School District	D
Philadelphia City School District	F
Detroit City School District	F
Houston Independent School District	F

Linking Diet, Activity, and Obesity to Academic Performance

School officials are often asked to modify the diet and activity environment to help improve the health of children. Health is important, but demonstrations that poor diet affects academic performance are likely to be a powerful motivation to change.

There is considerable research on malnutrition and school performance. Correcting malnutrition improves performance, but the effects of overnutrition have not been documented. It would be surprising if strong links do not exist.

There is the need for studies of both immediate and long-term effects of poor diet. David Figlio and Joshua Winicki tested short-term effects in Virginia schools. They examined whether schools at risk of not meeting state standards would increase lunch calories on days when standardized tests are scheduled, in hopes of improving scores. This is called "gaming the system." This study found that districts with at-risk schools did increase calories more on testing days than did other districts, mainly with "empty calories" (nonnutritious foods). Further, the districts that increased calories found the largest increases in test scores.[45] Many media accounts of this study suggested that eating junk food improves test performance.[46]

Several issues arise in interpreting this study. At-risk districts probably have disproportionate numbers of poor children. Given that malnutrition is most common in poor children and impedes academic performance, the increased calories, no matter their source, may have helped these districts by addressing the short-term malnutrition problem. The most important questions are whether performance would have improved just as much or more if the extra calories came from healthy foods, or if things other than the food might have caused the score increase (e.g., at-risk schools teaching to the tests, or the use of other gaming strategies that Figlio and Winicki discuss).

It is essential to test for the longer-term effects of unhealthy eating. A body improperly nourished cannot keep the mind alert, inquisitive, and sharp. Poor diet and inactivity produce lethargy and drowsiness, so attention and ability to retain information may suffer. In addition, it is possible that the poor self-esteem engendered by obesity generalizes to academic self-esteem. It is hard to imagine the mind at the top of its game when the body is in disarray. Studying this issue should be a national priority.

Can Existing Programs in Schools Solve the Problem?

Nutrition education by itself has not been consistently effective. Knowledge about nutrition can improve, sometimes accompanied by altered attitudes about eating, but there have not been many demonstrations of lasting changes in food intake.

There are exceptions, however.[47] For instance, developing an intervention program similar to one used in England,[48] the health ministry of Singapore created obesity programs for schools.[49] Nutrition education was woven into the school curriculum and special help was available for obese children. Rates of obesity dropped in both adolescents (ages fifteen and sixteen) and children (ages eleven and twelve).

Programs that have changed the school environment have been most successful. One study found that lower-fat dessert recipes were well accepted by children.[50] Another group of researchers were able to more than double the selection of low-fat milk in inner-city elementary schools in a Latino community.[51] The CATCH Trial (Child and Adolescent Trial for Cardiovascular Health) found positive changes in diet lasting three years in large numbers of children in four states who received a detailed intervention program.[52]

An innovative program has been undertaken by Simone French and colleagues at the University of Minnesota. Called TACOS (Trying Alternative Cafeteria Options in Schools), the program was designed first to assess the nutrition environment in schools, second to increase availability of lower-fat foods in a la carte areas of the schools, and third to develop student-based peer promotion programs to publicize the availability of the low-fat items. Only preliminary results are available, but they appear to be quite positive.[53]

One approach with consistently positive results has been to lower the price of healthy items. Much of this work has also been done by Simone French, Robert Jeffery, and colleagues at Minnesota.[54] Targeting both vending machine and cafeterias options, this group has shown that lowering prices of healthy foods increases how often they are selected.

Programs such as these are encouraging, but can be only part of the solution to eating problems in schools. Some programs are intensive and costly. Joined with this are positive but sometimes only modest results. In the CATCH program mentioned above, the difference in self-reported dietary fat intake was 30.3 percent compared to 32.2 percent in fifth-grade students who did or did not receive the program.

Nutrition education in the absence of environmental change is not likely to have significant effects (and sends mixed messages), and environmental change without nutrition education is likely to miss opportunities to teach children lessons they can use outside school. Teaching children healthy eating habits, coupled with changing the environment, is likely to have the greatest impact on overall lifestyle. Both education and environmental change are important.

The School Food Triad: Three Barriers to a Healthy Food Environment

Three barriers to healthy eating are fundamental to schools. These must be considered if schools are to become healthy places to eat.

Schools Do Not Consider Healthy Eating Relevant to Their Mission

What children eat has not typically been viewed as important to a school's educational mission. Providing food is often seen as a necessary service, much as custodial service might be, and is expected to generate a profit or at least break even. Ironically, earning money from selling energy-dense food is thought to promote education, as it helps buy a scoreboard, fund school trips, and so on.

Food service directors get stuck in a tug-of-war.[55] On one hand is their desire to serve healthy foods and to see children thrive. The American School Food Service Association, for instance, has excellent materials not only on school lunch programs, but on general nutrition information for children and parents.[56]

Tugging in the opposite direction is pressure from the schools to make money. Absorbing a loss might be acceptable if needed education were occurring and the cafeteria were considered a classroom, but residing outside the educational mainstream as it does, food service must focus on income.

A different conceptual stance is to view food as one key to making a school a top-rate educational institution and to agree that creating a healthy environment supercedes the need for income. Several changes then become obvious. Considering the cafeteria a laboratory for learning, where children eat in a healthy manner but also learn about nutrition, would be one move forward. Integrating nutrition education with both health education and physical education could generate consistent, powerful messages about the importance of good diet. The most important step of all, however, is to get better control over foods available in school. Schools making such conceptual and structural changes would stand out and would probably benefit from public reaction.

> In Duluth, Minnesota, the school food service director was forced to offer branded pizza (Pizza Hut and Domino's) to replace the frozen pizza they had been serving earlier. Local principals were hungry for revenue and had started competing for his "customers" by selling Little Caesars pizza in the school commons. The food service director was pleased that his move recaptured his "market share."[57]

Popular Foods Bring in More Money

As long as schools need the extra money and selling popular food provides it, there are heavy incentives for schools to continue current practices. Schools receive only $2.14 for each free meal they serve as part of the National School Lunch Program, often not enough to break even, while the profit margins on a la carte foods and items sold in vending machines can be 50 percent to 100 percent.[58] An example from a *Time* magazine article entitled "Flunking Lunch" is Northside Independent School District in San Antonio. The cost for an entire federal lunch is $1.75, while students pay $2 for just one slice of Papa John's pizza, which is more than double what the schools pay to buy it.[59]

If Unhealthy Foods Are Available, Children Will Eat Them

As described in Chapter 2, it is clear from research with both humans and laboratory animals that providing access to foods high in sugar, fat, and calories leads to overeating. Introducing healthier options into the picture does not have an appreciable effect on the appeal or consumption of the high-fat, high-sugar foods.

One study found that 76 percent of schools sell pizza, burgers, or sandwiches; 80 percent have high-fat cakes and cookies; and 62 percent sell French fries as a la carte items. But in addition, 90 percent have fruits and vegetables and 48 percent sell low-fat yogurt or low-fat cookies or pastry.[60] Still, the diet is in dire condition. For most children, for most of the time, healthy foods will be eaten if only healthy foods are available and if unhealthy foods are not available as competition.

The implication? Schools should not have unhealthy foods, at any time, at any place, in any amounts. Having healthier items added to a menu containing unhealthy favorites will help a few children, but most will go for the favorites.

An interesting case study is Orono High School in Orono, Maine. The school removed all unhealthy items from vending machines and replaced them with healthier choices. Principal Cathryn Knox noted, "Kids are hungry, and they will eat what you offer them. And the vending machines empty just as fast as when they had candy and chips."[61]

Moves by the food industry to offer some healthier items may be a legitimate attempt to help or may be a crafty means of dodging more drastic moves.[62] They know what children are selecting from machines, and our suspicion is that sales of unhealthy items will be unaffected by inserting a few healthier items. But in making what may turn out to be token changes, the food companies may fight off moves to expel all unhealthy products.

An important test of this will be an experimental program launched in the fall of 2002 by the USDA. This $6 million program, part of the 2002 Farm Bill and initiated as part of President Bush's Healthy U.S. campaign, will provide free fruits and vegetables to students in 100 middle and high schools in five states.

Two competing forces will be at work. The fact that there is no cost for the fruits and vegetables should boost consumption, according to work showing that lowering prices of healthy items leads to increased purchases in schools. Competing with this is the lure of the unhealthy foods, which may lead many children to ignore the healthy choices.

Learning which of these two forces prevails will be important. If the program has the intended effects, balancing the diet changes against the cost will be key.

The triad is powerful. Schools make more money on unhealthy foods; the money is important to the schools; and children are happy when they eat the brands of fast foods, pizza, snacks, and soft drinks they love.

Opposition to Commercialism in Schools

Just as there has been strong opposition to children's advertising, as explained in Chapter 5, many people and organizations object to the commercialization of schools. Objection ranges beyond food products, but food marketing is the most commonly criticized. The titles of several newspaper/magazine articles and reports by consumer groups show the growing awareness of this issue:

> "How Corporations Are Buying Their Way into America's
>   Classrooms"
> "Selling America's Kids: Commercial Pressures on Kids of the 90s"
> "Schools Teach 3 C's: Candy, Cookies, and Chips"
> "Captive Kids: A Report on Commercial Pressures on Kids at
>   School"[63]

Organizations have taken a strong stance on commercial activities in schools. Both national and local groups have been involved, including Commercial Alert, Consumers Union, Citizens' Campaign for Commercial Free Schools, Commercialism in Education Research Unit (at Arizona State University), and the Coalition for Public Education (part of British Columbia Teacher's Federation in Canada). These groups involve a broad range of individuals (parents, teachers, people from child advocacy and consumer protection groups, scientists), have websites, and offer ways to get involved.

Consumer Alert has been especially active at the national and even international level.[64] This group marshaled strong protest against Channel One and organized the ouster from the schools of ZapMe!, a company that used school-based computers to advertise to children and do market research on them. In 2002, Commercial Alert organized an international coalition of health advocates and professionals to protest the collaboration of UNICEF with McDonald's to sponsor "McDonald's World Children's Day."

One concrete step that can be taken in local communities is to form groups that can work with local press, community leaders, and schools to make the public aware of commercialism and to seek specific changes. For instance, Seattle parents gathered examples of advertising in schools and successfully halted school commercialism in their area.[65]

> "The kids we're reaching are consumers in training."
> —Joseph Fenton of Donnelly Marketing[66]

Early Signs of a Turning Tide

Senator Christopher Dodd of Connecticut and Rep. George Miller of California commissioned a study on vending machines in the fall of 2000 and found wide variance in the regulation of the machines from school to school.[67] Several senators have been working to introduce legislation restricting marketing and snack and soda sales in schools.[68] The USDA has recommended that all snacks sold in schools meet federal nutrition requirements, although those requirements are loose enough that candy bars can qualify.[69] Senator Tom Harkin of Iowa supported the Congressional bill subsidizing free fruits and vegetables in school cafeterias as an alternative to vending items.[70]

A report by the Government Accounting Office on state laws governing school commercialism found the laws variable and inadequate. As of November 2000, only nineteen states had regulations addressing commercialism in schools, some of which were designed to *promote* commercial activity. None of the policies were directed at more recent media-based commercialism (e.g., Channel One). Based on reports that children were lured to report personal information to databases, Congressman Miller and Senator Dodd introduced a bill to protect children's privacy from market researchers.[71]

Grassroots efforts make a difference. In 1999, New York parents brought a class-action lawsuit that resulted in an agreement that schools can sell only nutritious snacks during lunch. An important impetus for Philadelphia's turning down a ten-year, $43 million Coke school contract was opposition from parents.[72]

Success Stories
Sarah Church, Berkeley, California, High School Student
Sarah organized student opposition to commercialism in her school and aims to create a "national student movement against in-school advertising."[73]

Citizens' Campaign for Commercial-Free Schools in Seattle
This group halted a corporate partnership program proposed by the school board. The board then appointed group members to a task force to control other commercial propositions.[74]

5 A Day Power Plus Program in St. Paul
A team of scientists worked with twenty elementary schools in St. Paul, targeting a multiethnic group of children in the fourth and fifth grades. A program involving classroom instruction, parent involvement, changes in food service in the school, and industry support increased fruit and vegetable consumption in the children.[75]

High Schools with Food and Agriculture Programs and Courses
Some high schools have courses on food and agriculture where students learn about growing food, nutrition, and so on. Some are in rural, farm

areas, but others are in inner cities. Some schools sell the produce raised by students to local restaurants.

Some key examples are in Berkeley, California, where a number of schools have organic gardens that help children learn about growing and cooking food. In Philadelphia, a well-known restaurant, the White Dog Café, buys produce raised by students at a nearby inner-city school.[76]

Kentucky's Lt. Governor Fights Junk in School Vending Machines

Kentucky's Lt. Governor, Steve Henry, is a physician. He went to Carlisle Elementary School to explain why he supported House Bill 553, cosponsored by fifteen House members, which would eliminate most snack foods and sugared soft drinks from school vending machines. A study in Kentucky of 343 schools found that 88 percent had vending machines and 24 percent violated state regulations to not sell such foods until thirty minutes after the last lunch period.

Lt. Gov. Henry brought to the school a soft drink bottle filled with the undiluted sugar found in a soft drink, a pound of synthetic fat, and a model of a heart with clogged arteries. Nine-year-old Tommy Courtney said, "I didn't know that Fritos were bad for you" and "I'm not going to eat Fritos or drink pop anymore."[77]

The bill passed the Kentucky House but was defeated in the Senate. No matter the legislative outcome, such efforts are good first steps toward legislation that is almost certain to come and will help sensitize parents, teachers, and school officials to the food environment in schools.

Materials on "Nutrition Friendly Schools" in Pennsylvania

A collaboration between the Pennsylvania Department of Education and Pennsylvania State University produced an excellent kit for schools on creating a nutrition friendly environment. The videotape and booklet contain many helpful ideas and resources.[78]

Philadelphia Consortium Works for Healthier Eating in Schools

Galvanized by a proposed $43 million agreement between Coke and the Philadelphia school system and realizing that the food environment in Philadelphia schools should be improved, nutrition-minded people from various community organizations in Philadelphia came together to form the Comprehensive School Nutrition Policy Task Force.[79] With members from the school system, University of Pennsylvania, American Cancer Society, Greater Philadelphia Food Bank, and other groups, the task force works closely with schools to improve nutrition education and the food environment. Schools are encouraged to develop clever ways to teach children about healthy eating, and the task force offers financial incentives for schools who meet certain nutrition goals.

Health Promoting Schools in Australia

An impressive effort in Australia, the Health Promoting Schools program, has shown how the health of children should be seen as central to their learning and can be promoted by integrated efforts of families, schools, and communities. A health-promoting school "is a place where all members of the school community work together to provide students with integrated and positive experiences and structures that promote and protect their health. . . . This includes the formal and informal curricula in health, the creation of a safe and healthy school environment, the provision of appropriate health services, and the involvement of the family and wider community in efforts to promote health."[80]

West Virginia

West Virginia took earlier and more progressive action than any other state, banning the sale of junk foods in its schools.[81] As far back as 1974, state officials were concerned with mixed nutrition messages at schools and the negative effects of nonnutritious foods on the health of children.

Taking Action

A number of actions are available at local, state, and national levels to improve the food environment in schools.

Forge National Policy to Permit Only Healthy Foods in Schools

To its credit, the federal government has proposed that the food environment in schools become healthier. As three examples:

- The government's Healthy People 2010 report listed as one of its nutrition objectives to "increase the proportion of children and adolescents ages six to nineteen years whose intake of meals and snacks at school contribute to good overall dietary quality."[82]
- In 1985, Congress passed the Competitive Food Service rule, prohibiting the sale of foods with minimal nutrition in the food service area at meal times.[83]
- The Centers for Disease Control and Prevention issued guidelines for creating healthy eating environments in schools.[84]

However, both the spirit and guidelines from these government actions are violated routinely. Most schools do *not* offer healthy eating environments.

Current policies, guidelines, and regulations help, but not nearly as much as health leaders would like or children deserve. Pushing healthy food into schools, say through the National School Lunch Program or the USDA pilot program to offer fruits and vegetables at no cost, is worthwhile but must be coupled with policies to rid schools of unhealthy foods. Otherwise the pull of the good-tasting, heavily marketed, high-calorie foods will be too great.

State agencies and local school officials are granted the authority by the federal government to restrict competitive foods, but no specific action is required and most schools impose few restrictions. Stronger federal action is necessary.

Integrate Nutrition and Eating with the Educational Mission of the School

Children who eat well will be healthier. Healthier children are better students, will do better on standardized tests, and will reflect well on the school. Children win, parents win, and schools and their communities win.

The school cafeteria can be a classroom where children experiment with and learn to like healthy foods. Integrating the food environment with health and physical education classes and allowing children to be part of the food selection and preparation process can elevate nutrition to the role it must play in schools.

Some of the materials on nutrition and eating available to schools are produced or provided by the food industry and in many cases are biased or incomplete.[85] There exist unbiased, engaging, interactive materials that can be used in classrooms to teach children about healthy eating. An example is a program called Hungry Red Planet that was developed with funding by the National Institutes of Health and is available in versions for schools and home.[86]

Eliminate Fast Foods and Unhealthy Snack Foods from Schools

Manipulating where vending machines are placed, keeping the machines closed part of the day, and offering healthier items are good but inadequate steps. Unhealthy foods should not be sold in vending machines, school cafeterias, or school stores. This seemingly drastic move is consistent with recommendations from an expert consensus panel on school nutrition.[87] The little existing research and several anecdotal reports suggest that children adapt well to such aggressive changes. Cutting back on high-sugar and high-fat foods should be coupled with increasing the range of choices among healthy items by offering healthy foods and beverages in vending machines, school stores, canteens, and cafeterias. Such rules can be made at local, state, and federal levels. Local victories often lead to broader discussion and then subsequent state victories.

Control Unhealthy Foods in Reauthorization of the National School Lunch Program

For reauthorization of the National School Lunch Program, a bold and decisive move would be to require all participating schools to eliminate unhealthy foods and beverages from all locations. Merely considering this would generate a storm of opposition from the food industry, counters from health groups, and a sea of publicity that would raise public awareness of what is occurring in schools. This itself could mobilize people locally. If limiting unhealthy foods became federal law, children would eat what they are offered and improved diet would be the result.

A position far short of this has been proposed by some groups, namely to empower the Secretary of Agriculture to regulate competitive foods. This could be helpful or not, depending of course on the action the administration chooses to take. Thus far, there is no sign of any administration taking serious action on this issue. The history of the Department of Agriculture has been to permit the food industry considerable influence on nutrition policy.[88] Considering sentiments proposed by officials in recent administrations (see Chapter 1), there is no reason to be hopeful that providing this power to the Secretary of Agriculture would be helpful. There is a distinct possibility, in fact, that lax national regulation might supersede more strict state or local efforts.

Change the Nature and Price of What Is in Vending Machines and School Stores

If unhealthy foods are in schools, incentives should be established to steer children away from these foods and toward better options. The contents of vending machines and school stores, not the machines and stores per se, are the problem. Selling water, nonfat milk, and 100 percent fruit juices would help preserve income for the schools, let industry take part in education in a healthy way, and offer children a choice among healthy options. Snack food opportunities should be altered in similar ways to include healthy items such as fresh fruit.

Urge Schools and Companies to Stop Marketing to Children

There are signs of public pressure leading schools to forsake contracts with soft drink and food companies, so pressure from parents, the general public, and the press can be powerful. Pouring rights contracts, as described in Chapter 7, have been renegotiated, and many districts have allowed their contracts to expire under community pressure. Parents in New York and Philadelphia protested in the streets against vending contracts in local schools.[89] This negative publicity discourages both schools and companies from seeking contracts. Parents can work as individuals by writing and calling school superintendents, principals, and food service directors, along with state education, health, and other elected officials.

Some legislators have begun to propose bills requiring schools to limit commercialism in schools. These bills are dependent on constituent support.

End Tax Breaks for Contributions to Schools Coupled with Commercial Messages

Corporations should not be discouraged from supporting education, but opportunities to promote products should not be a *quid pro quo*. Tax law should not permit financial benefit to occur from these activities.[90]

Find Creative Ways to Replace Food and Soft Drink Money

If schools must partner with business to stay afloat, it should not be with companies selling unhealthy foods. Perhaps some national industry associated with positive activities (say sporting goods companies like Reebok or Adidas) or even a neutral image (computers) could be partners, or perhaps a coalition of local businesses could step in.

A number of states and municipalities have generated money through small taxes on soft drinks or snack foods, but the funds have not been earmarked for nutrition, physical activity, or obesity prevention.[91] Estimates are that a national tax of one cent per can of soft drink would raise $1.5 billion per year, more than enough to cover what schools now make from soft drinks and snack foods.

Encourage Community Groups to Embrace Nutrition as a Cause

School and community organizations could play an important role in sensitizing communities to the importance of nutrition. Nutrition and physical activity in schools would be a natural cause for parent-teacher organizations to tackle. Civic-minded groups such as the Junior League, Rotary, and local foundations might rally members around this cause.

Seek Change Through Legislation, Regulation, and, Perhaps, Litigation

Change produced by local efforts can have a striking local impact and can create victories that might then be replicated elsewhere. But more systematic and widespread change is necessary, as many schools might still find the sales of soft drinks and snack foods too compelling. Legislation and regulation are the natural choices to have broad impact.

We suggest national and/or state legislation to prohibit snack foods and soft drinks from schools. When legislation and regulation occur too slowly and public opinion alone is not enough to change institutions like schools, litigation may be necessary. This is a complex, thorny issue, as we'll discuss in Chapter 10, but the threat of legal action may be sufficient to motivate some school systems to change.

Require Schools to Be Open and Clear About Industry Connections

Schools must make thoughtful and transparent decisions about the degree to which money will be accepted from businesses in exchange for sales of products, promotion, or advertising space. These activities are considered inherently unethical by some and should cease. If schools feel they cannot operate otherwise, parent groups should be informed and made part of the process, school budgets should make clear the origins of their income, and some statement should be made to the community of the rules that govern these transactions.

Define Specifically How Poor Diet Affects Academic Performance

It is essential to establish the impact of overnutrition on academic performance. It is plausible that the lethargy produced by high-sugar and high-fat diets, spikes in insulin and "sugar lows," and the general disrepair of the body resulting from poor diet will have a negative impact on attention, motor skills, retention of information, and so on. Well-controlled studies on the topic are imperative.

Switch to Nonfood Fund-Raisers

The typical school fund-raiser has children selling candy (and more recently, pizza). Often the family buys some or most of the candy. Increasing candy consumption is a concern itself, but calculated into the human cost must be the glorification of candy through its association with causes, and the free advertising implicit in fund-raisers.

Alternatives are available. Fruit, wrapping paper, candles, family photographs, T-shirts, sweatshirts, ceramic tiles, and other items have been used. Alternative Fund Raising, Inc. works with a nursery to sell tree and shrub seedlings and other conservation and nature-related products. With such items, children might learn a very different message.

Teach Media Literacy to Inoculate Children Against Food Advertising

Current health education programs often teach children to understand advertising, to see through messages targeted at teens, and to resist exploitation. Buffering children from cigarette and alcohol advertising is often done in an attempt to teach "media literacy." Food advertising should be added.

Create "Food Free" Zones Within Walking Distance of Schools

Schools and the areas that surround them should promote health. Having donut shops, fast-food restaurants, and convenience stores near a school undermines what occurs in the school. Zoning laws could prohibit the operation of businesses selling food within a certain distance of schools.

Unite Teachers and Students

Teachers are a key part of the puzzle. As one teacher lamented, contracts with food and soft drink companies may be shrouded in such secrecy that teachers and even administrators may have little input.[92] Teachers should be nosy and find out about agreements the school is making. Teachers deserve to know—after all, they must deal with the consequences.

Studies have shown that healthy behavior can be successfully marketed, just like unhealthy behavior. Teachers can support school programs encouraging healthier eating and, of course, can model healthy eating themselves. Students can also mobilize and join forces to demand a healthier environment for themselves. Such action is likely to be of great interest to the local press and will capture the attention of parents who might not otherwise be interested.

Conclusion

A document including "The Ten Keys to Promote Healthy Eating in Schools" was developed by the USDA in conjunction with a number of notable groups: the American Academy of Family Physicians, the American Academy of Pediatrics, the American Dietetic Association, the National Hispanic Medical Association, and the National Medical Association.[93] The ten keys include a number of impressive ideas for changing the environment, but when we compare the list to reality, we see pie in the sky. It is possible that not a single school in the nation satisfies the ten criteria. Through documents like these, the USDA talks a good game and may in fact consider children's nutrition a priority, but until it breaks free of industry influence and can take decisive action, the nation will see little more than reports.

Why is the situation so bad? It would be convenient to blame the schools, but this ignores the financial and social realities schools confront. Schools have not had much choice. They need the money, want to keep children happy, don't want parents complaining, have other priorities, and may simply not realize how nutrition affects the academic well-being of their students.

Communities have not demanded that schools change because children's nutrition and the prevention of obesity have not been priorities. They have not been local priorities because state and national efforts have been weak, and the food companies have been allowed to roam free among our children. Something is dreadfully wrong.

That the USDA produced these ten keys is both shocking and wonderful. These might have been expected from nutrition activist groups, not a large, conservative government agency responsive to the food industry. We salute the USDA for this effort and suggest that these keys become guidelines and then regulations and that elected leaders provide the funds necessary to implement meaningful change.

7

SOFT DRINKS 102: Schools and Unhealthy Beverages

Soft drink companies have shown how deeply they care about the future of America's youth.

—NATIONAL SOFT DRINK ASSOCIATION[1]

In 1998, Coca-Cola held a national contest offering a prize to the school that could best devise a program for advertising Coke's new discount cards to children. Competing for a local $500 prize and the national prize of $10,000, Greenbrier High School in Augusta, Georgia, went all out.

The school's effort culminated in a "Coke in Education Day" where Coke officials were invited to lecture in economics classes and analysis of Coke products was done for chemistry. The crown jewel was to be a photograph of all 1,230 students, dressed in red or white shirts, assembled on school grounds to spell out "Coke."

As the picture was about to be taken, a senior named Mike Cameron pulled off his outer shirt to reveal a Pepsi shirt. He was lectured on discipline and suspended from school.[2]

Schools need money and the soft drink companies offer a way to get it. Coke, Pepsi, and the other companies dangle the bait and the schools must bite, even knowing a sharp hook lurks beneath the prize. If sports teams are to play, clubs to exist, and bands to have uniforms, the money must come from somewhere. Thus, alliances between schools and soft drink companies grow stronger with time.[3] The two parties have been creative at molding schools into marketing enterprises and have made soft drinks part of school life.[4]

Deeply Dependent Schools

Schools rely on the money from the sale of soft drinks and from contracts they sign with bottlers. This dependence is hard to break. Children expect their favorite drinks, communities count on the money when funding schools, vending machines become part of the school landscape, and partnerships between soft drink companies and schools are cemented into the country's education milieu.

These partnerships can be formidable, with schools often reacting strongly to proposals to end associations with the soft drink giants. In 2002, California State Senator Deborah Ortiz introduced legislation to ban the sale of carbonated beverages in schools. One of the earliest and most vocal opponents was the education lobby (superintendents and principals).

Legislation regularly appears before Congress to empower the Secretary of Agriculture to prohibit the sales of soft drinks, candy, and high-fat snacks in schools. The soft drink and sugar lobbyists fight off such moves, aided by the National School Boards Association and the National Association of Secondary School Principals.[5]

Connections between schools and the soft drink industry are not hidden. The industry boasts of these relationships with masterful public relations. For instance, the National Soft Drink Association presents data from a survey by the Trust to Reach Education Excellence that 92 percent of school principals say schools should form partnerships with local businesses and that 62 percent say their schools have entered into contracts with the soft drink companies.[6] The spin comes in interpreting these high numbers. The Association says:

Soft drink companies have had a strong and long-lasting commitment to America's education process for more than fifty years.

And

These partnerships are working well and serving the best interests of students and schools.

And

The soft drink industry has a long commitment to promoting a healthy lifestyle for individuals—especially children.

And finally

The revenue generated from the sale of beverages in schools is an important part of the education funding equation in the United States.[7]

We agree with at least this last statement. The soft drink companies *are* a presence in the schools and *have* become a regular part of the funding equation.

Sweet Persuasion: School Soft Drink Contracts

The Center for Commercial-Free Public Education estimated that 240 districts in thirty-one states have exclusive "pouring rights" arrangements or contracts with soft-drink companies. This may just scratch the surface, given the estimate from the soft drink association that 62 percent of all principals reported having contracts. Most without contracts have vending machines anyway.

The study of 610 secondary schools in Minnesota mentioned in Chapter 6 found that 98 percent have soft drink machines and 77 percent have contracts with soft drink companies.[8] In Kentucky, vending machines are in 44 percent of elementary schools, 88 percent of middle schools, and 97 percent of high schools. Eighty-three percent of Kentucky schools have exclusive contracts with bottlers.[9]

Schools see pouring rights contracts as a way to increase funding. This is increasingly necessary as communities are reluctant to raise taxes. Few school officials are savvy in negotiating corporate contracts and may find themselves supporting more than vending machines.

A case in point is Gulf Coast High School in Florida, which entered into a contract with Coca-Cola involving thirty-two vending machines. As part of the "Total Beverage Partnership Program," Coca-Cola "gives" the school educational support items such as Fruitopia software packages and Powerade coolers, squeeze bottles, towels, and clipboards. Coca-Cola, of course, owns Fruitopia and Powerade. Coke provides scoreboards, student awards, plastic tables and chairs, and umbrellas, all prominently displaying the product name. The school hopes to earn $124,150 in equipment, supplements, and commission within five years.[10]

Schools find themselves in a compromising position when contracts set minimum sales figures and when the school makes a percentage of what is sold. They must then market soft drinks effectively or lose money, leading in some cases to highly questionable, extreme behavior by school officials.

Colorado Springs Surrendering to Coke

In 1998, school officials in Colorado Springs, Colorado, signed a ten-year, multimillion dollar contract with Coca-Cola granting exclusivity for company products in all schools. In exchange, the school system agreed to sell 70,000 cases of Coke products in one of the contract's first three years. In 1997, the year prior to the contract, the system sold 21,000 cases of products. The school system had agreed to more than triple the sales of soft drinks.

Partway into the critical first three years, school officials grew worried because they were not selling enough Coke products. A letter was dispatched from John Bushey, the District Executive Director of School Leadership, requiring all school principals to allow students virtually unlimited access to soft drink machines, to move machines "to where they are accessible to the students all day," and to advertise Coke products through a calendar of promotional events. The letter went on to say, "Research shows that vendor purchases are closely linked to avail-ability" and "Location, location, location is the key." The letter also suggested that teachers should allow students to drink Coke products in the classroom. Bushey signed the letter as "the Coke Dude."[11]

The Colorado Springs experience shows the process by which a school system becomes a sales agent for a soft drink company. The administrators went from allowing machines in schools to aggressively encouraging students to increase soft drink consumption.

Principal Phillip Gainous of Blair High School in Maryland was par-ticularly proud of his Pepsi contract, the largest contract of its time, which netted the school more than $100,000 a year and paid for com-puter labs, a TV studio, floor buffers, and scoreboards. In order to keep the contract, Gainous was reportedly required to ignore state law by leaving vending machines running all day.[12] Noting that his school did not have the resources of schools in higher income neighborhoods, Gainous viewed the contract as a way to close the gap.[13]

Some schools pit Coke and Pepsi against one another in a bidding war, thus increasing their returns. In some cases, schools have brokered nonexclusive deals with both companies, although exclusive deals tend to be more lucrative.

The long-term benefits to schools, which vary according to the indi-vidual contract, may include money up front and a percentage of pro-ceeds from beverage sales. The lure is strong, especially in schools where money is tight. But what is the cost in terms of lost productiv-ity in the classroom, not to mention the health of the students?

Soft drink contracts in schools have given birth to a new business opportunity—consultants now specialize in brokering deals between soft drink companies and schools. An article in the *New York Times* characterized these consultants as clever and enterprising, not men-tioning that the people thought to benefit from the contracts (the chil-dren) might instead be victims.[14]

We see the tide beginning to turn. Parents, educators, and legislators are becoming more sensitive to the dangers of promoting soft drinks in schools, spurred in part by information on the impact of these bever-ages on children.

Are Soft Drinks Bad?

Not if you ask the soft drink industry. Responding to criticism of soft drinks in schools, the National Soft Drink Association says arguments for limiting soft drinks are "an insult to consumer intelligence," and that a link between soda and health problems is "not supported by the facts."[15] Also:

[S]oft drink consumption by children is not linked to pediatric obesity, poor diet quality, or a lack of exercise.

And

Soft drink consumption is not linked to adolescent obesity.[16]

A twelve-ounce Coke or Pepsi has more than nine teaspoons of sugar. Twenty-ounce versions, quickly becoming the default serving size, have fifteen teaspoons of sugar. No parent or school official would give permission for a child to take fifteen teaspoons of sugar several times a day, day after day. With soft drink consumption increasing dramatically over the years, all this sugar and all these calories must be going somewhere.

The country's primary nutrition organization, the American Dietetic Association (ADA) takes a surprising stance on soft drinks, given that dietitians work hard to decrease consumption of "empty calories." From the ADA's Nutrition Fact Sheet called "Straight Facts on Beverage Choices":

Regular carbonated soft drinks contain calories; milk and juice contain calories, vitamins, and minerals—all beverages can have a place in a well-balanced eating pattern.[17]

The fact sheet was paid for by a grant from the National Soft Drink Association. The soft drink association in turn uses statements from the American Dietetic Association as proof that soft drinks can be a part of a well-balanced diet.[18] Some members of the nutrition community are very critical of the ADA for representing their nutrition advice as unbiased and objective, while at the same time accepting money from the food industry.[19]

In a report entitled "Liquid Candy,"[20] the Center for Science in the Public Interest noted that soft drinks are the single greatest source of refined sugar in the United States, providing 9 percent of calories for boys and 8 percent for girls, triple the percentage from 1977 to 1978 for boys and double the percentage for girls. Another study estimated that soft drinks may contribute twice this percentage of children's calories.[21] As soft drink consumption rises, milk consumption falls. Children today consume twice as much soda as milk, the reverse of twenty years ago.

At least 75 percent of teenage children have soft drinks every day. In late 2002, scientists reported that more than half of the average child's calorie intake now comes from sodas, juices, and high-calorie drinks. Children who consume more soft drinks take in more calories overall, are less likely to eat fruit, and have increased risk for obesity.[22] Boys ages twelve to nineteen drink about twenty-four ounces of soft drinks daily while girls consume about eighteen ounces. Ten percent of teenage boys drink seven cans or more of soft drinks each day; 10 percent of girls have five cans or more.[23]

For the soft drink lobbyists to argue that there is no association between soft drinks and obesity requires us to accept several assumptions. The first is that people consuming extra calories from soft drinks will cut back calorie intake elsewhere and therefore maintain a stable weight.

Children who consume soft drinks are at much higher risk for obesity, perhaps because the body has trouble compensating for liquid calories. A study done at Purdue University had people increase their calorie intake by about 18 percent per day during two 4-week periods by using either jelly beans (solid calories) or soft drinks (liquid calories). The subjects could eat freely otherwise.

When subjects had the solid calories, they compensated by decreasing intake elsewhere during the day, thus there were no significant increases in eating or total calorie intake from prestudy levels. The picture was much different for liquid calories. Subjects who increased caloric intake with soft drinks showed no compensation. Total calorie intake increased from prestudy levels, and body weight increased significantly. The authors of the study concluded that "liquid carbohydrate promotes positive energy balance."[24]

Another study found that people do not compensate at meals for the extra calories consumed in sugar-sweetened drinks they drink either before or during the meal.[25] In addition, people getting an eight-ounce sugared drink during a meal did not report decreased thirst whereas people getting the same amount of water or an artificially sweetened drink did report decreased thirst. If sugared drinks are required in larger amounts to satisfy thirst, the calorie consequences of these beverages will be even more severe.

A study done in Denmark shows not only lack of compensation but how rapidly health can be affected by increased sugar consumption.[26] Scientists studied overweight volunteers who were given soft drinks sweetened with either sugar or artificial sweeteners but were allowed to eat freely otherwise. During this ten-week study the people having sugared drinks consumed an extra 500–700 calories per day from the soft drinks. Those receiving the sugared drinks did not compensate for the extra calories and gained 3½ pounds during the ten weeks. People with the noncaloric drinks lost two pounds. Those with the sugared drinks also had significant increases in systolic and diastolic blood pressure. These are troubling results, given that they occurred in such a short time.

The lobbyists' argument also requires us to believe that increased soft drink consumption beyond the already high levels would have no impact on obesity and that reducing consumption would not have a beneficial impact. It is hard to accept the no-impact argument. The twenty-ounce Coke or Pepsi has about 230 calories. A person adding one bottle per day to his or her diet would be adding about twenty-four pounds of extra calories per year. A person drinking Coke already would remove twenty-four pounds of calories by having one fewer bottle per day, assuming no other change in diet.

Common sense tells us that soft drinks contribute to weight gain. What of the science? The National Soft Drink Association website mentions one main research project on soft drinks and obesity.[27] This research, done by the Georgetown University Center for Food and Nutrition Policy (which appears to no longer exist), was paid for by the National Soft Drink Association. It found no relationship between soft drink consumption and obesity.

Other research paints a different picture.[28] In the soundest study to date, David Ludwig and colleagues at Harvard found that the consumption of sugar-sweetened drinks was strongly associated with obesity in children. For each additional daily soft drink serving in middle-school children, there was a 60 percent increased risk for the development of obesity, even after controlling for factors such as demographics, lifestyle, and diet.[29]

Several more studies are pertinent. One showed that children and adolescents who consumed the most soft drinks consumed the least milk and fruit juice and that children who consumed soft drinks had 10 percent greater calorie intake than those who did not.[30] Another reported that milk and juice consumption by children is positively associated with intake of several important nutrients, while soft drink consumption bears a negative association.[31] A study with young adults suggests that milk may protect against the development of obesity.[32] Finally, a study of children in grades four–six found that those who consumed the most soft drinks had the lowest intake of fruits and vegetables.[33]

> Increasing soft drink consumption is associated with decreased intake of milk. There are studies showing that (1) milk may protect against the development of obesity in children;[34] (2) increasing calcium intake is associated with lower weight in adults and children and less weight gain over time;[35] and (3) weight loss is higher in overweight people who follow a dairy rich diet.[36]

Concern has been expressed therefore, about "nutrition substitution." This is where one food, such as a sugared drink, takes the place of healthier alternatives. This substitution might explain why several studies have linked soft drink consumption with bone fractures in young girls (soft drinks substitute for milk). Another theory is that bone mass and calcium metabolism could be affected by phosphoric acid in cola and carbonated drinks.[37] Either way, one study showed that active girls who drank carbonated drinks (especially soft drinks) were much more likely to have bone fractures than those who didn't drink these beverages.[38]

Dentists are particularly upset about soft drinks in schools. Studies have linked erosion of tooth enamel with soft drink consumption.[39] In 2000, the American Dental Association House of Delegates passed an act opposing school contracts with soft drink companies.[40] The Michigan Dental Association has discouraged soft drink deals;[41] dentists in Toledo, Ohio, banded with parents to complain of a ten-year, $450,000-a-year soft drink contract the school district signed in 1999;[42] and the *Penn Dental Journal* urged schools to refrain from "auctioning themselves off to the highest bidder."[43] In 2002, the American Dental Association issued a press release opposed to targeting children in ways that would increase soft drink consumption:

Specific brand endorsements and marketing strategies, often found in exclusive soft drink contracts, may influence children's sugary beverage consumption patterns and increase the risk for decay.[44]

The evidence is clear—soft drink consumption is linked to obesity and other health issues because it leads to increased sugar and calorie intake and also supplants healthier drinks people might consume. This is especially troubling since soft drink intake in children has doubled in the past twenty years.[45]

The soft drink industry loses much credibility when saying that soft drinks do not contribute to obesity and should be part of a balanced diet. Soft drink consumption *must* decrease, particularly in children, and schools jump out as a logical place to begin the process.

What's in the Machines?

One of us (KB) testified before the U.S. Senate in 2002 urging the Senate to consider legislation prohibiting the sale of soft drinks and fast foods in schools. Subsequent testimony came from a spokesperson from the Grocery Manufacturers of America (the world's largest food lobbying group). This person said, ". . . 60 percent of schools today offer water and 100 percent juice as options in vending machines."[46]

This hardly seems worth the boast if 40 percent of schools have no water or juice in their machines at all!

The spokesperson also said, "Water is the fastest growing item in the beverage category."

Perhaps sales moved from a very low percentage to a slightly higher percentage, representing "fast" growth, but this seemed a statement that could be misleading.

When I (KB) returned from Washington, I went with my son to his public high school in Connecticut. We recorded every beverage choice in the school's thirteen soft drink machines; there were 170 buttons one could push to select a beverage. Only one of those 170 choices was for 100 percent juice, and 11 of the 170 buttons were for water. Juice, therefore, represented .5 percent of all choices and water was about 6 percent. Ninety-three percent of the choices were for soft drinks. A machine with a big picture of Minute Maid juice had no 100 percent juice, and four of seven buttons were for Yoo-hoo.

To see whether this was representative of other schools, we studied nine additional high schools, spread across both inner-city and suburban areas, serving poor and wealthy neighborhoods, and including both private and public schools.[47] Across all schools, with a total of 904 beverage choices, 100 percent juice drinks comprised 5 percent and water 7.5 percent of the choices. Not one of the 904 choices was milk. Poorer schools had more machines and more soft drink choices per pupil. Somewhat a surprise was that traditional drinks like Coke and Pepsi were outnumbered by other soft drinks, mainly sugared drinks such as Snapple Mango Madness, Snapple Kiwi Strawberry, Minute Maid Grape Drink, Minute Maid Orange Drink, Barq's Root Beer, and Yoo-hoo.

Of particular concern were drinks that might fool children. There were many choices of sports drinks like Powerade and drinks with "fruit" in the name such as FruitWorks Strawberry Melon and Fruitopia Fruit Integration. The sports drinks are quite high in sugar and calories, and the fruit-sounding drinks generally have little fruit juice.

For instance, Fruitopia's Orange Undercurrent and Fruit Integration have 10 percent juice, while Strawberry Passion Awareness, Peach Out, Kiwiberry Ruckus, and Cherry Vanilla Groove have 5 percent. Many of these soft drinks are owned by Coca-Cola or PepsiCo.

A Blind Spot for Sports Drinks

There are several examples of schools or even entire districts phasing out soft drinks but retaining sports drinks. This occurred with the Los Angeles Unified School District (discussed below).

Sports drinks like Gatorade and Powerade do have fewer calories per ounce than traditional soft drinks. But they are generally in twenty-ounce bottles, while some soft drinks can be purchased in twelve-ounce cans. Substituting a twenty-ounce sports drink for a twelve-ounce soft drink has a small calorie advantage in the case of Gatorade, but for Powerade, total calories increase. If children replace twenty-ounce soft drinks with twenty-ounce sports drinks, there is a calorie advantage, but noncaloric beverages and drinks with better nutrition would be preferable.

Product	Source of Calories	Total Calories
Gatorade (PepsiCo), 20 oz	Sucrose, glucose, fructose	125
Powerade (Coca-Cola), 20 oz	High-fructose corn syrup, glucose polymers	180
AllSport (PepsiCo), 20 oz	High-fructose corn syrup	175
Coke, 12 oz	High-fructose corn syrup, sucrose	150
Coke, 20 oz	High-fructose corn syrup, sucrose	250

Perhaps an argument can be made for sports drinks when children are undertaking strenuous activity, but with the exception of some children participating in organized sports, strenuous activity is not common in schools (see Chapter 4). Given that the calories come from sugar, we believe that sports drinks should be grouped with other soft drinks and that schools should sell neither, with the exception perhaps of machines placed near athletic facilities.

Early Signs of Changing Attitudes

The tide may be turning against exclusive contracts as school districts question their effects. Two Colorado districts turned down an agreement with Coke, and a school board president noted that, "Responsible parents don't encourage their children to increase their consumption of caffeinated drinks, and the school district shouldn't either."[48] Philadelphia rejected a $43 million contract with Coke,[49] while Santa Fe passed on a $2.4 million Pepsi contract.[50]

Several schools have reversed contracts, and some districts, including Madison, Wisconsin, have allowed theirs to expire.[51] In all, about forty schools or districts have resisted exclusive and lucrative contracts during the past few years.[52] Rick Nichols, a writer for the *Philadelphia Inquirer*, estimated that each student in the Doylestown, Pennsylvania, district would have to spend $50 annually (based on the required 9.5 million purchases during ten years, amounting to 1.7 soft drinks daily per high school student) to meet the contract. Considering that only about half of that money would be returned to the schools, Nichols sent a check for $25 to the school district to support a "Coke-free high school student."[53]

In February 2001, state lawmakers in St. Paul, Minnesota, introduced a bill to ban soft drink sales to students during school. However, the Minnesota Soft Drink Association and the Minnesota School Boards Association criticized the bill as severe, both concerned with a loss of revenue.

Maryland State Senator Paul G. Pinsky introduced "An Act Concerning Captive Audience/Stop Commercialism in Schools Act of 2001," aimed at removing corporate advertising from Maryland Public Schools.[54] Maryland also is considering a law that requires most vending machines to be switched off during the school day, although many local districts ignore federal and state laws that already dictate when machines can operate. In fact, local contracts have included stipulations required by the soft drink companies such as: "If the Board of Education actively enforces the policy in which vending machines are turned off during the school day, the commission guarantee will be suspended."[55] The U.S. Department of Agriculture (USDA) attempted to ban candy and soda sales in schools more than twenty years ago, but a federal appeals court rejected the ban in 1983.[56]

In March 2001, the Coca-Cola Company announced it would decrease its marketing tactics in schools; end some school contracts; and include water, milk, and juice in vending machines.[57] The Center for Commercial-Free Public Education saw this as only a "partial victory," noting that Coke, the parent company, only "urged" local bottlers to decrease pressure on schools.[58] Only 20 percent of Coke's vending machines were to have logos replaced by noncommercial graphics by 2002, a fact Coke attributes to the high replacement cost.[59]

The president of Coca-Cola Americas, Jeffery Dunn, said the company would discourage using minimum sales numbers as a condition of support, but a spokeswoman for Coca-Cola enterprises said the bottlers would comply only if schools stopped asking for pouring rights contracts.[60] After the official Coke announcement, some local bottlers continued to sign pouring rights contracts and the easy cash continued to lure many schools. The senior vice president of public affairs for one of Coke's largest bottling companies noted that it "will continue to participate in [contracts] because we are proud of our long-term partnerships with schools to support positive youth development programs."[61]

Coca-Cola, to its credit, announced a change in school contracts and has created "Project Mother," a program to develop dairy and fortified nutritional drinks for children and teenagers. A Coke spokesperson says that the company also plans to change its marketing strategy.[62] Coke, with its marketing domination, can take a step in the right direction if soft drinks can be replaced with healthier drinks.[63]

Some schools, however, including Phillip Gainous's Maryland Pepsi school, have seen efforts to sell healthier drinks fail.[64] In addition, some Coke bottlers offer schools bigger commissions on soft drink sales because soft drinks are cheaper than juice to produce. Other Coke bottlers, such as the second-largest U.S. bottler, say they have begun boycotting the agreements because of negative publicity. Coke has an Education Advisory Council to work out its new policy.[65]

Having healthier drinks in addition to soft drinks is a start, but not likely to be sufficient. If the soft drink companies could sell more healthy drinks, they would be doing so now, but these are not what children select. The soft drinks taste good and are promoted with a budget that towers above that for healthier drinks. Soft drinks need to be removed from schools.

Heroes and Success Stories
North Community High School in Minneapolis
North Community High School removed all soft drink machines but one, added fruit and vegetable juice machines, and changed prices ($1.25 for soft drinks, $1.00 for fruit and vegetable juices and sports drinks, and $0.75 for water). Soda pop sales declined and water, sports drink, and juice sales increased. The school did not lose money. Retaining sports drinks could be questioned, but otherwise this school gets high marks for innovation.[66]

Orono High School, Maine
School administrators wanted vending companies with healthier options. Coke and Pepsi offered to include healthier drinks, but the school went with a local, family-owned company with an "all-healthful product line." The school gave up revenues for exclusive rights with larger companies, but deemed the students' health more important. The reaction from the students has been positive.[67]

Program Increases Low-Fat Milk Intake in Schools
A study found that marketing low-fat milk in six inner-city schools in a Latino community produced a 32 percent increase in sales, which remained at a four-month follow-up. There was no increase in control schools.[68]

Los Angeles Unified School District

In August 2002, the Board of Education for Los Angeles Schools voted unanimously to ban soft drink sales from all schools. This affects 677 schools and 736,000 students. This is a great start, but again, sports drinks are left untouched and the ban is in effect only during school hours. Still, this major victory signaled the nation that school boards are questioning whether money should trump the health of children.[69]

Taking Action

Many of the actions discussed for food in Chapter 6 apply to soft drinks. Among these are offering beverages with the health of children the prime goal, becoming political and urging companies to stop marketing to children, finding ways to replace money now generated from soft drinks, developing media literacy programs, and encouraging legislators to be active in protecting the diet of children. There are also avenues for action specific to soft drinks.

Eliminate Soft Drinks from Schools

Soft drinks should not be sold in vending machines, school cafeterias, or school stores. The rationale is similar to that for foods as discussed in Chapter 6. If high-sugar drinks are available, children will choose them. Increasing healthy choices may help a little, but such choices are there now and children select the sugared drinks. Children do not need soft drinks. There are healthy alternatives like milk and bottled water, and, of course, water fountains are a good option.

Children should have choices, but from among healthy products. Prudent public health practice structures the environment so citizens have lowered exposure to hazards. It is important to make it easy for children to make healthy beverage choices.

As discussed in Chapter 6, changing the balance of healthy and unhealthy foods may not lead to lost revenue, but if needed revenue declines, creative means of replacing the funds must be developed.

Change Prices

Prices can be modified in ways that encourage the consumption of healthy beverages (see Chapter 6). Eliminating unhealthy beverages entirely would be the optimal move, but to the extent such beverages are in schools, there should be heavy incentives for children to select healthier alternatives.

Dispute Industry Claims That They Help Education

Claims by the soft drink industry that they promote education are hard to accept. The industry does not complain of losing money in schools, hence what they invest must be nicely compensated by product sales and the marketing opportunities with millions of young customers.

It is more the case that soft drink companies drain resources from the community. Children are the ones dropping quarters and dollars into machines, so the money schools earn comes from children and their parents, but with the soft drink companies taking a substantial cut.

Challenge Soft Drink Companies to Honor Their Word

The soft drink industry presents itself as having a commitment to education and health. The industry could prove this true by withdrawing its products from schools and by helping fund American education without attaching strings.[70]

Create Nutrition Advisory Councils in Schools

The TACOS program from the University of Minnesota (described in Chapter 6) includes establishing a Nutrition Advisory Council made up of students, parents, teachers, administrators, and food service personnel.[71] Such a group can work with school officials to develop policy. The council would generate visibility and credibility for the planning process and would demonstrate local ownership of changes in a school's nutrition environment.

Conclusion

Soft drinks in schools are likely a major barrier to improving the diet of American children. Having these products in schools helps companies sell high-sugar drinks, pushes drinks that displace other healthy beverages children might be consuming, and creates an objectionable climate of commercialism in schools.

The soft drink industry claims to be helping American education. But, for the reasons outlined in this chapter, one could argue that they are a major force holding back education. The companies must leave schools entirely, or at least be true to their word and support education without commercial motives.

PORTIONS THE SIZE
OF CLEVELAND

Experts cite increasing portion sizes as one factor that pushes up calorie intake in the population. It is often stated, for instance, that the old large size of French fries at McDonald's is now the small. A twelve-ounce can of cola seemed large compared to the eight-ounce bottle that preceded it, but now it is small next to the twenty-ounce plastic bottle. There are countless more examples of expanding portions.

Some eating places are notorious for large portions: the steakhouse where your meal is free if you finish the forty-eight-ounce steak, restaurants with a mound of fried seafood, diners with giant stacks of pancakes, and, of course, the all-you-can-eat buffet. Massive portions are mainly a U.S. phenomenon; the buffet is quite rare outside the United States, as is the concept of a doggie bag.

Expanding portions are not confined to restaurants. They are in convenience stores, vending machines, corner markets, supermarkets, our homes, and even our cars. Automakers have installed larger cup holders in newer models to accommodate the growing size of drinks.[1]

This expansion is clear in the way we describe food; servings often are labeled *Big*, *Mega*, and *Super*. This is not a ploy by food companies to make us think we get more—there really is more.

We will show how portions have increased, and then address the issue of whether it matters. If larger portions lead people to eat more, growing sizes will increase calorie intake and the nation's weight will rise, but if people naturally regulate what they eat, people served portions of any size will eat the correct amount. Science shows that the first explanation is more correct than the second.

People eat more than they need; after all, there is an obesity epidemic. Average daily calorie intake has increased by at least 200 calories per day since the 1970s, enough to lead to substantial increases in weight. Physical activity is declining and therefore cannot compensate. People eat what they do for many reasons (recall the discussion in Chapter 2), but one reason appears to be portion size.

"Nelson, Party of Four: Your Muffin Is Ready": Ballooning Portion Sizes

Portion sizes for foods and beverages are larger than ever, in some cases orders of magnitude larger than what existed only forty years ago. Food companies, of course, make more money the more they sell, and profit margins tend to increase when people buy larger sizes; thus, the financial interests of the food companies are in lockstep with ever-increasing sizes.

Food Language

A person visiting America for the first time might guess how we eat from our speech. Words and phrases like *dainty, petite, tiny, delicate, tasteful, just enough, the right amount,* and *healthy sizes* are not part of American discourse. Instead we use *Big* and all its synonyms to describe what and how we eat:

Big Mac	McDonald's
Extreme Gulp	7-Eleven
Biggie Fries	Wendy's
Big Grab	Frito-Lay
Bacon Ultimate Cheeseburger	Jack in the Box
Whopper	Burger King
The Beast (85-oz. drink)	ARCO

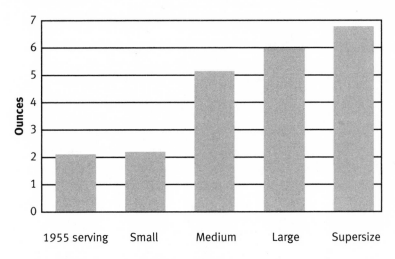

Figure 8.1 McDonald's Fries and Size Inflation

Words like *Big*, *Whopper*, *Ultimate*, *Extreme*, and *The Beast* are at the far edge of describing size. Similar terms describe how we eat. *Big Grab* implies handfuls of chips, cheese curls, Doritos, or Fritos, and *Big Gulp* describes fast, heavy drinking.

Growing, Growing, Gone

Portion sizes grow and grow. Gone is any association between what is offered and what a person might reasonably need. This is true of many, many foods, but we can begin with French fries, hamburgers, and soft drinks.

Supersize is a widely known word, so let's explore what it represents. Figure 8.2 shows the calories and fat grams from the largest serving of French fries at Wendy's, Burger King, and McDonald's.[2]

A serving of French fries (a mere side dish) can provide almost a third of a day's total calories and 36 percent to 47 percent of the daily allowance for fat. The largest serving at McDonald's is triple the size of what the chain sold in 1955.

Hamburgers have followed the same trend as fries. An article on obesity in *U.S. News & World Report* noted the growth in burgers:

	Weight	Calories
Typical hamburger in 1957	1 ounce	210
Typical hamburger today	6 ounces	618[3]

And, a plain hamburger is not the typical order at fast-food chains. Accompanying the meat can be cheese, bacon, and sauces. Jack in the Box serves a Bacon Ultimate Cheeseburger with 1,120 calories and a staggering seventy-five grams of fat (more than ten grams of fat above the total recommended for an entire day).

The food companies boast openly about the portions, using mighty words to describe what they serve. The companies scramble to see who creates the biggest sounding, biggest tasting, and biggest selling version of most foods. Consider the following press release from Jack in the Box:

SAN DIEGO—*Big burgers rule at Jack in the Box restaurants, now home to perhaps the meatiest and cheesiest burger in the fast-food industry—the Triple Ultimate Cheeseburger.*

Consisting of three beef patties, two slices of American cheese, one slice of Swiss cheese, mayo-onion sauce, and a jumbo bun, the Triple Ultimate Cheeseburger is a two-fisted burger sure to satisfy the heartiest of appetites.

"The Triple Ultimate Cheeseburger is definitely not for the faint of heart," said Tammy Bailey, senior product manager for Jack in the Box. "In focus groups we discovered that our target audience, men ages eighteen to thirty-four, want more meat and cheese. So we designed the Triple Ultimate Cheeseburger for cheeseburger purists who don't want a salad on their burger."

	Calories	% of RDA Calorie Levels for a Full Day	Fat Grams	% of RDA Fat Levels for a Full Day
Wendy's Great Biggie Fries	530	27%	23	36%
Burger King King Fries	600	30%	30	47%
McDonald's Supersize Fries	610	31%	29	45%

Figure 8.2 Fries and a Day's Intake

Though this is Jack's first triple-decker, it's not the chain's first behemoth burger. Over its fifty-year history, the chain has introduced such heavyweights as the Bacon Ultimate Cheeseburger and the Ultimate Cheeseburger, but none have matched the meaty magnitude of the Triple Ultimate Cheeseburger.[4]

Fast-food restaurants are not the only ones with large portions. Family-style restaurants and even fine-eating establishments can have meals with very large portions. The common denominator at family-style restaurants like TGI Friday's, Outback Steakhouse, Applebee's, and Red Lobster is large serving sizes.

Beverage sizes have also increased dramatically. Soft drink containers morphed from eight ounces to twelve ounces to sixteen ounces and then to twenty ounces as the standard serving size. Pepsi now has a twenty-four-ounce bottle, and one-liter bottles are more common. One consumer noted, "It's pretty scary when we're using the same volume measure for putting liquid into a 200-pound person and a 2,500-pound car."[5] Beverages sold from the fountain machine at 7-Eleven also demonstrate rising portion sizes.

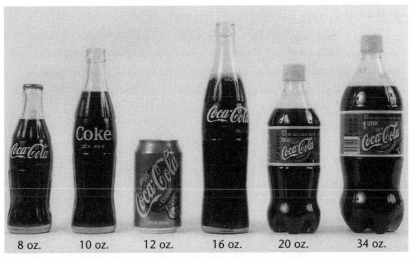

Figure 8.3 Growth in Beverage Sizes (Photo courtesy of Matt Brownell.)

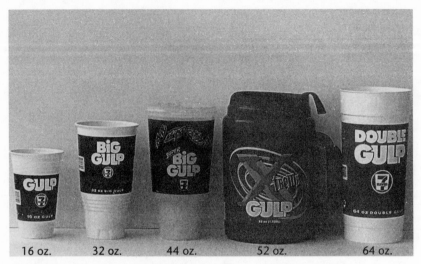

Figure 8.4 From Big to Double Gulp

With labels like *Big*, *Super*, and *Extreme*, what is a store to do next? Are bigger sizes possible? Are bigger words available? We think so and wonder if 7-Eleven might consider the five-gallon "Insane Gulp" for their next advance. Think of the exercise in lifting that bucket! While this is said tongue-in-cheek, there are no signs that portion sizes are diminishing.

Large portions have enveloped the entire food landscape. Candy bars come in King Sizes (a King-Size Snickers has 505 calories),[6] potato chips are in larger bags, pastries are served in bigger sizes, and so on. Lisa Young and Marion Nestle of New York University wrote an excellent article showing how an array of foods have been affected by the rising tide, as indicated in Figure 8.5.[7]

Comparing the United States to Other Countries. It is interesting to compare our portions to those in other countries. When foreign foods enter the United States, they often become "Americanized." The French croissant doubles in size when baked in America. A Canadian chain increased its serving sizes by a third when opening a franchise in the United States.[8] French fry servings in London contain about 125 calories less than those in the United States, and an English steak weighs

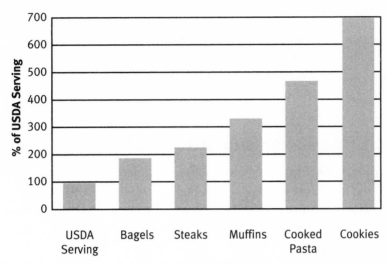

Figure 8.5 Portion Sizes for Common Foods (% USDA Recommended Size)

eight ounces (545 calories) compared to the U.S. version at twenty ounces (1,360 calories).[9] Our portions shock foreign visitors.

Paul Rozin and colleagues at the University of Pennsylvania did a fascinating study comparing cookbooks, restaurant guides, supermarkets, and restaurants in the United States and France.[10] Restaurant portions are 25 percent larger in the United States. Guides recommending restaurants from the United States more often use the word *large*, mention portion sizes, and recommend all-you-can-eat establishments. Individual portions of foods in U.S. supermarkets are 37 percent larger, and French cookbooks call for smaller amounts of meat in comparable recipes. Yet, people spend longer when eating at McDonald's in Paris than in the United States.

A Study on Children's Portions. We assume that the large portion size mind-set in restaurants spills over to children. Our colleague Marlene Schwartz coordinated an analysis of children's menus at the nation's five leading fast-food restaurants and five leading family-style restaurants.[11]

These researchers obtained portion size and nutrient information and found that the meals provide more calories, more fat, and less fiber than recommended for children. The meals at family-style restaurants are especially high in calories by virtue of having large portion sizes. Fruit and vegetables (other than potatoes used for French fries) are essentially absent from all menus.

Do Large Portions Increase Eating?

A study by the American Institute for Cancer Research found that 67 percent of Americans report that they eat whatever is on their plates, regardless of portion size.[12] Larger serving sizes then lead to greater intake. This observation is consistent with carefully controlled research studies.

Barbara Rolls and her colleagues at Pennsylvania State University did a series of studies on this issue. In one study, people were allowed to eat whatever they wanted when served submarine sandwiches of different sizes. When subjects were given a twelve-inch sub instead of an eight-inch version, calorie intake increased 11 percent in women and 20 percent in men. The size of the sub did not affect how the people rated how hungry or full they were after the meal, suggesting that people may not compensate for the larger serving by being less hungry later.[13]

Another study by the Rolls group looked at serving people different portions of macaroni and cheese for lunch one day each week for four weeks.[14] The serving sizes were 500, 625, 750, or 1,000 grams. Some people were served the food on a plate while others were given the amount in a serving dish and could serve themselves. Food intake was 30 percent higher when people were given the largest compared to the smallest serving, regardless of how the food was served.

Brian Wansink, marketing professor at the University of Illinois, has done very creative studies to see whether people consume more when container sizes increase. Even if containers of different sizes have the

Moviegoers eat 49 percent to 61 percent more popcorn when given a larger container.[15]

same amount of food, Wansink believes there are several reasons why consumers would take more from the larger container. He would predict, for instance, that people would pour more Pepsi, root beer, or Sprite from a two-liter bottle than a one-liter bottle, even if each contained one liter of beverage. Wansink proposes several reasons:

1. Controlling the amount dispensed from a larger container may be more difficult.
2. People are more willing to "finish up" products in a large container because it takes up more household space.
3. A product in a small container might seem more like a scarce resource and therefore be conserved.
4. Larger packages are perceived to bring lower unit costs for what they contain.
5. It is harder to monitor how much is eaten if it comes from a larger container.[16]

Wansink hypothesized that people would take and eat more when given larger portions. Among the results from his research:

- People asked to prepare foods using cooking oil or spaghetti use more if the oil or pasta are in larger containers.
- People eat more M&M's, as much as 70 percent more, when served from a large container.

"People use more from larger packages—typically between 9 percent and 36 percent more—because, deep down, they perceive that per-unit cost is cheaper in large packages."
—Brian Wansink, University of Illinois Marketing Professor[17]

Lessons from the Food Companies. Company after company increases portion sizes and more recently sells foods as individual servings (e.g., single serving bags of chips, candy, or items such as Hot Pockets). It appears that both are encouraging more buying and more eating. This is clear from an article in the *Wall Street Journal* that reported:

- ConAgra sells six-packs of individual cups of popcorn fried chicken at Wal-Mart. ConAgra is targeting children ages four through sixteen and wants consumers to see their 3.5-ounce products as a better deal than the 3-ounce Chicken McNuggets at McDonald's.
- Chef America, Inc. added 10 percent more filling to its microwave sandwiches Hot Pockets while not increasing price, which boosted sales by 32 percent.
- The Costco wholesale chain has pushed food companies to offer larger multipacks of single serving foods. When Frito-Lay agreed to replace its thirty-six packs of three-ounce bags of chips with a forty-two pack, sales increased by 36 percent.
- Costco increased sales 30 percent by selling Nabisco fruit snacks in packs of eighty for $9.99 instead of forty for $6.99.
- The best-selling individual food items most often come in larger than usual serving sizes.[18]

7-Eleven introduced gummy candies in a five-ounce clear plastic cup called the "Candy Gulp." It fits into cup holders in cars and became the chain's leading candy seller. Seeing the potential, 7-Eleven worked closely with Nabisco and now has cups filled with Nabisco's Chips Ahoy and mini Oreos and with Hershey's Reese's Bites and Kit-Kat Bites.[19]

Do People Correct for the Extra Calories?

There is now abundant evidence that people do not compensate for larger portions by eating less subsequently, at least in the short-term. In Chapter 2, we discussed studies with both animals and humans that looked at the impact of increasing either sugar or fat in the diet. In animal studies, for instance, increasing access to sugar leads to significant weight gain. The animals do not adjust their diet to get a healthy mix of nutrients and do not eat less to keep weight stable.

Once again, the work of Barbara Rolls and colleagues at Penn State helps us understand the impact of the eating environment. More than a decade ago, they tested whether people would eat differently if given water, a drink with artificial sweetener, or a sugar-sweetened drink before or during a meal.[20] When people had the sugar-sweetened drink, either before or during a meal, they did not decrease food intake to compensate for the extra calories, and hence took in more calories overall. Those who were given an eight-ounce sugar-sweetened drink with the meal did not report reduced thirst whereas those having the other two beverages did. This could lead to even greater consumption of calorie-containing beverages.

More recently, Rolls and her group tested thirty women and twenty-four men who were given an afternoon snack and then later had dinner.[21] The snack was potato chips served in different amounts. When people were given a six-ounce bag of chips compared to a three-ounce bag, women ate 18 percent more and men ate 35 percent more, showing once again that larger portions increase eating. What people ate later at dinner was unaffected by the size of the earlier snack, so there was no compensation for larger amounts eaten earlier.

A longer-term study was done by a team at the National Institutes of Health led by Jack Yanovski.[22] These scientists studied weight gain between Thanksgiving and New Year's Day in 195 adults, but then checked on them a year later. The average person gained weight over the holidays, but in the subsequent year, few of them lost the added weight. Fully 165 of the 195 people had not lost the holiday pounds. The weight gain could have been caused by large portions, more access to calorie-dense foods in general, declining physical activity, or other factors, but the lack of compensation is striking.

The ubiquity of large portions may also thwart the body's ability to regulate. If exposure to large portions happened infrequently, the body might compensate over the long-term and maintain a reasonable weight. In today's conditions, a person who eats a large meal will encounter large snacks even before the next meal, which itself is likely to have large portions. There is no "time-out" from the toxic environment, so the body has little time for regulation.

Why Do Large Portions Increase Eating?

There are both biological and social reasons. Humans overeat in response to abundant food because biology is programmed for this mission (see Chapter 2). James Hill and John Peters state it nicely: the body has strong biological mechanisms to protect against weight loss and weak ones to prevent weight gain.[23] Eating more in response to large portions has a strong biological impetus, while little more than sheer willpower helps with compensation.

Modern life places people in situations where this calorie-inclined biology is easily activated. People are in repeated contact with supermarkets, convenience stores, work cafeterias, vending machines, gas stations with mini markets, and restaurants, most with large portions. The following phenomena then converge:

- Larger portions lead to greater eating.
- Foods offered in large portions tend to be higher-calorie foods.
- Higher-calorie foods taste better, also leading to increased consumption.
- Better-tasting foods are eaten in larger quantities.

Another issue is that Americans are paying more attention to the *types* rather than the *amounts* of foods they eat. Seventy-eight percent of adults believe that avoiding certain foods is more important than how much one eats.[24]

Distortion of the Portion: Perceptions of What Is Right to Eat

People are served too many calories but do not define it as such. One survey found that most people in the United States believe that the amount they are served in restaurants is "just right."[25] The definition of what is just right has changed dramatically, both because portion sizes are growing and because people have difficulty judging how much they eat and what constitutes a serving.

Can People Estimate Portions and Serving Sizes?

Portions may contain multiple servings, yet 62 percent of Americans believe that restaurant portions are the same size or smaller than those served ten years ago; 80 percent said that their portions at home are the same or smaller. This does not fit documented increases in average calorie intake (Chapter 2).

One cannot blame people for misjudging servings. Estimating food amounts is not easy. Back in 1982, one of us (KB) worked on a study where people entering a weight-loss program (many had kept food records) were asked to estimate the quantity and calories in servings of ten common foods.[26] Estimates were sometimes high and sometimes low, but the errors were considerable—64 percent average error in estimating the quantity of foods and 53 percent in estimating calories. Many other studies have shown large errors in estimating food portions.

A major problem is that people rarely know how much food is in a serving. While the food guide pyramid explains serving sizes, only 1 percent of those who responded to the American Institute for Cancer Research's 2000 survey could correctly identify serving sizes for a range of foods.[27]

Understanding serving sizes is hard when portions are so large. The study by Young and Nestle mentioned above found that with the exception of one item (sliced white bread), all foods they studied were served in amounts exceeding U.S. Department of Agriculture (USDA) and Food and Drug Administration (FDA) standard portions (e.g., some cookies were seven times a serving and muffins three times a serving).[28]

With estimating serving sizes so difficult, it is not surprising that Americans underestimate their daily calorie intake by up to 25 percent.[29] Combine this with the fact that people often eat according to what they are served, and the stage is set for overconsumption.[30]

Changing Our Portion Size Definitions

Americans have redefined the normal serving. What was the large serving of fries is now the small. Most people do not feel they need "small" servings, and small does not exist on many menus. "Regular" connotes normal but often means a large size. For many adults, a child's size might be most reasonable.

Hungry people may not feel that a regular or small portion will be satisfying. Large becomes the default, and supersize, biggie size, or something similar is a treat. *Regular* has become a euphemism for *very large*, *large* a euphemism for *massive*, and words like *extreme*, *ultimate*, and *supersize* euphemisms for something the size of Cleveland.

Who Is Responsible?

Once again we face the question of supply and demand. If consumers simply demand large portions, the food companies can rightly claim they respond to the market. This evokes the standard argument that packaging, labeling, and marketing persuade people to buy a specific brand but do not increase consumption overall (see Chapter 10).

An opposing view is that people have biological vulnerabilities that promote overeating when large portions are available, a strong desire for value, and the capacity to be persuaded by advertising. This offers an opportunity for food companies to drive portions (and profits) higher. If enough companies do this, demand rises because supply is pushed to the extreme. Consumer exploitation becomes an issue if two conditions are met: harm comes to the buyer and there is intent by the seller to sell more of harmful products.

Certainly people are being harmed by larger portions. They eat more, do not compensate adequately, and gain weight. Some people are exceptions, but enough people obey this rule that we face a public health crisis.

Whether the companies manipulate conditions to promote overeating is difficult to prove, but will probably become clear in the near future. The national spotlight on obesity and increasing criticism of the food industry should encourage insiders to come forward with relevant information. The recent lawsuits against the food industry will reach discovery phases in which food companies may be forced to produce some of this information.

Risking prejudgment, we find it hard to believe that food companies have not packaged and marketed foods in larger portions to promote increased eating of their products, with the knowledge that overall eating increases. From a business perspective, there would be no reason to do otherwise.

> Fast-food companies have specific marketing campaigns directed at "heavy users," defined as those who visit more than twenty times a month. This group comprises 20 percent of the customer base but makes 60 percent of visits to the restaurants. Most often single males, some spend as much as $40 a day. A senior official from Kentucky Fried Chicken said, "We used to have this great sign around here that said something like, 'Marriage and kids are bad for your business.'" Worried that internal use of "heavy user" has both weight and addiction connotations, companies now use terms like "core customers."[31] Large portions, taste, convenience, and perceived value are likely the key factors underlying the heavy use.

Based on the actions of the industry thus far, one sees a well-funded effort to market large sizes. The industry invented *supersize* and many equivalent terms, has increased container sizes, and uses *value* time and time again in its marketing. Companies compete with each other to offer the biggest sizes, or in the words of Jack in the Box, to excel in "meaty magnitude."

Customers consistently rate value as a high priority when buying food. The most profitable way to provide value is to increase portions (rather than decrease prices). Research indicates that profits on most items increase when manufacturers increase the size of the item.[32]

What Can Be Done?

This trend toward bigger portions will not be reversed easily. The food industry will resist because profits are at risk, and consumers may balk if they risk losing the perceived value of large sizes.

Value is good, but "more product for less money" opportunities exist mainly with unhealthy choices. If value existed more often for healthy foods, price incentives would match public health priorities. Changing the economics of food is discussed in detail in Chapter 9. Here we offer suggestions specifically pertaining to portion sizes.

Calibration Education

Most people have little idea of what constitutes a reasonable portion of food because they are not calibrated to serving sizes. There is no reason to expect otherwise, as there is little education on this issue, people are not served reasonable amounts when eating out, containers of packaged foods bear no relationship to suggested serving sizes, and language associated with foods makes larger sizes seem the norm.

One particular problem is that serving sizes listed on food labels may differ substantially from those used by health authorities in nutrition guidelines.[33] What is listed as a serving of pasta on a box might be twice the serving used in the food guide pyramid. Having universal definitions of serving sizes is the first step.

Americans, beginning with children, must be better informed about serving sizes. As nutrition is taught in schools, serving size amounts should be discussed in any instruction on healthy eating. In Chapter 6, we recommended that the school cafeteria be a learning laboratory. Food models that match up with the day's menu could begin educating children about servings. Serving sizes could be displayed on vending machines, in school stores, and the like. Educating adults might be done with changes in labeling and advertising practices, as discussed below.

Show Reasonable Portions in Advertising

Advertisements can make lasting impressions, and people see so many ads that showing reasonable portion sizes might help readjust population perceptions of serving sizes. Similarly, ads portraying people eating rapidly, eating large amounts, offering children large portions, or using the amount of food as a distinguishing feature should be avoided.

To make this change will require a concerted and organized effort of the food industry. Self-policing by the industry may be one means to this end (as will be discussed in Chapter 11), but if not sufficient, government oversight may be necessary.

Encourage Companies to Repackage Foods

Foods meant to be eaten in a single bout should be packaged to coincide with recommended serving sizes. A company making this change would run counter to industry trends, which may create an initial strategic disadvantage. But if the change were made with fanfare and the company, by virtue of being first, could show its responsiveness to the nation's health needs, the public might respond. Brand loyalty improvements may offset revenues sacrificed by selling smaller portions. A company could probably get trusted figures in the health field to endorse the concept and, in turn, become more trusted itself.

As an example, if snack-size bags of chips were available in smaller portions, a parent might pack a school lunch knowing a child would need additional food to complete the lunch. If the smaller bag were a reminder about healthy eating, parents might pack fruit or another healthy food to fill the void. The company with the smaller portions then becomes known and trusted for being concerned with the health and well-being of its customers.

Relabeling Foods

Food labels contain serving sizes and the number of servings per container. We recommend that the number of servings per container be given more prominence and be listed on the front of the container where weight is now displayed. For instance, a large cookie might list the number of ounces and then below have "seven USDA servings." If the USDA declares that a serving of soft drink is eight ounces, a twenty-ounce bottle would list "2.5 USDA servings."

At the very least such labeling would educate people on recommended serving sizes for various foods, but it may also help curtail eating. We mentioned research showing that large numbers of people eat according to portions. Knowledge of serving sizes may help people stop eating earlier.

Require Food Labeling on Restaurant Menus
Nutrient information of foods purchased in stores is available on labels. The same opportunity should exist in restaurants. Information posted in the restaurant is not sufficient—it should be on menus. The number of servings of each food should be displayed prominently. Requiring this of restaurants is important, given how many meals Americans eat outside the home.

Encourage Better Personal Choices
Educational campaigns aimed at adjusting perceptions of serving sizes may help people make more informed food choices. Strategies for avoiding overeating in response to large portions could be emphasized (sharing an entrée at restaurants, avoiding upsizing, ordering children's sizes, etc.). Also needed may be training in media literacy, similar to that described for children in Chapter 5.

Learning to eat in response to internal signals rather than to portion sizes may also be helpful. Working with people wanting to lose weight, Linda Craighead and colleagues at the University of Colorado have developed an "appetite monitoring" program in which people are taught to be sensitive to internal cues of hunger and fullness. This program draws attention away from how much food is available and focuses instead on internal signals. It is showing good results.

Activism
Speak up. Food providers pride themselves on giving consumers what they want. They say time and time again that they are in business to offer choices, but sadly, the choice is between the monster, gargantuan, and Cleveland sizes. Let them know that reasonable serving sizes are important.

Schools with programs on nutrition could be encouraged to emphasize portion size. The National School Lunch Program could educate children about serving sizes in the context of offering food. Nutrition education for mothers in the Women, Infants, and Children (WIC) program could better deal with portion sizes. Government officials, if made aware of these possibilities, may be willing to take action, especially if the public demands it.

Conclusion

Portion size increases conspire to drive up food intake and appear to contribute to increasing obesity. Food companies claim to "provide people what they want" and take no responsibility for manipulating portion sizes in ways that increase overall eating. The companies have redefined what people consider small, medium, and large, but accept no responsibility.

We can now answer several key questions:

Have portion sizes increased? *Yes*
Do people underestimate what they eat? *Yes*
Do people underestimate what constitutes a portion? *Yes*
Do individuals compensate by eating less later? *No*
Is anyone to blame? *You decide*
Can anything be done? *Yes*

The nation must demand more of the food industry to reverse the damage that has been created. Portion sizes are not a trivial issue and should be considered in developing a national nutrition agenda.

9

THE INEXORABLE ECONOMIC MARCH TO OBESITY

The epidemic of obesity cannot be understood or reversed without recognizing the fundamental role of modern economic conditions. The way food is produced, priced, and sold; the value people place on taste and convenience; changing employment patterns; and advances in technology are central to the obesity epidemic. Each is affected in profound ways by economics.

Many broadscale factors are at work. Technological advances that "grow" the economy may also grow the waistline. Technology provides more calories to the population at lower cost than was ever possible and simultaneously shrinks the demand for physical work. Government policy in agriculture, economics, taxation, export and import, transportation, processing, marketing, and education, all affected by the economy, in some cases create conditions that promote obesity.

Micro factors we confront every day also matter. "For just another 39¢ you can get _____" symbolizes a system that optimizes calorie intake. There are few financial incentives to eat a healthy diet.

The problem can be stated simply—unhealthy food is convenient, accessible, good-tasting, heavily promoted, and cheap. Healthy food is harder to get, less convenient, promoted very little, and more expensive. This alone would predict an overweight nation.

We will discuss four economic factors that affect diet, activity, and weight—fundamental economic changes in food and activity costs, costs of healthy and unhealthy foods, poor access to healthy foods and physical activity in disadvantaged groups, and price inducements to overeat. Obesity is not an intended consequence of economic development, but a consequence nonetheless.

Food, Eating, and Economic Development

The economy and technology make food cheap. Combine this with growth in income, and we see why it is easier than ever for people to eat a lot. Changes in agriculture are part of the picture.

Agriculture in developed countries has undergone startling change in the past 100 years. Vastly increased crop yields; reduced price of production; irrigation of previously unusable land; genetic engineering; and widespread use of fertilizers, pesticides, and antibiotics have transformed the basic economics of food. Food can be stored, shipped, and engineered in ways that enlarge the divide between the people who raise food and the people who use it.

In the United States, massive agribusiness companies (Archer Daniels Midland, Monsanto, ConAgra, Cargill, etc.) may someday own the genetically engineered seeds that get planted, the fertilizers and pesticides that get applied to the soil, the antibiotics and hormones used to make animals grow, the farm itself, and even the final food products.

This vertical integration has some advantages, namely that more food is now produced for less money. The percent of personal income needed to feed oneself has declined sharply.[1] There are also significant downsides. Shrinking genetic diversity in plants and animals, resistant strains of bacteria developing from the heavy use of antibiotics, and the effects of pesticides and fertilizers on the environment are all major concerns arising from the food "monoculture" that has developed.[2]

Economics also affect diet through the enormous power wielded by big agribusiness and food companies. They contribute large amounts to political campaigns and influence government nutrition policy at all levels, sometimes in ways that undermine the health priorities of the nation.[3] It has been most difficult to keep these interests at arm's length when establishing national nutrition policy.

Economic and Technology Changes Affecting Diet

Scientists have developed sophisticated economic models to explain changes that have occurred in food intake.[4] Economists Darius Lakdawalla and Tomas Philipson note:

With the exception of one sharp upward movement at the time of the early 1970s oil shock, the relative price of food has been declining consistently. . . . the expansion of the food supply through agricultural innovation has outpaced any increases in demand.[5]

Stated another way, agriculture produces more calories than the population needs. The population has enough money to buy the calories and the food industry must sell them. They do so by:

- packaging foods in larger portions
- increasing inducements for buying more food (package meals, etc.)
- intensifying advertising
- targeting new groups for sales (youth, minorities, etc.)
- developing new sites for selling food (schools, drugstores, gas stations, etc.)
- engineering foods to maximize taste (enhancing flavors, adding sugar and fat)
- reducing prices

As food becomes cheaper, more accessible, and more heavily advertised, a number of factors inherent to modern living steer people toward some foods over others. Lower prices permit people to eat for pleasure and even recreation, rather than just survival. Most people treat themselves with foods that are high in sugar, fat, or both. The most heavily marketed foods, and those most convenient and accessible, tend to be the least healthy.

Increasing work hours and the addition of so many women to the workforce leave time to prepare meals in short supply and more valuable, thus placing a premium on fast and convenient food. Convenience becomes part of the unconscious cost-benefit analysis people make when choosing where and what to eat. Eating out increases, and with it comes deterioration in diet (see Chapter 2). What is eaten at home is also likely to be convenience foods.

Technology also permits the manipulation of food into forms that would impress even Dr. Frankenstein. Sugar, fat, and other nutrients are blended together with flavors to produce items that do not look, smell, or taste like anything humans have ever encountered. Water is married with sugar, colors, and flavor, and a new soft drink is born. Marshmallows, not the most natural food to begin with, are dried and put in cereal; chicken becomes nuggets; cheese is fried; corn is popped and covered with caramel; and ice cream is crammed with pieces of candy and bathed in chocolate. We have chocolate French fries and purple ketchup. Freakish or not, people value these foods because they taste good.

Imbalance in Costs for Healthy and Unhealthy Foods

In a consumer survey by the Food Marketing Institute and *Prevention* magazine, over half of consumers agreed that "It costs more to eat healthy foods."[6] This perception is supported by facts. Several studies in Canada reported that it is difficult for consumers to afford a healthy diet, particularly single adults.[7] The National Population Health Survey found that almost 10 percent of households were not financially able to purchase enough food or were forced to purchase low-quality, low-nutrition foods.[8] Food insecurity was linked to obesity, depression, poor/fair health, and various chronic conditions.

These average statistics reflect what one sees in day-to-day food choices. Apples range from $1–$2 per pound (usually one to four apples, depending on size), compared to a Big Grab bag of Doritos for $.99, or two Big Macs for $2 when McDonald's runs a special. Tomatoes can be $1–$5 per pound (usually one to four tomatoes), while a large bag of cheese curls may be $1.49.

Foods reduced in fat, sodium, and other ingredients tend to cost more than their nonmodified counterparts.[9] Consumers tend to substitute one food for something similar to what they are replacing, so healthy options will cost more. With extreme care, it is possible to modify diet and not experience large cost increases,[10] but most often price is a barrier to healthy eating.

Price Incentives to Eat More

A person we know stopped at a McDonald's on a trip with her family and at the counter had the following exchange:

> Customer: "I'll have an apple pie."
> Cashier: "You can get two for a dollar."
> Customer: "I just want one. How much for one?"
> Cashier: "89 cents."
> Customer: "OK, I'll have two."

It is human nature to stretch precious resources as far as possible. Getting more of one important resource (food) and expending less of another (money) is both reasonable and reinforcing. Multiple opportunities exist to get food for less money—stores run sales, large sizes are ubiquitous and tend to have lower unit prices, and so on. However, this is truer for packaged foods than for fresh foods like fruits and vegetables. There are few promotions with raw oats or lower costs per pound of fruit the more one buys.

When a person leaves the supermarket, the disparity is even more pronounced. Price incentives for healthy food exist but are greatly outnumbered by those for unhealthy foods. It is common to see two Whoppers or two Big Macs for as little as $2.

It is common for fast-food restaurants to lower prices or to increase what can be purchased at a given price to bring in more customers. A typical example was the move by McDonald's and the countermove by Burger King to offer a variety of menu items at low cost. The McDonald's Mickey D's Dollar Menu was first, bested by a penny with the 99¢ BK Value Menu. Consider the following low-priced promotions by Burger King and McDonald's:

99¢ BK Value Menu	Mickey D's Dollar Menu
Grilled Sourdough Burger	Big 'n' Tasty
Onion Rings	McChicken Sandwich
Two Crispy Tacos	Chicken Fajita
Soft Drink	Mickey D's Medium-Size Drink
Side Garden Salad	Mickey D's French Fries
Ice Cream Shake	McSalad Shaker (side salad)
Five-Piece Chicken Tenders	Bottled Spring Water
Bacon Cheeseburger	Sundae
Chili	Snack Size Fruit & Yogurt Parfait
Baked Potato	Two Pies
French Fries	Three Store-Baked Cookies[11]

Both restaurants do offer some healthier items on the low-cost menu. This is a positive move because people who wish to choose healthier foods can save money, and the economic incentives line up with public health priorities. The majority of items, however, are traditional fast foods.

Putting foods together into "value" packages is also less common for healthy foods. For decades restaurants have offered meals combining options (the classic is a hamburger together with fries, cole slaw, and a drink) for a lower price than if the items were purchased separately. Asking for a cheeseburger at a restaurant with package meals will usually evoke, "Would you like the meal?"

Fast-food restaurants have made package meals an institution. One can order by number ("I'll take a number five"). These meals typically include the featured entrée (say a Whopper, Quarter Pounder with Cheese, or a Wendy's Double with Cheese), fries, and a soft drink.

Such meals are a value only for customers who would have ordered those sizes of those items anyway. A person who wants only a burger and drink often decides on the "value meal" because the fries seem almost free. Another person may want the entrée, small fries, and a large drink, but the packaged meal with the large drink carries large fries. One could probably ask that a smaller package of fries be inserted, but with no money being saved, it is hard to pass up the larger size.

And then there is supersizing. "For only 39¢ extra, you can get . . ." is a well-known phrase in America. Across thousands of places like fast-food restaurants and movie theaters, one is asked to consider the large popcorn, drink, or fries. The extra cost seems small, but of course the people selling the food are expanding profits.[12] You pay an additional 39¢ for the giant popcorn, but the incremental cost to the theater may be only a few pennies.

The National Alliance for Nutrition and Activity did a clever analysis of upsizing.[13] They examined the extra cost and the additional calories for foods available from well-known food sellers (see Figure 9.1). With many types of foods, one can greatly increase calories for a relatively small increase in price.

What is not known is the degree to which package meals and up-sizing promote excess calorie intake. It *is* known that intake increases

Product	Cost and Calories	Impact
Cinnabon		
Minibon to Classic Cinnabon	48¢ buys 370 extra calories	24% more $ = 123% more calories
7-Eleven		
Gulp to Double Gulp (Coke)	37¢ buys 450 extra calories	42% more $ = 300% more calories
Movie Theater		
Small to Medium Unbuttered Popcorn	71¢ buys 500 extra calories	23% more $ = 125% more calories
Baskin Robbins		
Kid's Scoop to Double Scoop	$1.62 buys 390 extra calories	129% more $ = 260% more calories
McDonald's		
Quarter Pounder with Cheese to Medium Value Meal	$1.41 buys 660 extra calories	61% more $ = 125% more calories
Source: National Alliance for Nutrition and Activity		

Figure 9.1 Bargain?

as people are served more food, as described in Chapter 8, but this is different—people are ordering the sizes rather than having someone else serve them. The two possible outcomes:

1. People who order large sizes and package meals were going to eat that much food anyway.
2. Package meals and large sizes encourage increased calorie intake.

Given all that is known about human eating, the rise in obesity coinciding with such practices, and the fact that industry is structured to maximize profits, we believe that the second argument is probably more likely.

The Personal Economics of Eating

Some people (a minority) find value in healthy foods and are willing to pay the extra cost, but nutrition does not drive most food choices. Study

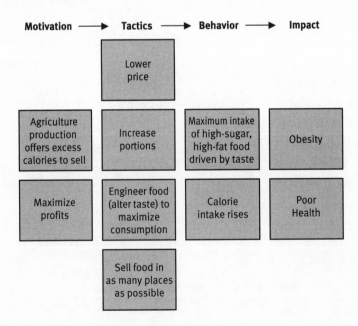

Figure 9.2 Food Industry Economics and Obesity

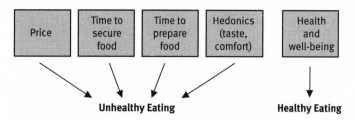

Figure 9.3 The Personal Economics of Eating

after study shows that taste is the primary determinant of what people eat, with cost and convenience also ranking high. Good taste most often resides in unhealthy foods. When people create their internal balance sheet, unhealthy foods have high value and low cost, but healthy foods have high cost and lower value, making conditions ripe for overeating.

The benefit/cost ledger for children is especially slanted. Good health and the prospect of preventing disease later in life are not relevant to most children. The instant gratification offered by good taste and the opportunity to use advertised products trump healthy eating.

Economic conditions, changes in agriculture, and modern lifestyles create personal economies for most people where foods high in fat, sugar, and calories are the logical choice. People are making rational, predictable decisions within the distorted environment that surrounds them.

Poverty and Obesity

Poverty brings with it multiple levels of disadvantage, health disparities among them. Recall from Chapter 2 that obesity is one such disparity. Hunger, once the predominant problem, is still a very real issue, but obesity is now a greater threat to the health and well-being of America's poor.

With issues such as poverty, eating, and obesity, we face yet again the question of environment and personal responsibility. We have made the case repeatedly in this book that the environment promotes obesity in all groups of Americans. But if the environment places some groups at especially high risk, issues of inequity arise. There is no question that the environment is structured in ways that make obesity a massive burden to the poor.

> Because of limited resources, soup kitchens confront the ethical dilemma of feeding more people worse food or fewer people more healthy food.

Inequitable Access to Healthy Food

The American stereotype of poor neighborhoods includes fast-food restaurants and small markets or bodegas with high-calorie packaged foods. If true, risk for the poor would be elevated simply by virtue of where they live.

There is truth to this image. Researchers in Australia found that people living in the poorest neighborhoods have 2.5 times the exposure to fast-food restaurants as do people in wealthier areas.[14] This has been found in a number of other countries, including the United States.

> A British study found that in 1988 a shopping cart of healthy food cost 18 percent more than a cart of unhealthy food. By 1995, the difference was 51 percent. The price gap was the most significant at corner stores and smaller convenience stores frequented by low-income families. The researchers concluded that lower-income families are "priced out of a healthy diet."[15]

One group of researchers looked at food-buying opportunities in Mississippi, North Carolina, Maryland, and Minnesota.[16] Supermarkets were much more common in wealthier areas, and there were four times more supermarkets in white than in black neighborhoods. A study in which 330 low-income families were interviewed in Hartford, Connecticut, found that the inability to travel to a large supermarket was related to difficulty with feeding the family and decreased likelihood of buying perishable items like vegetables and dairy products.[17] Hartford had thirteen chain supermarkets in 1968 and now has two.[18]

A study in North Carolina found that only 8 percent of black participants lived in a neighborhood with at least one supermarket, compared to 31 percent of whites. In addition, whites were three times as
likely to have cars, making it easier to get to places where healthy food
is available and affordable.[19]

The Los Angeles Experience. In May 2002, The Center for Food
and Justice at Occidental College released a report on food conditions
in inner-city Los Angeles.[20] The researchers tracked changes that had
occurred since the 1992 riots in Watts, after which the five-year
"Rebuild LA" plan was put into motion promising that consumers in
south central Los Angeles would have access to services and goods similar to those found in wealthier suburban areas.

The report reached an unmistakable conclusion—the promise had
not been fulfilled. The food situation, particularly lack of access to
healthy foods, was bad before the 1992 watershed and then grew worse.

The erosion of food shopping opportunities is so strongly embedded
in social conditions that even a major city commitment to change, such
as the Rebuild LA initiative, could not reverse things. Among the key
findings from the report were (1) the average supermarket in LA
county serves 18,649 people, while the number is 27,986 in low-
income areas; (2) the higher the concentration of poverty in a given
area, the less likely there will be supermarkets; and (3) there are
more supermarkets in white than in African American and Latino
communities.

The Occidental report also asked whether chain supermarkets are
viable in the inner city. Information from one chain (Top Valu) answers
this question. While the average customer spends less per trip through
the checkout line in inner-city stores ($15–$20 versus $20–$28 for the
chain in general), higher population density in the inner city brings in
more customers. Top Valu reported that it makes twice the amount per
square foot in the inner city compared to the industry average.

Supply or Demand? Results like these leave open the question of
whether the food supply determines eating patterns or demand drives
the supply. Scientists at the University of North Carolina found that the
presence of at least one supermarket in a black neighborhood was linked

with a 25 percent increase in those who limited the amount of fat in their diets; the figure was 10 percent in white neighborhoods.[21] Supermarkets are more likely than small stores to have healthy foods at cheaper prices.

> The UK-based Child Poverty Action Group found that approximately 2 million UK children live in families that cannot afford to buy healthy foods. While the richest 10 percent of households spend 14 percent of their income on food, the poorest 10 percent spend 21 percent.[22]

Additional evidence that the food supply hurts poor people comes from an analysis completed by the Economic Research Service of the U.S. Department of Agriculture.[23] This study found that people using food stamps may get enough to eat, but their diets are very high in fat and sugar.

Demand could explain this finding, but so could a poor food supply. Here is where the report made an interesting comparison. People in the Special Nutrition Program for Women, Infants, and Children (WIC) had significantly less added sugar in their diets than did food stamp participants. The WIC program, also for low-income individuals, supplies juices and cereal to participants.

One cannot conclude from these studies that having more healthy foods in poor areas would eliminate the obesity problem, but limited access is likely contributing to obesity and improved access to healthy foods may help. Further, assessing blame to the poor for demanding unhealthy foods is not justified.

Do Federal Food Programs Help or Hurt?

America does a great deal to feed the poor. The three main food programs, listed below, spend a combined $31 billion per year. Low-income families may be enrolled in all three programs, plus qualify for Temporary Assistance for Needy Families ($12 billion annually). In addition, children may receive food through Head Start. Annual federal funding for food programs is:

Food Stamps	$18 billion
National School Lunch Program	$ 8 billion
WIC	$ 5 billion

The school lunch figures include breakfast served in the program, while WIC is the special supplemental nutrition program for women, infants, and children.

Douglas Besharov and Peter Germanis of the American Enterprise Institute and the University of Maryland have placed each of these programs in the context of what the others offer. In late 2002, Besharov wrote an editorial on this topic in *The Washington Post*,[24] and Besharov and Germanis published a 2001 book on the WIC program.[25] Their analysis, motivated perhaps by an agenda to cut government food programs, does help us think about food programs and the obesity problem.

We discuss WIC, Food Stamp, and Head Start programs here. A detailed discussion of the National School Lunch Program (NSLP) is in Chapter 6.

WIC. WIC is designed to correct nutritional inadequacies in low-income pregnant and postpartum women and their children (under age five) by providing nutrition education, counseling, and healthy foods. It serves 7.3 million women and children per year. Free food is given to families each month, worth about $120 for infants and postpartum mothers and around $35 for children ages one through four. The food includes formula, enriched juice, and fortified cereals for the infants, and fruit juice, milk (sometimes whole milk), cereal, eggs, peanut butter, and dried peas or beans for others. In his *Washington Post* article, Besharov says:

A food package like this makes sense only if it is the family's major source of food, which almost certainly is not the case. It would be better to use the package to introduce low-income families to more healthful foods, such as fruits and vegetables.[26]

At best, WIC has modest success at improving diet. It has a small but positive effect on the diets of some pregnant women, leading to improved birth outcomes, but as Besharov and Germanis note, WIC may reduce the number of women who breast-feed their babies, which may contribute to obesity. They recommend that WIC specifically seek to prevent obesity through education, counseling, and food preparation classes and that WIC cover children older than age four because overweight worsens as children grow older.

Food Stamps. The Food Stamp Program serves 20 million people each month. A household of four can qualify for up to $465 per month for the purchase of food. To prevent people from buying nonfood items, people are given coupons that can be used in food stores only. Unused coupons cannot be redeemed for other purposes, so rather than wasting them, the tendency is for people to redeem them for foods they might otherwise not have purchased. And, there is no incentive to use stamps for healthy foods.

Head Start. The Head Start Program, launched during the Johnson administration in 1965, and now Early Head Start, are child development programs serving low-income children. Head Start serves three- and four-year-olds and their families, and Early Head Start serves children from the mother's pregnancy to the age of three. The goal is to increase readiness for school. Two teachers work with classes limited to seventeen to twenty children, and parents are encouraged to be involved. Children work on cognitive and social skills, and there is also a focus on health issues such as immunization, hearing and vision testing, and nutrition. Head Start serves many meals to many millions of people.

The comprehensive services approach, pioneered in Head Start, grew from the philosophy that both mind and body must be healthy for either to thrive.[27] The emphasis on nutrition came early with recognition that malnourished children had difficulty learning, so meals were added to the program. Head Start enjoys strong bipartisan support in Congress, parents are deeply appreciative, and programs sharing many of the features of Head Start have proven very cost-effective.[28] As with WIC, overnutrition is a key issue in Head Start.

The Total Picture. Federal food programs may promote obesity, but at the very least, do nothing to prevent it. This is a massive lost opportunity. Such programs may promote obesity in two ways. The first, as with Food Stamps, is to provide the opportunity to buy unhealthy foods. Food Stamp coupons can be used to buy healthy foods, but because such foods cost more, are less available, and don't taste as good, the poor are "incentivized" to eat poorly.

Second, programs like WIC and NSLP, using rules dating back as far as 1946, can provide excess calories to children and families. This is a residual effect of past concerns with malnutrition. Besharov notes that through the NSLP, schools must provide 25 percent of the RDA of calories for breakfast and 33 percent for lunch, leaving only 42 percent for dinner and snacks. The focus must change from enhancing to controlling calorie intake and to emphasizing balanced nutrition.

Any one program is likely to offer calories and saturated fat beyond optimal levels, but Besharov notes that many families are involved in more than one program. In the absence of national policy and accompanying oversight of nutrition programs, the aggregate effect of federal food programs will pass unnoticed and a unique opportunity for obesity prevention will be missed.

The Economics of Physical Activity

At the same time food costs drop, the cost of being physically active is rising. The opportunity costs in particular have grown so extreme that physical activity in the population has plummeted (see Chapter 4).

Few people perform physical work as part of employment, so one must use leisure time to be active. Most leisure time activities are themselves sedentary, plus leisure time is in short supply and multiple activities compete for attention (time with family, chores, a second job, entertainment, and even rest). Economists Philipson and Posner argue that:

The price of calories has fallen because food prices have declined and income has grown and, consequently, a rise in weight would be a natural consequence, but it would be due to a rise in calorie consumption. An equally important change has been in the amount of physical exertion required when supplying labor.[29]

> People were once paid to exercise—work required physical labor. Now people are forced to be inactive, must make conscious choices to do otherwise, and must pay for the opportunity.

Economics craft institutions into energy-saving enterprises. A company that minimizes physical labor saves costs. Schools may be in favor of physical education, but boosting PE time in the curriculum increases opportunity costs—the time must be used for subjects perceived to be more important.

A major contributor to calorie imbalance is the dwindling work needed to perform day-to-day functions. We interact many times each day with devices that save us energy. Some devices like washing machines and elevators save energy in great amounts, but even the small savings from devices like electric toothbrushes and TV remote controls become sizable when added up over a year, a decade, and a lifetime. These devices have become standard equipment for living. Day by day, year by year, calories get banked (as body fat) because we are not forced to spend them.

As with nutrition, physical activity is more difficult for the poor. One study found that declining income was associated with less physical activity, partly because the poor lacked places and opportunities to exercise and were in worse health.[30] Safety, lack of child care, and insufficient resources are all barriers to activity among the poor. These researchers found what is intuitively obvious, but often ignored—that the fewer places there are to exercise, the less exercise there will be.

Should Obesity Be Addressed with Economic Changes?

There really isn't much question. Economic factors are powerful determinants of eating and activity, economic conditions favor obesity, and hence economic changes must be part of an overall obesity strategy for the nation. Confronting the economics of food and activity is not the path of least resistance—there are controversial issues to be debated. But taking easy paths to avoid dispute is a trap that has ensnared the nation for years.

One cannot understand the obesity epidemic without considering economic factors such as the per capita price of food in comparison to other needs (housing, transportation, etc.), relative prices of healthy and unhealthy foods, and the value to families of obtaining food quickly. If there is one truth in this war on obesity, it may be that the economics of food and physical activity must change.

Will the Free Market Support Healthy Eating?

There are mixed signals. The number of supermarket shoppers claiming high concern with nutrition dropped from 60 percent in 1996 to 46 percent in 2000. The annual supermarket industry trade show in 2000 emphasized products like cheesecake snack bars and high-fat microwaveable calzones.[31] Taco Bell abandoned its healthier Border Lites option and McDonald's its McLean Deluxe, yet McDonald's has introduced a fruit and yogurt option, Frito-Lay is working on healthier snacks, and so on. One could be optimistic or pessimistic.

Currently the free market does not promote healthier eating. Change might occur if consumer demand increases dramatically for healthier food, which may be driven by food sellers offering good-tasting choices at reasonable prices. There may be ways to stimulate this process on both supply and demand sides.

There are examples now of healthier stores and restaurants establishing a foothold. Health food stores are a bit more in the mainstream, and the number of restaurants with healthy menus, anchored by Alice

Waters's legendary Chez Panisse in Berkeley, California, are on the increase. Both Wild Oats and Whole Foods stores are expanding, sales of organic foods are increasing, and several restaurant chains are hopeful of getting established.

The big players in the food industry see what's coming and want to cover all bases. General Mills bought two organic food companies (Muir Glen and Cascadia Farms); Philip Morris bought Boca Burger; and Darden, a large restaurant group (owners of Red Lobster and Olive Garden), announced its entry into the healthy foods business with a concept called Seasons 52.

Several restaurant chains offering healthier foods are establishing themselves in the marketplace. HeartWise based in Chicago; O'Naturals in Falmouth, Maine; Health Express USA of Florida; and Topz of Southern California are examples. HeartWise is a particularly interesting case. HeartWise predicted sales of around $1.1 million in 2001, based on operation hours of only 6 A.M. to 5 P.M., Monday through Friday. A Chicago HeartWise restaurant now serves 1,000 customers a day and the company's goal is to open 1,000 restaurants in total. Rosemary Deahl, CEO and founder of HeartWise, responding to our request for information on the menu, explained her philosophy:

My goals are simple. I want to have information available to everyone who chooses to see it. Every item available in my restaurants will have no hydrogenated fats (right now we have two products that do and we are asking two very large companies to reformulate for us. If they can't, we will replace them.) All items will have less than 30 percent of their calories from fat. Our chicken and turkey will be free range and hormone- and antibiotic-free. We are working with a bread company now to add more whole grains to the breads we are currently using. We use brown rice because we believe that the carbohydrates you eat should come from whole grains. We are striving to be GMO [genetically modified organisms] free— that will be an ongoing process. We serve no beef. Our best-seller is a sloppy joe and it is made with a soy mixture. By the time the next store is open we will have printed nutritional labels to put on every item. We have them now in a book at the restaurant. We want to be known as the place that is truly healthy and not healthier seeming.[32]

This represents striking progress and is a distinct change from most foods available in restaurants. The fact that the business is successful shows that good taste can be packaged with good nutrition.

The food industry will offer healthier foods if the profit is agreeable. Allowing the free market to operate in an unfettered way may produce a preponderance of healthier foods at some time in the future, but there may be ways to help the process along (discussed later). Lowering the price of healthy foods such restaurants use to prepare their dishes is one such way.

The Free Market and Physical Activity

There are a few encouraging signs that businesses related to physical activity, mainly the national health club chains like Bally's, are at least speaking about opening franchises in inner-city areas.[33] If this talk turns to action and the businesses succeed, stereotypic attitudes about poor neighborhoods (interest does not exist) may be proven false. As we mention below, incentives may help fitness businesses to move more quickly into the areas with greatest need.

The Furor Over Taxing Foods

Whatever methods one favors for dealing with obesity, every approach other than looking the other way will cost money. Given the intractable nature of obesity, the number of people affected, and the strength of the forces that promote weight gain, small efforts are not likely to help. Generating funds to support initiatives on diet, activity, and obesity prevention is a bridge that must be crossed. It is in this context that food taxes enter the picture.

In a 1994 Op-Ed piece in the *New York Times*, we began public discourse of taxing high-calorie, high-fat, or high-sugar foods as one means for addressing the obesity epidemic.[34] This elicited a firestorm of controversy. The storm still rages. However, the intervening years have seen a decline in the hostility toward the tax concept. The topic has become a legitimate part of the nation's obesity deliberations and is debated in the press, at scientific meetings, and among political leaders. It raises many complex issues.

We begin with two emphatic points. First, obesity is a complex problem and is likely to thwart any single solution, including food taxes and subsidies. These approaches must be examined in the context of multiple points of attack.

Second, we do not favor a tax unless the revenue is earmarked for programs to improve diet and activity. Taxes, even quite small ones, have the potential to generate considerable revenue that if used wisely, might be a powerful tool for improving the nation's diet and physical activity. Taxation as a deterrent to behavior is less appealing than using tax revenues to encourage positive changes.

Taxes, no matter what their purpose, generate strong feelings. Proposals of a new tax can be greeted with considerable ill temper. Primary objections are:

- A food tax would be manipulative and evokes images of a "nanny" or Big Brother intruding in people's lives to tell them what to eat.
- Taxes would interfere with personal liberties and freedom of choice.
- Additional bureaucracy is undesirable.

We would add:

- Taxes on food may be regressive (affect poor people disproportionately).
- Decisions on what would be taxed could be arbitrary.
- There is the possibility of unintended consequences.

These criticisms are defensible and must be considered. Taxes can have important social effects if used correctly. An example is high taxes on cigarettes. There is clear evidence that such taxes drive down smoking rates and are especially effective at preventing smoking from taking hold among teenagers.[35]

The question then is whether taxes might be effective in the national effort to improve diet, increase activity, and prevent new cases of obesity.

Conceptualizing Taxes

Taxes can have multiple purposes:

- to raise general revenue (income earmarked for an unrelated purpose)
- to generate revenue earmarked for diet, activity, and obesity prevention initiatives
- to function as a disincentive to unhealthy eating without regard to how revenue is spent
- to function as a disincentive with revenue earmarked for diet, activity, and obesity prevention efforts

These approaches will vary in the likelihood of garnering public support and in helping address the obesity crisis.

Successes and Failures

The revenue-generating approach is now used in a number of states and municipalities, where small taxes on soft drinks or snack foods have been enacted. These taxes have been put in place to raise general revenue or to support programs such as road maintenance and litter control, and they have been small enough that the public and food companies have not objected strenuously.

Studies have not been done to see if the small taxes affect consumption of the taxed items. It seems unlikely. The taxes were not put in place to affect food choices and, of course, were not coupled with public health campaigns that would encourage healthier food choices. The success from these taxes is in the money they generate. Michael Jacobson from the Center for Science in the Public Interest and one of us (KB) reported that eighteen states and one major city have taxes on soft drinks, candy, chewing gum, or snacks foods, raising about $1 billion annually.[36] Arkansas, for instance, raises $40 million annually from a tax of about 2¢ per twelve-ounce can of soft drink. Were these taxes instituted more widely and the money earmarked for nutrition and the prevention of obesity, the resources available for this task would increase exponentially.

The Spotted History of Snack Taxes. Several states have enacted larger food taxes, not to change eating practices but to repair budget deficits. These taxes have been similar to the "sin taxes" imposed on tobacco and alcohol that have become so common. The foods taxes, however, did not stick.

California enacted an 8.25 percent snack food tax in 1991 in part to remedy a $14.3 billion deficit problem.[37] It was repealed less than a year later. Retailers received a list of approximately 5,000 taxable and nontaxable food items. The distinctions were arbitrary, with popped popcorn and Milky Way bars being taxed but unpopped popcorn and Milky Way ice cream bars left untaxed. Cupcakes were taxed but only when at room temperature (frozen cupcakes were exempt), while muffins, considered bread, were not taxed. M&M's sold as candy were taxed, but those sold for baking were not. An entire cake was tax-free, but a slice of the same cake was taxable. Only a small percentage of California's stores were able to use electronic scanners, leaving cashiers to puzzle through what was taxable.

The California tax was a bureaucratic morass. Retailers had to reprogram or purchase new cash registers. Opponents criticized the tax as regressive, stating that it penalized those who did not have the facilities to prepare fresh foods. Partly due to the "Don't Tax Food" initiative, led by an assemblyman, the California Grocers Association, and others who lobbied aggressively against the tax, 60 percent of Californians voted for repeal in 1992. Following the repeal, store owners reported that snack food sales rose 16.7 percent above those of the previous year.[38] The tax generated revenues of approximately $200 million, and snack sales dropped an estimated 10 percent during the period the tax was in effect.[39]

Maryland also experimented with a snack tax, levying a 5 percent tax in 1992. Frito-Lay noted a drop in demand for snack foods in Maryland and reported $500,000 in lost sales due to the tax. The Snack Food Association, an international trade association comprised of about 850 members representing snack manufacturers and suppliers to the snack industry, lobbied strongly against the legislation.[40] The Maryland General Assembly repealed the tax in 1997.[41]

Maine enacted a tax on "nonnutritious" foods in 1991, but the 5.5 percent tax was repealed in 2001.[42] The Snack Food Association and the Don't Tax Food Coalition of Maine led a citizen initiative supporting repeal of the law.[43] Washington, D.C., had taxed individual snack food products at 5.75 percent since 1993 but repealed the tax in 2000.[44]

These snack taxes succeeded in some ways but failed in others. Arguments that the taxes were arbitrary, confusing, and regressive, combined with general public distaste for taxes and heavy lobbying by the food industry, brought down the taxes.[45]

From a nutrition standpoint, the taxes appeared to be successful. Sales of snack foods declined, to the point that the biggest player, Frito-Lay, complained of lost income in Maryland. A 10 percent drop in snack food sales was estimated in California. No studies were done to track overall nutrition changes in these states during those times, so it cannot be said that total food intake patterns changed. We suspect, however, that most nutrition experts and health professionals would agree that a decline in snack food sales is a positive development.

The experiences from California, Maryland, Maine, and Washington, D.C., show that large snack taxes (in the range of 5 percent to 10 percent) can generate considerable revenue and appear to drive down sales of these foods. It is possible that similar taxes (or ones imposed on other foods such as soft drinks and fast foods) put forward in a different context would meet less resistance, have many more advocates, and be less vulnerable to repeal. Three changes would be necessary.

1. The aim of the taxes to decrease consumption of unhealthy foods must be made explicit.

2. The revenue must be earmarked for nutrition initiatives the public will embrace (e.g., improving the nutrition environment in schools).
3. The way taxes are applied must be less arbitrary, easy for stores to manage and the public to understand, and undertaken with maximum health benefit as the goal.

Under these conditions, the public might accept the concept of food taxes. If people see a public health goal rather than a state needing to rectify a budget deficit and hence develop confidence that the funds would be used for worthwhile purposes (such as creating a healthier environment for children), grassroots support may offset opposing pressures from the food industry. Under the right conditions, there probably is a future for food taxes.

Public Opinion on Taxes

Two recent studies addressed public opinion on various expenditures that might be made to improve diet and physical activity. Eric Oliver at Princeton and Taeku Lee at Harvard used public opinion polling to test attitudes on obesity and on public policy initiatives like taxing food. Among their findings:

Number Who Agreed or Agreed Strongly

Snack foods should be taxed	33 percent
Get rid of snack foods in schools	47 percent
Food advertising should be regulated	57 percent
Willing to pay $50/yr in taxes to support more parks for exercise	53 percent
Willing to pay $50/yr in taxes to support nutritious school lunches	64 percent[46]

Beth Olson from Michigan State University did a public opinion survey of Michigan residents and found similar figures:

Number Who Agreed

Tax fast food	26 percent
Tax less healthy food from stores	31 percent
Tax $ should be used for community recreation facilities	89 percent
Tax $ should be used for nutrition/ activity education for adults	60 percent[47]

A third opinion poll asked consumers about small taxes, this time using specific numbers. Forty-five percent of a nationally representative sample said they would support a 1¢ tax per pound on soft drinks, chips, and butter.[48]

These three polls show that more than half the public is opposed to dramatic actions such as taxing foods, regulating advertising, and changing foods in schools. Interpreting these numbers is a classic example of the half-full/half-empty glass. Without similar polling from previous years, it is not possible to say whether support for these actions is growing, but judging from the tone with which these issues are discussed in the press, the mail we receive, and the interactions with groups we speak to, we believe the landscape is changing rapidly. We suspect the figures are more favorable than would have been the case ten or even five years ago and, considering that the three polls are now several years old, might be an underestimate of today's support.

Critics of policies like food taxes may note that a majority of people oppose taxes, but 33 percent to 45 percent in favor of taxes represents a formidable (and probably growing) force. In addition, polls on taxes have not distinguished large from small taxes and have not discussed the tax idea coupled with the funds being earmarked for a worthwhile cause, such as preventing obesity in children. The number in favor might rise even more if some promoting of the taxes were done and if the taxes were placed in a public health context.

The food industry clearly perceives a threat. As discussed in Chapter 10, the websites of its organizations and lobbying groups are filled with attacks on these and other policy ideas. The Snack Food Association, for instance, lists one of its recent priorities as "Leading the fight to successfully repeal discriminatory taxes on snacks in several states."[49] The industry reaction is further evidence of growing public support for policy change.

Would Food Taxes Be Regressive?

Poor people may eat more of the foods likely to be taxed, so they might be most affected by a food tax, much as they are by cigarette taxes. The concern that poor people would then pay an even higher percentage of their income for food is a legitimate one, particularly if the tax were substantial (small taxes would have negligible impact) and if consumption of the taxed foods did not decline.

An additional concern that has not been raised is that poorer people would have little opportunity to avoid the tax because they are trapped in situations that do not offer healthier (nontaxed) choices. This is precisely why we believe that a food tax has the potential to be regressive and is much more defensible if prices of healthier foods are reduced simultaneously (see the subsidy proposal below).

A regressive tax is more reasonable if it generates revenue for a progressive subsidy. If lowering prices on healthy foods has the largest impact on those with the least money (a progressive subsidy), poorer people would benefit most. The desired effect of a tax/subsidy combination, therefore, would be to have a positive impact on diet but not increase the overall cost of feeding a family.

It is important to remember that the food system as it now exists is regressive. Lower income groups have least access to and can least afford healthy foods. Therefore, they are forced toward inexpensive, unhealthy foods because of the way food prices are currently structured.

What Would Be Taxed?

There is an easy answer—the foods where reduced intake would have the greatest impact on obesity and other diet-related diseases. Defining these foods, however, is a process that could be straightforward or enormously complex.

The complex approach would be to classify every food as taxed, untaxed, or subsidized. There is great debate now among nutrition experts about which foods contribute to disease or are protective, so the act of forcing every food into one of three categories would be extremely controversial and difficult to do fairly.

If this approach were attempted, we would favor a metric that would classify foods according to a ratio of the nutrition they provide to their calories. Fruits and vegetables, for instance, would score high and be considered healthier foods because they offer substantial nutrition and tend to be low in calories. A soft drink, for example, may have no nutrition (beyond sugar) and be high in calories. Therefore it would be scored low.

Even this seemingly straightforward approach would be complicated. Diet soft drinks and water would each have no nutrition and no calories and so would score the same. A food high in nutrition and high in calories would score the same as a food low in both. Also, defining what constitutes "nutrition" for the numerator would be complex itself. Whether to include fiber, how to judge sugar and fat content, and other issues introduce complexity that, while not insoluble, would make it difficult to reach quick agreement.

A Broad-Brush Categorical Approach. A more sensible and somewhat less controversial approach would be to focus on categories of foods where consensus is possible on the need to increase or decrease consumption. There is now broad consensus among political leaders, health professionals, and the public that increased consumption of fruits and vegetables would be desirable. Consensus might be possible that the nation's health would benefit if consumption of snack foods, soft drinks, and fast foods decreased.

If a tax/subsidy approach is to be pursued, the first iteration might be to subsidize all fruits and vegetables with revenue generated by a tax on soft drinks, snack foods, and fast foods. This is not free of difficult decisions (e.g., it would not make sense to tax yogurt sold at McDonald's), but the number of difficult decisions would be far less than if all foods were to be discussed.

This broad categorical approach is possible only if special interests (food and agriculture groups) are excluded from the decision making because of conflicts of interest. Deciding whether snack foods should be taxed with the Snack Food Association at the table or whether soft drinks should be taxed with the National Soft Drink Association and Sugar Association at the table is akin to asking Philip Morris and R.J. Reynolds to help decide whether cigarettes should be taxed (see Chapter 10). Political courage is a necessary ingredient for change.

Would Taxes Work?

The potential for a tax to change behavior and/or generate revenue is one consideration, but so is the likelihood that a tax will have "political legs." A highly effective tax that would never be enacted has little value. Figure 9.4 shows different approaches that might be taken.

The figure shows two dimensions on which taxes might be considered—the size of the tax itself and whether the revenue generated would be earmarked for a relevant purpose. What is known about food taxes thus far suggests that:

- **Small soft drink and snack food taxes are acceptable to the public.** Small taxes have been implemented in a number of places around the United States, some existing for many years.
- **Small food taxes generate considerable revenue.** The Arkansas tax of 2¢ per soft drink yields $40 million per year. California's 7.25 percent soft drink tax generates about $250 million per year. A national tax of 1¢ on each twelve-ounce soda could yield approximately $1.5 billion in annual revenue. Charging a 1¢ per pound tax on fats and oils would generate $190 million in revenue, on candy would generate around $70 million, and on chips and snacks around $54 million.[50]
- **Food tax revenue has not been earmarked for improving diet and activity.** Although numerous taxes have been implemented, there is not a single case where the revenue has been earmarked for programs related to nutrition, physical activity, or obesity prevention.

- **Larger snack food taxes (5 percent to 10 percent) thus far have not endured.** It is difficult to know whether public resistance, lobbying from the food industry, or problems with implementation have been the stimulus for the repeal of these taxes. Large taxes have not been tried with public health as the stated goal.
- **Larger snack taxes appear to decrease snack food sales.** Based on initial data from the snack tax in California, where the 8.25 percent tax was associated with a 10 percent drop in demand, the elasticity of snack food was estimated at -1.21, indicating that snack food demand may be quite sensitive to relatively small price increases. Better studies are needed to define changes in purchases at different levels of price increases.
- **Taxes are more acceptable with revenue earmarked for relevant causes.** Cobbling together information from public opinion polls suggests there may be a considerable increase in support for food taxes if the revenue would be used for a cause relevant to diet and obesity. This supposition should be tested directly. We believe support will be highest for taxes with funds earmarked for children.

Referring back to the chart showing different approaches to food taxes (Fig. 9.4), Approach 1 (small taxes with earmarked money) may be the way to begin. This would introduce the concept to the public,

		Small Tax	Large Tax
Money Earmarked for Diet and Activity Initiatives?	**Yes**	Approach 1	Approach 2
	No	Approach 3	Approach 4

Figure 9.4 Possible Aims of Food Taxes (Small Taxes to Generate Revenue vs. Large Taxes as Disincentives and to Generate Revenue)

and if the earmark programs were successful, higher taxes might be acceptable at a later time. Approach 2 (large tax with earmarked funds) might ultimately have the greatest impact, both because the funds generated would be maximized and because a larger tax might decrease consumption of the taxed foods. Acceptability of such taxes will be the key. Approach 3 (small taxes, no earmark) has little appeal, and Approach 4 (large tax, no earmark) is quite undesirable because it might be perceived as punitive and regressive, and in the past it has been unpopular.

Lessons from Tobacco and Alcohol. The literature on cigarette and alcohol taxes is vast and is based on studies done in many states and countries. The results have been clear. As taxes and hence prices increase, scientists can estimate precisely what will occur with per capita consumption, the number of people engaging in use of the substance, and the impact on health and well-being.[51]

A sampling of studies on tobacco shows striking findings:

- A British study reported that 100,000 additional people would live to age sixty-five as a result of doubling the federal cigarette tax in Britain.
- Scientists estimated that a 12¢ increase in cigarette taxes in New York State would prevent almost 29,000 premature smoking-related deaths in the subsequent generation.
- The 1989 25¢ tax in California produced a 5 percent to 7 percent decline in smoking and raised $600 million in the first year.
- Researchers in London estimated that tax increases raising the world price of cigarettes by 10 percent would prevent 5 to16 million tobacco-related deaths and that using taxes is one of the most cost-effective ways of dealing with tobacco.[52]

As we stated earlier, tobacco and alcohol do not map on perfectly to food. At the very least, one must eat, whereas smoking and drinking are discretionary. Taxes do have a significant impact on consumption of tobacco and alcohol, and if the same is true of food, taxes may be a powerful means at the nation's disposal to improve diet and prevent future obesity. The section that follows shows the role we believe taxes might play in the overall effort to improve diet and activity.

Changing the Price Structure of Food

Given that the economics of food should be the reverse of what they are, changing the price structure of food may be the single most powerful means of affecting the prevalence of obesity. This could be done by lowering the price of healthy foods, increasing prices of unhealthy foods, or both.

Lowering Prices of Healthy Foods

Price and convenience (along with taste) are the leading determinants of food choice in the population. The high cost of healthy foods relative to that of unhealthy foods is a clear barrier to improving the nation's diet. Lowering the price of healthy foods must become a national priority.

Lowering prices would make healthy eating choices more appealing for purchase by consumers, but similar benefits may also occur at different points in the food chain. If demand for healthy foods increases, more stores, restaurants, vending machine companies, and fast-food chains would offer these as choices because of "pull" from the population. The competition within these industries could lead to technological advances in preparing, packaging, and delivering these foods, thus helping with convenience and taste.

The degree to which prices must decline is a figure economists must generate, but there is a large body of evidence on the price elasticity of food, beginning with work of the late James Tobin, Nobel Prize economist from Yale. Data could be assembled from national food consumption surveys, tracking information from supermarkets, and proprietary data from the food industry to create a blueprint for price changes.

The main question is how much reduction on specific foods is necessary to increase consumption and thereby improve public health. The point at which benefit is optimized relative to cost would be the target, factoring in how much increase in consumption of a given food is possible (given taste, availability, etc.) and how likely that food will contribute to health improvement.

There are important questions to answer. In addition to assigning values to foods as described above, there are questions of where in the food chain a subsidy should occur (growers, wholesalers, retailers, etc.) and how a lowering of prices would be supported. We will rely on those in agriculture and economics to answer the first question. Support from sources other than food taxes would generate less controversy than supporting a subsidy with a tax. A tax on unhealthy foods, however, would have the dual potential of raising money and discouraging use of the foods with higher prices.

Will Lowering Prices Increase Consumption? This can be answered in part with common sense. Stores run sales continuously. If people bought the same amount of a product no matter the price, price reductions would be counterproductive. When fruits are in season and prices decline, consumption increases. When the orange crop in Florida is devastated by freezing weather, prices increase and consumption declines.

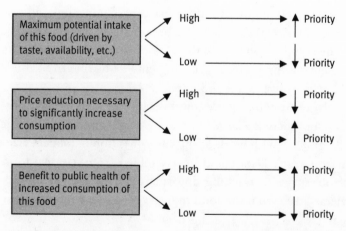

Figure 9.5 Factors to Balance in Decisions on Foods to Target with
Price Reductions

A number of studies support this commonsense observation. As mentioned in Chapter 6, Simone French, Robert Jeffery, and colleagues at the University of Minnesota have done a number of clever studies in which the prices of healthy items in vending machines and cafeterias were dropped.[53] Significant increases in sales occur as prices decline.

A study we did in a restaurant came to similar conclusions. Lowering the prices of healthy food items (certain sandwiches, salads, and soups) increased sales. A smaller increase was produced by posting health messages. When price reductions and health messages were used together, sales increased less than for price reductions alone. We speculated that health messages may have a paradoxical effect if consumers believe a "healthy" food will taste bad.[54]

Generate Revenue for Needed Programs with Small Food Taxes

Throughout this book, we have suggested several initiatives that might be supported with revenue raised from small taxes. Helping schools offset the lost revenue from prohibiting snack foods, soft drinks, and fast foods is one example. Another is to create an advertising "superfund" that could be used to develop compelling messages aired in prime TV time for children.

These are but two ideas. Other initiatives may take higher priority as the nation begins to develop new ways to address the obesity crisis. Having a revenue stream from the small taxes may encourage creative thinking about new initiatives because there is a greater likelihood for funding.

Which foods should have the small tax assessed? Taxes on snack foods and soft drinks have been enacted already. Fast foods are another possibility because of growing public concern with the industry. Most people would agree that national consumption of these foods should decline.

The snack food, soft drink, and fast-food industries will likely cry foul, say they are unfairly targeted (as did the tobacco industry years ago), and state emphatically that they cannot be blamed for the obesity epidemic. Imposing a tax on their products does not require proof that the products are entirely responsible for obesity, just that the public agrees they contribute.

In addition, any policy action carries at least minor inequities. Not all snack foods are equal in nutrition or calories, so some segments of the snack food industry might claim that they are treated unfairly. In designing a tax policy, care should be taken to minimize inequities, but the presence of any inequity cannot be used to invalidate the general approach. Yielding to this predictable maneuver by the food industry will guarantee paralysis (see Chapter 10).

Raising Prices of Unhealthy Foods

Reducing the price of healthy foods is a top priority and is likely to be acceptable to more parties than is a food tax. There are three conditions, however, under which raising the price of unhealthy foods might be desirable. The first is the possibility that healthy foods will not be eaten in sufficient amounts no matter how low prices drop. The second is that more healthy foods are eaten but intake of unhealthy foods does not decrease, leading to a paradox that total calorie intake could increase! Only experience will tell whether the reinforcing nature of unhealthy foods can be offset by price reductions in healthy alternatives, but if not, disincentives may be necessary. If taxes push the cost of unhealthy foods significantly higher, the disincentive may lower consumption.

The third condition would arise if subsidies for healthy foods or other diet and activity initiatives are effective in changing diet, but the government does not allocate funds to support the effort. Revenue generated by a tax on unhealthy foods could be used to support the reduction in price for healthier foods and also fund programs for changing diet and activity in the population.

Provide Buying Incentives for Healthy Foods

Offering price incentives for healthy foods could be a powerful tool. For instance, if a pound of tomatoes costs $3, but the price lowers to $2 for more than one pound, the pursuit of value might push consumers toward tomatoes. As we mentioned before, such incentives are quite common but are applied more often to unhealthy than healthy foods.

With foods like fruits and vegetables where spoilage is an issue, buying too much of one product can lead to waste, thus some of the price reduction is forfeited. Perhaps incentives could be structured such that a customer buying one type of vegetable would receive the usual price, but buying two or more types would reduce the price of all. A person buying carrots, squash, and green beans, for instance, would receive reduced prices on each.

Sensitize Consumers to Inducements to Buy Unhealthy Foods

Price incentives offer the consumer the choice of buying the same amount of product for less money or more of the product for the same money. How humans react to these contingencies is important. If a consumer is set on buying a bacon cheeseburger, fries, and a drink and can group the foods for less money, she or he wins when buying the package. But if incentives draw people to unhealthy foods, promote larger sizes, or encourage more frequent eating of fast food, the incentives are harmful. Studies we mentioned in Chapter 8 suggest that offering package meals, low-cost opportunities to raise sizes ("supersizing"), or offering bigger sizes at "value" prices lead people to eat more.

Education plus offering an alternative (enhanced value packages for healthy foods) should be undertaken to weaken the perceived value of unhealthy foods. A person ordering a cheeseburger and drink at the drive-thru window and told there is better value if fries are included in a package meal should recognize there is virtue in saying no. Consumers must be sensitized to the obvious—that companies want you to eat as much as possible. Both adults and children can be alert to the tricks of the food trade and develop means of resisting the pressure.

Increase Access to Healthy Foods for the Poor

Food inequity does not appear to result from low demand for healthy foods or poor patronage of large supermarkets when they do exist. The stores are not there. There are barriers to stores locating in poor areas, including difficulties locating sufficient space for large stores, complex marketing challenges with diverse populations of customers, and negative stereotypes about the inner city.[55]

Financial incentives may provide ideal opportunities to make healthy eating opportunities available to all. Local, state, and federal incentives could be offered to large supermarkets (or even smaller stores with primarily healthy foods) to locate in poor areas. Such incentives could be structured in different ways and may need to change depending on local conditions. Loan guarantees, reduced tax rates, lowered costs for purchasing property, and other incentives might all be considered.

The report from Occidental College mentioned earlier provided additional ideas on increasing the density of supermarkets in the inner city. These include assistance with matters such as zoning approvals and building permits as well as community involvement in planning. To this last point, the report recommends "accountable development" in which neighborhood and community groups get involved in discussions between the city and developers.[56]

Changing the food landscape for the poor may pay especially high dividends with children. Helping parents gain better access to healthier foods will be a move forward, but more can be done to help children. We found in a small survey of Connecticut high schools that inner-city schools had more soft drinks available per pupil than did schools in wealthier areas. More financial help may be needed for schools serving poor areas to rid themselves of soft drinks, fast foods, and snack foods. Supporting nutrition education and physical education may also be especially important for these children.

Emphasize Obesity Prevention in National Food Programs for the Poor

There is considerable opportunity to improve American eating conditions with modifications of federal food programs. These programs touch millions of people each day and represent established vehicles for reaching those at highest risk for obesity. Optimizing their impact will involve making changes in philosophy, policy, and some existing approaches.

The first necessary step is for obesity prevention to be a priority in the four main food programs (WIC, Food Stamp Program, National School Lunch Program, Head Start). Obesity is a major threat to the health and well-being of the people served by these programs. There are special opportunities for prevention given the power of these programs to help children.

A number of changes might be possible in each of the relevant programs.[57]

WIC

- Emphasize diet quality while controlling calories
- Offer more frequent and better nutrition counseling
- Provide healthier foods
- Encourage breast-feeding more strongly

Food Stamps

- Add incentives for purchasing healthy foods
- Provide cash rather than coupons to prevent overbuying

National School Lunch Program

- Emphasize diet quality while controlling calories
- Use only healthy commodities
- Use school cafeterias as learning laboratories
- Integrate school lunches with nutrition and physical education

Head Start

- Emphasize both nutrients and calorie control
- Provide better nutrition education for parents
- Encourage breast-feeding more strongly

As a final note about Head Start, it is housed in the Administration for Children, Youth, and Families, which also houses the National Child Care Office. Obesity recommendations relevant to WIC and

Head Start could also be integrated into planning for child-care programs.[58]

Make Physical Activity More Affordable and Accessible

Increasing physical activity must be a priority if obesity is to become less of a public health problem. This is discussed in detail in Chapter 4.

Some economic changes could be used to help correct the increasingly sedentary lifestyle of the nation. Changing major transportation initiatives to include support for walking and biking options would be a start. This could be done through the massive transportation reauthorization legislation (Transportation Equity Act—see Chapter 4).

There are additional ways to structure economic conditions to encourage physical activity. Low-income neighborhoods have special problems with a lack of facilities, unsafe streets, and lack of leisure time in which to be active. Tax incentives for exercise facilities to be built in low-income areas could be very helpful. A number of approaches are possible:

- State or federal funds could be used to encourage cities and towns to build and maintain parks, basketball and tennis courts, and other facilities in low-income areas. Maintenance of facilities and supervision of children are important to consider in allocating funds.
- Private enterprises, such as health clubs, skating rinks, and skateboard/rollerblade parks, could be offered tax incentives to build in particular neighborhoods.
- Funds could be provided to schools to stay open late for use of athletic facilities and support made available to supervise and organize physical activities (e.g., aerobics classes, sports leagues, dance groups).
- Support could help communities organize to be active. Examples would be parents escorting large groups of children

walking or biking to school, walking clubs for adults, or sports leagues for adolescents.

Means of enhancing work site physical activity programs are discussed in Chapter 4. Financial incentives for businesses to create opportunities and facilities for physical activity as well as for employees to take part could be very helpful. Business could also be encouraged, perhaps through matching funds, to direct their philanthropy toward the activity environment of the community. Businesses might be able to work together. For example, if a series of businesses clustered together along a corridor, companies could join together to build a bike path giving employees access to work from different neighborhoods.

The Importance of Understanding the Economics of Obesity

As a nation, we simply must know more about the economics of obesity. Understanding the supply and demand of why healthy foods are scarce in poor neighborhoods, why more companies do not offer time for employees to exercise, and why states do not build bike paths are but a few of the questions that need to be answered. The most important task of all is to identify the complex reasons that have shaped America into a voracious nation.

Other nations of the world are in transition. Some are quickly approaching the United States in consumption of unhealthy foods, declining activity, and the obesity that follows, but others are much earlier in the process. Identifying key economic underpinnings of obesity may be especially helpful to forewarn developing countries of what may come.

Creating Cost-Benefit Analyses of Policy Change
There are few cost-benefit analyses of public health approaches to diet and physical activity. Resources are finite, so finding the best returns

on investments is important. An example of a first step might be the reporting of costs in projects with positive effects. A campaign in Clarksburg, West Virginia, for example, used paid television and radio announcements to encourage a switch to lower fat milk.[59] The market share of nonfat or 1 percent milk increased from 18 percent to 41 percent after the seven-week program. The cost was about 22¢ per resident. This campaign applied to 200,000 people would cost the same as one coronary bypass operation.[60]

The challenge is then to interpret figures like these from West Virginia. Whether such a program merits expansion (is sufficiently cost-effective) depends on many factors including the long-term maintenance of the changes, the effects of this change in milk consumption on health, spillover effects to other health behaviors, and, of course, what the cost and benefits are to alternative programs. Evaluation of matters such as these must be built into any new initiatives.

While evaluation and cost-effectiveness seem like obvious priorities, they are typically left behind when new programs begin. People feel the need to "do something" with available funds and therefore balk at reserving portions of the funding for evaluation. This feels good at the moment, but is costly in the long-term because little is known about which programs should be embraced or abandoned, goals have not been defined, and there is little way to know how one program compares to another in return for the investment.

Conclusion

Economic factors are central to the obesity epidemic. The costs of poor diet and being sedentary are too low and the costs of eating better and being active too high. Why this occurs is complex, with technology and broad economic changes being key factors. Technology delivers more calories to the population for less money, manufactures food to maximize taste (with sugar and fat the primary vehicles), and makes physical exertion increasingly unnecessary.

The reaction of the population to these conditions—to eat more, exercise less, and gain weight—is perfectly understandable given the circumstances. If a nation's goal was to maximize obesity, an excellent approach would be to arrange economic conditions that (1) promote the behaviors leading to weight gain; (2) allow an industry to profit immensely from products that contribute (political clout would then minimize chances for change); and (3) permit that industry free access to all potential customers including children.

Changing the economics of food and physical activity are essential to reining in obesity. Exhorting people to behave differently, criticizing parents for doing a poor job with their children, and supporting small programs with the "first here, then there" approach will not be sufficient. More fundamental changes are necessary, because fundamental economic factors are central to the obesity epidemic.

PART 3

....

CHANGING THINGS

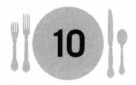

THE FOOD INDUSTRY AND A NATIONAL NUTRITION CRISIS: Trustworthy Ally or Troubling Adversary?

Proposals to change the food environment present the food industry and the nation with serious challenges. The industry must fight off unwanted legislative, regulatory, and legal action that could damage business while at the same time it engages in practices such as marketing to children that are increasingly unpopular. The nation must decide how to deal with the food industry.

Food companies confront the paradox of claiming public health as their priority while knowing that profits increase when people eat more. If the nation moves to a healthier diet, some segments of the industry will benefit and others will suffer. But for the industry as a whole, lower food consumption will lower earnings. Business acts in self-interest and industry leaders must protect their jobs, so significant changes in diet are frightening.

The nation and its leaders are at a crossroad and must decide soon whether the food industry should be trusted as an ally or kept at arm's length.[1] Numerous decisions must soon be made that involve interaction with or exclusion of the food industry. In speaking about inclusion, collaboration, and involving all stakeholders, the industry infers that its business aims are consistent with public health priorities, and for the most part the industry is taken at its word.

Without active discussion, the nation will default to current practices. Industry will be involved in key decisions, exercise its lobbying might, and be invited to the table by national leaders wanting to be friendly with business.

Decisions on dealing with the food industry must be made at many levels. Legislators, themselves subject to lobbying, must decide how bold they can be with policy decisions. Food service directors in schools must weigh nutrition and health against pressures to serve popular foods. School superintendents and principals must balance profits from snack foods and soft drinks against the well-being of their children. Is the food industry friend, foe, or both?

It might seem that some segments of the industry are easier to embrace than others. The fruit and vegetable growers, for instance, might be more obvious health allies than the snack food manufacturers. The industry defies easy classification, however. Foods may start off healthy but get altered. Vast quantities of potatoes are used to make French fries; fruit becomes gummy fruit snacks; and chicken becomes nuggets, tenders, strips, and other fried products. Companies often control many different products; Campbell Soup Company owns both V8 and Godiva; Unilever owns Birds Eye and Breyer's; Coca-Cola owns Minute Maid juices and Coke; and General Mills owns Green Giant and Häagen-Dazs. Planters is owned by Nabisco, which is owned by Kraft, which is owned by Philip Morris. The good guys become hard to distinguish from the bad guys—if such a distinction is even worth pursuing.

As we discuss later, the food industry is not a monolith and never should be considered all good or all bad. When we refer to the "food industry," we think less about individual companies and more about categories of foods (such as soft drinks and snack foods) and about the industry lobbying groups.

The industry comprises hundreds of companies selling thousands of products but speaks through a small number of powerful voices. The Grocery Manufacturers of America (GMA) describes itself as the "world's largest association of food, beverage, and consumer product companies" with sales by its constituents of more than $460 billion just in the United States.[2] The National Soft Drink Association "represents hundreds of soft drink bottling firms, franchise companies and support industries" and claims $52 billion in U.S. sales.[3]

These voices have made it clear how the industry is responding to the obesity crisis and calls for change. They lobby, testify at Congressional hearings, have websites, publish journals, react swiftly to outside threats, and more. It is partly through their actions that the behavior of "the food industry" takes an organized, coherent form.

Friends at the Top

Tight connections between the food industry and key government officials are legendary.[4] Players from the food industry appointed to posts in the United States Department of Agriculture (USDA) are one example. This practice is sensible from one perspective—these are the people who know about food—but conflict of interest becomes a problem.

This milieu of influence became quite public during the Clinton administration, when Michael Espy, under pressure from the White House, was forced to resign in 1994 as Secretary of Agriculture. Espy was accused of taking unlawful gifts from food and agriculture businesses. He was indicted but later acquitted of the charges. Circumstances surrounding the Espy controversy included:

- A Tyson Foods executive was convicted of making illegal gifts to Espy.
- Tyson's chief lobbyist was found guilty of lying to the FBI about these favors.
- Tyson admitted guilt and paid $6 million in fines and costs.
- A California agriculture cooperative was convicted in federal court of "showering" Espy with gifts, including fancy restaurant meals and an all-expenses-paid trip for Espy and his girlfriend to the U.S. Open tennis tournament.
- Espy's top aide was sentenced to twenty-seven months in prison for lying about thousand of dollars he received from two people in Mississippi who had large farming subsidies from the government.[5]

This is not to say that impropriety exists now or was once widespread, but there is considerable potential for conflict of interest. The food industry has much to lose if government policies change the food landscape.

An arm's-length approach is the opposite of what occurs now. In October 2002, Health and Human Services Secretary Tommy Thompson and USDA Secretary Ann Veneman met with leaders from the National Restaurant Association and the National Council of Chain Restaurants on combating obesity. The industry is invited in.

"I am calling on the leaders from the food and beverage industry to aid us in our fight against obesity."

—HHS Secretary Tommy Thompson

"Bringing various industries together to promote balanced diets and healthier lifestyles is important as we look at more aggressive ways to fight obesity in America. At USDA, our goal is to work together in partnership with all sectors to strengthen our ability to reach consumers about these important lifestyle decisions."

—USDA Secretary Ann Veneman[6]

A similar stance was expressed by Derek Yach, the executive responsible for tobacco and obesity programs at the World Health Organization (WHO). After a private meeting of WHO officials with executives from large food companies (Coca-Cola, McDonald's, Unilever, etc.), Yach said, "We recognize that we must work with food and related sectors since they are global, they understand consumers in diverse markets, and are successful in selling products in poor, middle, and rich countries."[7] He therefore assured the industry that they would not be excluded from the decision-making process.

HHS Secretary Thompson swings ever further toward the industry. In November 2002, he held a meeting with the Board of Directors of the GMA. The GMA reported that Thompson urged the food companies to "go on the offensive" against industry critics and that he lauded the industry for "doing wonderful things" to help educate people on diet and exercise.[8]

What is evident thus far is a trusting, probusiness stance that is likely to have serious repercussions. Time may prove this probusiness approach preferable to holding the industry at bay and being skeptical of their motives and actions. Time may also prove the opposite, and officials appear unprepared for this possibility. There is little recognition that the food industry may be undermining public health and stifling policy changes. Attitudes of government leaders toward the industry may become a very real barrier in addressing the obesity crisis.

Should They Join the Team?

The food industry wants in the game and presents a "Mom and apple pie" rationale. They argue for partnerships, coalitions, and involvement of stakeholders. This sounds appealing and offers some advantages, making it tempting to invite them in. The industry has enormous resources, talented people, the world's best food technologists, and impressive marketing expertise. Perhaps more important, fighting the food industry courts conflict with a powerful, well-funded lobby that is not afraid to attack.

The industry says that exclusion equals demonization, raising two main issues. One is whether the industry deserves demonization, and the other is whether demonization is inevitable as this social movement takes form.

Political scientists Rogan Kersh and James Morone have addressed this issue in tracing the history of important health movements such as efforts to curb problem drinking, drug use, and smoking.[9] They point to an "evil industry" as one essential element that allows an issue such as tobacco to be transformed from a personal to a political problem, which in turn permits changes in public policy:

[A] popular cry goes up against an industry peddling poison. Invariably, reformers in private and public realms lament the evil corporate empire that

coins money out of human suffering. Worse, the greedy industry lures
helpless children into self-destructive habits.[10]

Demonization may help put a problem on the political map, but feelings that the demon deserves to be punished can lead to controversial actions like prohibition and criminalization. Kersh and Morone note that concerns with strict actions such as criminalization and prohibitions are warranted, given the history of the war on drugs and prohibition with alcohol. With tobacco, the concept has worked much better. Prohibiting smoking in public places, enforcing rules on advertising and sales to minors, and implementing taxes have had a major impact on smoking rates in the United States, to the point where these and other actions have produced some of the most impressive public health victories of recent years.

While demonizing has a downside, so does colluding with an industry whose tactics might stall, divert, and compromise important public health actions. This is precisely what happened with tobacco, and one can find many signs of this happening with food today. "Involvement of stakeholders" can be a euphemism for caving in to influence.

The industry wants in, and in these early stages, is being invited—by elected and appointed leaders, those who run government agencies, organizations in the health professions, and researchers needing funding. At the very least, this provides a window into the industry's strategy. There is also the opportunity to anticipate what will come next.

Perhaps more important, there is an opportunity to avoid the "work with them versus fight them" dichotomy and address instead the conditions under which working together could be beneficial. Working together, however, must be free of influence and must be in the ultimate interest of the nation's health.

The food industry is at a crucial time where its actions are being scrutinized as never before. The nation and its leaders will come to expect specific actions from the industry as proof of its commitment to public health. A new chapter in the way the nation deals with obesity is about to begin, and the food industry has the opportunity to mastermind its own happy ending.

A Centrist Approach

There is a more centrist position between demonization and glorification, between drastic action like prohibition and no action at all. It is a position that views industry, because of its history, with skepticism and leads not to sales prohibitions but to considered actions that will protect public health.

Many who view the tobacco companies as demons would not support a ban on cigarettes but are in favor of taxing tobacco products, prohibiting advertising to children, restricting where smoking can occur, and so on. While a complete ban on tobacco might have had more impact, these other actions have become acceptable to the public and are working.

A centrist position with food may offer the best opportunity to garner wide support and still make a difference. Many of the suggestions in this book are grounded in this centrist philosophy. The food industry may make some changes voluntarily and in other cases may need more encouragement through regulation and legislation. The nation cannot afford weak, inconsistent, and superficial action grounded in fears that the food companies will be angry.

Food-Tobacco Connections: Can We Avoid a Repeat Performance?

Striking parallels exist between the beginning of the war on tobacco and where the nation stands now with food. First let us address a key issue—that food and tobacco are not the same. We agree that they are not the same.

People do not have to smoke, but they must eat. There is a better defined addictive process with nicotine than with food. Selling cigarettes to minors is illegal; selling food is not. The tobacco industry, with a single product and a few companies selling it, is much less complex than the food industry, with many companies and many thousands of products. There are important differences.

There are, however, instructive similarities in the ways these two industries have responded to public health alarms about their products. There may be key lessons to learn.

By 1964, there was sufficient scientific evidence to prompt Surgeon General Luther Terry to issue the first Surgeon General's Report on Smoking. Many years passed and many millions died before decisive action was taken to ban smoking in public places, hold the companies responsible for the death and disability caused by cigarettes, and truly monitor advertising directed at children. Repeating this history with food and obesity would be tragic.

Food and Tobacco Connections and Interactions

Connections between the tobacco and food industries are numerous and in some cases are hidden quite masterfully. Great public mistrust of the tobacco industry now exists. The food industry risks the same unless they avoid repeating tobacco's mistakes and can distance themselves from the tobacco industry.

Who Owns Whom. The tobacco industry controls important parts of the food industry. Nabisco, a massive company once connected with R.J. Reynolds, is now owned by Kraft, as are Planters, Oscar Meyer, and many other companies. Kraft in turn is the largest food company in the world, but itself is owned by Philip Morris. The extent to which Kraft's political and business strategy is governed by Philip Morris and how Kraft responds to the obesity crisis will be important to follow.

Cloaked Connections in Trade Organizations. Food and tobacco money are intertwined in organizations that fight for wholesome-sounding causes. One example is the Center for Consumer Freedom (discussed in detail below). This group, reportedly started with tobacco money, is now a coalition of restaurant and tavern owners. We are not certain whether this group still receives tobacco money, but it attacks people who argue for policy changes to improve nutrition. It also has fought strongly against proposals that would restrict smoking, especially at bars and restaurants. Tobacco and food companies become allies when smoking and eating occur in the same location, such as restaurants. Dressed up to appear to defend consumers and basic freedoms, the Center for Consumer Freedom opposes actions that would hurt food or tobacco companies.

A telling example of this phenomenon is in a report by researchers on tobacco and food money supporting the Massachusetts Restaurant Association. This association represents more than 7,000 restaurants and groups in the food service industry throughout the state. It downplays connections with the tobacco industry, yet has worked with the industry to defeat legislation that would restrict smoking in workplaces, public spaces, restaurants, and bars. Philip Morris and R.J. Reynolds are dues-paying members. Such organizations exist in other states. The authors of this report conclude:

The close political association between the Association and the tobacco industry has been mutually beneficial. The Association has helped to conceal the tobacco industry's state and local political activity in exchange for a variety of resources.[11]

Historical Parallels of Food and Tobacco. David Kessler, former head of the Food and Drug Administration and now Dean of the Yale Medical School, chronicled the war on tobacco in his book *A Question of Intent*.[12] Kessler, Stanton Glantz, Kenneth Warner, and other pioneers have shown clearly how the tobacco industry operates. These leaders showed how companies paid highly esteemed scientists (presumably to secure their allegiance), obscured scientific information, formed "citizen action" groups that claimed to protect consumer freedom, waged a very expensive public relations campaign against antismoking efforts, devoted great resources to lobby government officials here and abroad, paid for product placement in television and movies, and targeted children with advertising.[13]

The response from society, after some years of inaction, was to be furious with these companies and fight them in every way possible. The fight has come through public outrage, legal action, legislation, and regulation. Thirty years ago, one could not have imagined states suing tobacco companies, limits on advertising, very high taxes, investigative reports, and even popular movies chronicling the misdeeds of the industry. Will the same happen with food?

The food industry has established a presence in our lives far beyond what most people realize. In her book *Food Politics*, Marion Nestle notes case after case of how the food industry has influenced national dietary guidelines, has helped support the nation's major professional nutrition association (American Dietetic Association), and has been a relentless marketer of foods poor in nutrition.[14] The industry makes no pretense about advertising to children. It is powerful and well organized. We can look at its behavior to see if we are witnessing a repeat of what tobacco did many years ago.

In 1954, the tobacco industry ran a full-page ad entitled "A Frank Statement to Cigarette Smokers." It said:

We accept an interest in people's health as a basic responsibility, paramount to every other consideration in our business. . . . We always have and always will cooperate closely with those whose task it is to safeguard the public health.[15]

Today, the Grocery Manufacturers of America states:

The food and beverage industry we represent has long advocated for comprehensive, long-term strategies for improving the health and fitness of all Americans.[16]

The National Soft Drink Association claims:

The soft drink industry has a long commitment to promoting a healthy lifestyle for individuals—especially children.[17]

The "Frank Statement to Cigarette Smokers" also said:

We believe the products we make are not injurious to health.

As late as 1994, the CEOs of the seven largest tobacco companies testified one after another in Congressional hearings that nicotine is not addictive, while internal documents obtained later indicated the industry knew otherwise.

I do not believe that nicotine is addictive.
                    —THOMAS SANDEFUR (BROWN & WILLIAMSON)

I believe nicotine is not addictive.
                    —WILLIAM CAMPBELL (PHILIP MORRIS)[18]

The National Soft Drink Association states:

. . . soft drinks do not cause pediatric obesity, do not reduce nutrient intake, and do not cause dental cavities in children.[19]

The soft drink industry group may or may not really believe this, but its strident claims in the face of contradictory science are hard to defend (see Chapter 7).

Interesting parallels also exist in the recognition by tobacco and food industries that children must be cultivated as customers. Both industries developed considerable skill at luring children to their products.

The base of our business is the high school student.
                    —LORILLARD TOBACCO COMPANY INTERNAL MEMO[20]

They got lips? We want 'em.
                    —R.J. REYNOLDS TOBACCO COMPANY INTERNAL MEMO[21]

We always, always have kid-related programs.
                    —MCDONALD'S VICE PRESIDENT[22]

Who Can Be Trusted?

The food companies say the right words. Food industry websites have information on nutrition and physical activity, they support coalitions that promote changes in diet and exercise, they say they are working to develop healthier products, and they state with no ambiguity that they are committed to the health of the nation. Can they be taken at their word?

The words sound familiar, and once again, tobacco's history may give us helpful insight. Kenneth Warner from the University of Michigan wrote an editorial for the *American Journal of Public Health* on how this history unfolded with cigarette companies.

To read the cigarette manufacturers' websites, one would think the industry must be a wholly owned subsidiary of the Public Health Service. The sites warn about the dangers of smoking, say smoking is addictive, list chemicals added in manufacturing cigarettes, encourage smoke-free environments for nonsmokers, and offer smokers Web-based quitting resources. Industry leader Philip Morris sounds downright altruistic in its enunciated commitment to youth smoking prevention: the company wants "to work with those who share our goal of reducing youth smoking. If collaborative efforts to solve this problem are successful, and this leads to a smaller adult consumer base in the future, we say 'so be it.' " The other major producers—runner-up R.J. Reynolds, bronze medalist Brown & Williamson, and last-place Lorillard—all pledge allegiance to youth smoking prevention as well.

This is the face of the "new" tobacco industry, they tell us, committed to public health and to America's children. They have finally come clean, they would have us believe, after half a century of targeting kids and deceiving the public about their products' dangers. Their social commitment extends well beyond the issue of smoking, they inform us. Each company devotes millions of dollars to a variety of causes, including feeding the hungry, aiding victims of natural disasters, and protecting women who are victims of abuse (of the nonsmoking kind). In 2000, industry behemoth Philip Morris, with domestic tobacco revenues of $23 billion, spent $115 million on such worthy endeavors—and then spent an additional $150 million on a national advertising campaign to inform the public about the company's largesse.

Consistent with the spirit of a liberal society, of course, these companies defend their right to market cigarettes, a legal product, to the tens of millions of adult Americans who "enjoy" smoking.

If readers detect herein a hint of sarcasm, they will forgive the author if he does not credit them with unusual perspicacity. Any industry watcher appreciates that this industry has consistently articulated one position while knowing its diametric opposite to be true, to devastating effect. As recently as 1994, the companies' chief executive officers all swore before Congress that they did not know that smoking caused disease or believe it was addictive. Their scientists and lawyers knew and had been telling them so for decades.[23]

We must not repeat the dreadful history that occurred with tobacco. It is simply not reasonable to allow the food industry to stake out this moral high ground while toiling to increase sales of snack foods, soft drinks, fast foods, candy, and so on, particularly to children. The industry will be believed when its words and actions correspond.

So yes, eating and smoking are different. But it is difficult not to notice that modern food companies may be owned by tobacco companies and that money from the two industries is mingled in organizations that fight for both. We must ask whether the behavior of the food industry differs from that of Big Tobacco and whether we should ignore the lessons handed to us by history.

Legislators, the press, and the public were flabbergasted when tobacco industry CEOs testified that nicotine is not addictive. This helped sensitize the nation to how badly industry leaders can behave when money and power are at stake. Decades from today, history will look back on how legislators, the press, and the public are responding right now to claims by the food industry that they support public health, to statements that their products are not contributing to obesity, and to their pleas not to be demonized. We hope a positive history is about to be written.

McDonald's and Frito-Lay: Two Cases in Point

The food industry is responding in many ways to the rising volume of criticism. One way is to introduce healthier foods. Major announcements in 2002 by McDonald's and Frito-Lay (owned by PepsiCo) are interesting case studies on how companies are reacting to changing public opinion and how the nation might respond. These announcements could represent positive, groundbreaking developments, or superficial, diversionary tactics aimed at deflecting criticism.

The McDonald's Announcement

McDonald's made dramatic news by promising to change the oil used to cook fried food items. The most notable item is French fries, but other key foods like chicken nuggets, fried chicken sandwiches, and hash browns are also affected. The new oil will have a 48 percent reduction in trans fatty acids, reduce saturated fat by 16 percent, and increase polyunsaturated fat by 167 percent. A spokesperson from McDonald's says, "It's a win-win for our customers because they are getting the same great French fry taste along with an even healthier nutrition profile."

This was a blockbuster move. McDonald's worldwide serves 46 million people *each day*, and in the United States uses 7 percent (3.2 billion pounds) of all potatoes grown for its fries and hash browns.

The McDonald's announcement was embraced by high-profile health experts such as Dean Ornish, who stated, "From a nutrition standpoint, this is going to have a major and immediate impact." The President of the American College of Nutrition said, "I applaud McDonald's for its leadership in this area and urge others to follow their lead."

In the spring of 2003, McDonald's announced the change in oil was delayed indefinitely, reportedly because of concerns that sales would be adversely affected.

The Frito-Lay Announcement

In September 2002, Frito-Lay announced it was eliminating trans fats from Doritos, Tostitos, and Cheetos and unveiled Lay's Reduced Fat Chips and Cheetos Reduced Fat Snacks. The press release contained the following:

"We're taking several steps that will change the way America snacks," said Al Bru, President and Chief Executive Officer of Frito-Lay North America.

Along with Frito-Lay's world class food scientists, the company has partnered with Kenneth Cooper, MD, MPH, one of the world's foremost experts on health, nutrition, and exercise and founder of the Cooper Aerobics Center, to create breakthrough new products and enhance existing products to meet the nutritional needs of today's consumers.

"The obesity epidemic has spurred Americans to take action and embrace proper nutrition and physical activity," said Dr. Cooper. "I'm delighted to partner with Frito-Lay to help them develop more healthy snacks and to promote fitness and wellness." [24]

What Does It Mean?

These announcements received widespread publicity and are noteworthy in that high-profile figures in the health community, Dean Ornish and Kenneth Cooper, are lending their names to the effort. The tone of media coverage was generally positive, based perhaps on the support of the health celebrities. The happiness with McDonald's and Frito-Lay makes sense at first glance—foods eaten by millions of people will be healthier. There may, however, be a negative consequence, perhaps intended, perhaps not.

The positive reactions to the McDonald's and Frito-Lay announcements rest on a fundamental assumption that may be simple, appealing, but wrong: namely, that consumption of fast foods and snack foods will not increase because of these changes. If consumers must eat fried foods and Frito-Lay snacks and do not eat more, having healthier versions is a clear improvement. We worry, however, about the "SnackWell's paradox."

When Nabisco introduced their lowered-fat SnackWell's product line, some (and perhaps many) people feasted on cookies feeling they had been issued a free pass. SnackWell's cookies were not reduced in calories; the deterioration in taste from reducing fat was countered with added sugar. Concerns were raised that foods like SnackWell's might increase rather than decrease calorie intake.

One can gain weight just fine with SnackWell's cookies, or with McDonald's changed-fat foods, or with modified Doritos, Tostitos, and Cheetos. It all depends on how much people eat, something that is difficult to predict. McDonald's new versions of their fried foods will not have fewer calories—one fat is simply being replaced with another.

We cannot predict how the public will respond to the McDonald's and Frito-Lay changes, but if the free pass mentality prevails, people may believe the new foods are healthy in an absolute sense and therefore enjoy a license to eat more. If they eat more, they will weigh more. It is nice that fat is being changed or reduced, but the net impact on health must be the prime consideration.

Frito-Lay and McDonald's may have altruistic motives and may be leading the way such that other companies must follow. They are certainly taking a risk by changing core products—if people eat less fried food at McDonald's or fewer of Frito-Lay's key products, these companies could be hit hard.

McDonald's and Frito-Lay are not known for marketing blunders, so it would be surprising if these decisions were made without understanding how consumers will react. We reserve judgment, but feel it is important to examine whether the overall impact will be increased consumption of the changed foods.

As with exercise initiatives discussed below, we applaud efforts by these companies to make their foods healthier. At the same time, it is important to examine the complex motives for change. We hope that such initiatives will provide public health benefits and that companies will remain motivated to find creative ways to provide healthy choices for consumers.

Food Industry Tactics

Judging from stated positions of the food industry thus far, we can infer how the industry intends to position itself with respect to legislative and regulatory actions designed to improve the nation's diet. Beyond the goodwill they seek by connecting with professional health organizations, sports enterprises (e.g., Pepsi Center in Denver, NASCAR sponsorships, Tostitos Fiesta Bowl), and world events like the Olympics, they make campaign contributions, support powerful lobbying groups, and use their political muscle in many ways.

In addition, the industry is employing a number of strategies when it perceives legislative, regulatory, and public relations threats. We will list the main arguments and give our response to each. The press, legislators, and the public can expect to hear these arguments with increasing frequency.

The main points made by the industry are exemplified by statements of industry lobbying groups such as the Grocery Manufacturers of America (www.gmabrands.com), the National Soft Drink Association (www.nsda.com), and the Sugar Association (www.sugar.org). Their websites contain press releases, accounts of testimony before legislative bodies, and other material that make the industry's positions quite clear. What follows are the arguments we believe are most central to the industry strategy.

Claim Commitment to Public Health

The food industry is quick to say that public health is a priority, as indicated by quotes shown earlier in this chapter. One more example is a quote from Walt Riker, Vice-President of Social Responsibility & Communications at McDonald's:

McDonald's has sponsored physical fitness programs and nutrition education for decades. McDonald's takes nutrition very seriously.[25]

Once again the behavior of the industry can be interpreted in different ways. The commitment to health may be genuine, or it could be a clever way to preempt critics by claiming to have common goals and insisting on involvement in government decisions about nutrition.

Influence Public Policy Directly

Within a short period of time, one of us (KB) took part in an academic meeting on the politics of obesity, testified before the New York State

Assembly, took part in a meeting of the U.S. Department of Agriculture, and testified before a Senate committee on Capitol Hill. The same spokesperson from the grocery manufacturer's group (GMA) was at each of the meetings, saying things like "GMA believes the food and beverage industry has a very important role to play in helping to improve fitness and nutrition."[26] A spokesperson from the National Soft Drink Association also testified at one of the meetings.

The prime way to influence policy is to be part of policy decisions, and it is understandable that the food industry wants in. A great deal rides on these policies. Much caution should be exercised before granting the industry its wish list of access.

Seek Influence Through Campaign Contributions

Groups of all types court favor from politicians by making campaign contributions. If these failed to affect voting, contributions would have stopped long ago. Many millions of dollars are spent by specific companies and by industry associations and lobbying groups such as the National Food Processor's Association, National Cattlemen's Beef Association, International Dairy Foods Association, Grocery Manufacturers of America, and the Snack Foods Association. Both "hard" and "soft" funds are directed at members of Congress, especially those on agriculture and nutrition committees.[27]

The Center for Responsive Politics estimated that the various sectors of the food industry made more than $34 million in campaign contributions just in election year 2000.[28] This does not count the large contributions from tobacco companies that own food companies.

Claim That Advertising Affects Brand Share, Not Consumption

This old and tired argument has been used by many industries, tobacco and food included. Despite claims to the contrary, internal documents from the tobacco industry show concerted efforts to increase smoking.[29] Some segments of the industry admit freely that their aim is to increase consumption. Several quotes from the Snack Food Association (SFA) website are illustrative. For instance, SFA states that it "Promotes increased snack consumption by sponsoring National Snack Food Month in February, along with other promotions." In addition:

SFA and the National Potato Promotion Board (NPPB) initiated National Snack Food Month in February 1989 to increase consumption and build awareness of snacks during a month when snack food consumption was traditionally low. The result has been a substantial increase in snack food sales during this month. The promotion kicks off on Super Bowl Sunday and publicity is generated throughout the month of February.[30]

SFA is a player. In its own words, the SFA "represents over 800 companies worldwide. SFA business membership includes, but is not limited to, manufacturers of potato chips, tortilla chips, cereal snacks, pretzels, popcorn, cheese snacks, snack crackers, meat snacks, pork rinds, snack nuts, party mix, corn snacks, pellet snacks, fruit snacks, snack bars, granola, snack cakes, cookies, and various other snacks."

The food industry advertises directly to children and has spent billions of dollars doing so. It is very difficult to believe that advertising only helps children make choices between McDonald's and Burger King, Coke and Pepsi, Skittles and Twix, and Lucky Charms and Cap'n Crunch, and that their desire for fast food, soft drinks, candy, and sugared cereals is unaffected.

Focus Attention on Physical Activity

A key industry strategy is to emphasize the importance of physical activity. Time and time again, food companies say that physical inactivity is a major contributor to obesity, sometimes implying that food is not important. A spokesperson from the National Soft Drink Association said that obesity "is about the couch and not the can."[31]

Industry puts its money where its mouth is when emphasizing activity. As we mention below, the industry is quick to sponsor activity-related programs. An example is the innovative program we discussed in Chapter 4, Colorado on the Move. Another example is the Kidnetic program from the International Food Information Council. Supporting physical activity is good, but care must be taken to avoid having the spotlight removed from food.

Divert Attention from Food

It is in the interest of the food industry, of course, not to have food considered the cause of an epidemic and for food not to be the main target for change. As we have mentioned, emphasizing physical activity is one means of drawing attention away from food, but several other strategies also are becoming evident.

Claim That Nutrition Information Is Confusing. The food industry paints a picture of a nutrition morass, saying that information on nutrition is so unpredictable and perplexing that consumers do not know what to eat or where to turn. Consumers hear that fat is bad, but some fat is good. One day a food hurts you and the next day it prevents a major disease. A spokesperson for the Grocery Manufacturers of America, for example, states:

. . . consumers are potentially more confused about food and its role in enhancing health than ever before.[32]

Nutrition information does change rapidly, and confusing messages are common. This should not create policy paralysis, however, and should not block the nation from favoring some foods over others. In its most basic form, nutrition is straightforward and some actions are completely justified. Calorie intake in the country is too high, consumption of high-calorie foods with little nutrition should decrease, and intake of fruits and vegetables should increase.

While these actions are obvious based on common sense, policy gets stalled when interest groups claim lack of consensus. There may never come a time when nutrition knowledge is complete, when the science is perfect, and when all parties agree on what should be eaten.

Decry Demonization of a Food or the Food Industry. Industry lobbyists cry foul when certain foods or companies are singled out. They claim that no one food is responsible for the epidemic of obesity.

. . . it is too simplistic to attribute the origins of obesity to a particular food.

—National Soft Drink Association[33]

Dumping the obesity issue on fast food is completely missing the issue. People don't only eat fast food. They eat at home or white tablecloth dining. We as Americans tend to look at quick scapegoats.
—BURGER KING SPOKESPERSON ROBERT A. DOUGHTY[34]

. . . programs will go a lot further in attacking this obesity problem than making accusations and finger pointing.
—GROCERY MANUFACTURERS OF AMERICA SPOKESPERSON[35]

This is a clever approach, but it may hurt the industry. No one we know, even the most florid food fanatics, would claim that any one food or company is totally responsible for an epidemic of disease. The industry, therefore, attacks a position that no one embraces.

The dangerous inference made by the industry, however, is that they do not contribute to the problem, are blameless, and should not be forced to change. Here is where they will lose public support. Americans have a long history of taking action when there is contributory blame. A company releasing toxic chemicals into the groundwater can claim it is not responsible for the nation's water pollution, but it is fined for contributing.

As the public becomes more aware of the actions of food companies, especially those targeting children, it seems inevitable that contributory blame will be assessed. Whether they will be sued successfully, fined, or penalized in some other way remains to be seen, but they will certainly be forced to change.

Claim There Are No "Good" or "Bad" Foods

The food industry says time and time again that no food is good or bad, using the position of the American Dietetic Association (ADA) to defend its stance (see Chapter 1). This is a variant of the demonization argument.

The American Dietetic Association has stated that the entire diet, rather than specific foods, should be scrutinized. Identifying the extra calories that might be contributing to an adolescent being overweight or obese will probably be more effective in changing his or her diet than portraying individual foods as good or bad. . . . We must take a total diet approach and forever abandon blaming one nutrient or food as the cause of America's weight gain.

—GROCERY MANUFACTURERS OF AMERICA[36]

The claim that nutritive sweeteners have caused an increase in chronic disease (e.g., obesity, cardiovascular disease, diabetes, dental caries, and behavioral disorders) is not substantiated . . . persons can include sugars in their diets and still consume a healthful diet. . . . The ADA counsels that there are no "good foods" and "bad foods," just good diets and bad diets. In other words, all foods have a place in a balanced diet.

—SUGAR ASSOCIATION[37]

As we noted in Chapter 1, this position has several negative consequences. It implies that no food or types of foods (such as soft drinks, candy, or snack foods) should be singled out and that programs aiming to change their consumption would be unfair. This paralyzes discussion, leads to nutrition guidelines without teeth, and deflects blame from the industry. The argument is destructive from a public health perspective—some foods should be eaten more and others eaten less. Implying otherwise leaves no constructive option.

Say That Restricting Access to Foods Will Backfire

This industry reacts to ideas like taxing foods or removing soft drinks from schools by stating that restricting access to foods increases desire and will be counterproductive. If this argument were correct, of course, we would expect the food companies to stop selling their products in schools. The students, crazed with desire for the restricted foods, would stampede the 7-Eleven after school and eat themselves silly. Profits would skyrocket.

Hyperbole aside, the industry cites one study to support their claim.[38] This lab study looked at the consumption of snacks after a meal in girls and boys ages three to five. Girls, but not boys, ate more snacks if their mothers reported restricting access to snack foods at home. However, restricting could mean no snack foods around the house or having the foods available and then denying access. We do not feel this study can be used as evidence that creating a healthier food environment in places such as schools will have a negative effect.

A perilous corollary of the restriction concept is that people benefit from having access to candy, snack foods, fast food, and soft drinks. There is clear scientific evidence that the more food is available the more people eat, that increasing energy density (calories) leads to more eating, and that taste is a prime determinant of how much is eaten (see Chapter 2). Snack foods and soft drinks are high in calories and taste good. Having them in schools makes them more available. Here science agrees with the obvious business truth (companies would remove these foods from schools if doing so would help sales).

Play the Choice and Freedom Cards

The food industry often cites threats to personal freedom and choice when condemning proposals for change.

Consumption of food is one of the most fundamental liberties people can enjoy.
—MIKE BURITA, CENTER FOR CONSUMER FREEDOM[39]

The personal liberty argument has been used by the tobacco industry for years. By restricting access to, availability of, or price for something like cigarettes or food, personal freedoms are restricted, so the argument goes.

The argument goes further to say that people deserve choices and that limiting choice has undesirable effects. In response to questioning about soft drinks and snack foods in schools during Senate hearings, Lisa Katic of the GMA said:

I feel very strongly that "just say no" to these kinds of foods in schools does not give children the tools they need to make choices throughout their life. You know, it's something that they really need to be educated on and that needs to start in the classroom.

*If you take foods away . . . they're going to go somewhere else to get it.
. . . So if they don't learn how to include it in the diet, they never learn.
They have to learn, when, how much, when it's appropriate. And if that's
not offered in the school, they don't have the right tools to navigate the food
environment as they get older.*[40]

Time will tell whether this argument has currency with the public,
but the industry will have to convince people that unhealthy foods in
schools help children develop healthier diets. If this were correct, one
could argue for cigarette machines in schools so children learn to make
the right choice about tobacco.

Personal freedom and choice are concepts that play well in America,
so the industry may be using the best available approach to defend their
practices. Appealing to emotions surrounding freedom, however, may
ultimately hurt the food companies because public skepticism is increasing—people are asking just how it is that promoting unhealthy food in
schools enhances freedom and preserves the nation's democratic ideals.

Warn of the Slippery Slope
If food now, what's next? The road of regulating and restricting goes
downhill fast, according to this view.

*When we begin controlling what people can put into their mouths, there is
no end to what might be next.*
—MIKE BURITA, CENTER FOR CONSUMER FREEDOM[41]

There are several problems with this argument. The first is the
assumption that coercive people want to usurp personal liberties and
will pick any arena in which to exercise that power. Those arguing for
changes in the food environment, so the feeling goes, will quickly move
to another area where they can limit choice. The second is the fact that
no action, on any issue, would be possible if the nation were paralyzed
with fears of the slippery slope. No change, no matter how important,
could be made because it might lead to subsequent changes.

Emphasize That Parents Must Teach Children Healthy Habits

Sure they should but look at what interferes. Parents try their best, but it is no contest between them and pressures to eat unhealthy food. Children see thousands of food advertisements. Their favorite cartoon characters, sports stars, and movie heroes are used to sell them fast food and soft drinks. A few parents prevail in the face of this pressure, but they seem to be dwindling in number. Even our dietitian friends are horrified to see how little control they have when their children start watching television, go to friends' houses to play, and begin school.

By implication, saying that parents must educate their children about nutrition places blame on them when their children are overweight. This deflects responsibility and is not likely to be helpful. In addition, this approach of counting on parents is a failed experiment. We have been relying on parents all these years and what is there to show—an epidemic of obesity. Should we educate them more? Of course, but how would this be done, how much would it cost, and what hope would there be for its success?

Parents *can* help their children, and as a society, we must make this task as easy as possible. A wise society creates safe and healthy environments for its children. We have taken bold steps to protect our children from cigarettes. We do not allow free access to cigarettes and then say that parents must teach children to make choices. Parents may be part of the solution, but without changing the environment, they stand no chance of being the sole remedy.

Silence Critics by Suing or Intimidating Them

In her book on the politics of food, Marion Nestle points out that the food industry can play "hardball" by suing people who criticize it.[42] She notes two highly visible cases as examples. One was McDonald's suing a tiny activist group in England that distributed leaflets critical of the company. A British judge ruled against the group on some counts, but awarded McDonald's only $1 in damages and ruled that just criticisms had been made that McDonald's exploited children through advertising.

The second case cited by Nestle involved Oprah Winfrey being sued by a group of Texas cattle ranchers for $10.3 million in lost business when Winfrey did a show on mad cow disease. The cattle ranchers lost the case in what was considered a crushing defeat, but Winfrey was said to have spent $1 million for her own defense.

An illustrative case of the food industry dealing with a scientific critic has now occurred with Nestle herself. She has written and spoken extensively on food issues, and among the topics she covers is her opinion on sugar and its role in obesity and other diseases.

The Sugar Association had a Washington, D.C., law firm send Nestle a certified letter accusing her of making statements that were false, misleading, disparaging, defamatory, distorted, and damaging. The letter from the law firm to Nestle, and Nestle's response, are printed in Figures 10.1. and 10.2 (see pages 270–273).[43] Nestle did not back down. The fact that the letters are now posted on the Internet allows people to see firsthand how the industry chooses to handle criticism in at least some cases.

Front Groups for Tobacco and Food

The tobacco industry funded a number of groups that helped wage war on the antismoking movement. The groups were launched in states where the most aggressive antismoking legislation was being considered and often had words such as *choice* and *freedom* in their title. They argued that the health "police" were crusaders looking to stomp out individual rights. The way to protect civil liberties, of course, was to fight off any action that would curtail smoking.

The groups probably helped stall early efforts to curb smoking, but then became a liability to the tobacco industry. When their funding became evident, these groups lost credibility with government leaders, and when exposed by the media, made the tobacco industry look even more manipulative and deceitful.

The same phenomenon is occurring with food. The most vocal and perhaps well-funded group is the Center for Consumer Freedom (formerly known as the Guest Choice Network). According to a history of this group assembled by the group PR Watch:

- Its founder, Rick Berman, approached the Philip Morris tobacco company for $600,000 to begin the organization. The group began in 1995 with funding entirely from Philip Morris.
- The group now represents alcohol distributors and thousands of restaurants and bars, including Cracker Barrel, Hooters, Olive Garden, Outback Steakhouse, Red Lobster, and TGI Friday's.
- The group has fought strenuously against minimum wage increases (to protect restaurant profits), limits on smoking in public places, and efforts by Mothers Against Drunk Driving and other groups to toughen blood alcohol limits.
- Fighting these changes is done while invoking freedom, consumer "choice," and individual rights as recurrent themes.
- The group has attacked a broad range of people and groups, including the American Medical Association; National Association of High School Principals; National Safety Council; National Transportation Safety Board; the U.S. Department of Transportation; researchers from institutions such as Harvard, Princeton, and Yale (guess who this might be!); the Centers for Disease Control and Prevention; and New York Mayor Rudy Guiliani (who proposed confiscating the cars of drunk drivers).
- In a 1999 interview with a trade publication for restaurant chains, *Chain Leader*, Berman said, "Our offensive strategy is to shoot the messenger" and "Given the activists' plans to alarm beyond all reason, we've got to attack their credibility as spokespersons."[44]

Here is what the Center for Consumer Freedom says about itself:

The Center for Consumer Freedom is a coalition of more than 25,000 restaurant and tavern operators working together to preserve the right to offer our guests a full menu of dining and entertainment choices. As promoters of choice—the right of adults to make personal decisions about what we eat and drink—we've stepped out of the "he said, she said" product debates. We've engaged instead on the higher moral ground of freedom to make personal choices about what we eat and drink.[45]

RE: Inaccurate Sugar Statements

Dear Dr. Nestle:

We represent The Sugar Association, Inc. ("SAI"), an organization that is committed to integrity and sound scientific principles in educating consumers and professionals about the benefits of pure natural sugar. We understand that you are a professor at New York University School of Education and Chair of its Department of Nutrition and Food Studies and that you have recently published a book entitled *Food Politics*, which you are currently promoting. It has come to our attention that during the course of this promotion, you have made numerous false, misleading, disparaging, and defamatory statements about sugar. While we are perplexed as to why or how a professional educator of your stature would disseminate such distorted and damaging statements, we must demand that you stop making such statements about sugar.

There are numerous examples of such statements, some of which we will provide below. First, you continually repeat the false and inaccurate statement that soft drinks contain sugar. For example, in your March 4, 2001, interview with WBUR, a National Public Radio affiliate in Boston, you said that: "Soft drinks are a really easy target because they're sugar and water and nothing else." As commonly known by experts in the field of nutrition, soft drinks have contained virtually no sugar (sucrose) in more than 20 years. The misuse of the word "sugar" to indicate other caloric sweeteners is not only inaccurate, but it is a grave disservice to the thousands of family farmers who grow sugar cane and sugar beets.

Second, in this same news interview, you state that the U.S. Department of Agriculture ("USDA") changed its Dietary Guideline on sugar from "limit your intake of added sugars" to "moderate your intake of sugars" based on political pressure without revealing the lack of scientific support for the initial "limit" language. Specifically, you said that: "In the last dietary guidelines for Americans, the word 'limit' was removed by [that is] 'limit your intake of added sugar' was removed by the Department of Agriculture under pressure from sugar lobbying organizations . . ."—without mentioning that the language was removed because public law mandates that the Guidelines be based on the preponderance of scientific evidence, which did not support the recommendation to limit sugar intake. *continued*

Figure 10.1 Letter from Venable Attorneys at Law to Marion Nestle

Third, your inferred claim that sugar is physiologically addictive is false. As you know, sugar is not addictive. Sugar is pure carbohydrate, and as such, is no more addictive than any other food.

Finally, you clearly connote that sugar has been scientifically proven to be a prime contributor to heart disease, obesity and other diseases besides dental caries. This ignores and directly contradicts the conclusions of the most recent authoritative government publication on the subject—a December 2001 research brief published by the USDA in *Family Economics and Nutrition Review*, Vol. 13, No. 1 (2001), entitled "Current Knowledge of the Health Effects of Sugar" by Ann Mardis, M.D., MPH. This review is consistent with the conclusions of other authoritative reports including the FAO/WHO report on Carbohydrates in Human Nutrition (1999), WHO Technical Report Series 894 Obesity: Preventing and Managing the Global Epidemic (2000), and the COMA report on Dietary Sugars and Human Disease (1989).

SAI has provided you with truthful and non-misleading facts concerning these issues, including a February 21, 2002, letter from its President and CEO, Dr. Richard Keelor. To ensure that you have all of the facts, we enclose a copy of the Mardis article.

The purpose of this letter is to appeal to your sense of fairness and academic integrity. We share your goals of providing important nutrition information to the public and to address the problems of chronic disease and childhood obesity through awareness of good nutrition, exercise and a healthy lifestyle. However, such goals should not be achieved through disinformation, or at the expense of an important natural, simple and low caloric source of carbohydrate. We ask that you be guided by the most current scientific evidence and government statements and that your writings and comments be reflective of them. We also ask that you be more precise and accurate in your definitions and cease making misleading or false statements regarding sugar or the sugar industry. If not, the only recourse available to us will be to legally defend our industry and its members against any and all fallacious and harmful allegations.

Sincerely,

Jeffrey S. Tenenbaum

Dear Mr. Tenenbaum,

I was surprised to receive your letter of March 27, 2002, stating that I have made "numerous false, misleading, disparaging, and defamatory statements about sugar." Your statement is incorrect and appears to be based on both a misunderstanding of carbohydrate science and a mischaracterization of my views and opinions.

1. Your letter notes, correctly, that soft drinks do not contain *sucrose* (a disaccharide sugar composed of one molecule each of the monosaccharide sugars, *glucose* and *fructose*). Soft drinks are for the most part sweetened with corn syrup, a mixture of *glucose* (a monosaccharide sugar), *fructose* (a monosaccharide sugar), *maltose* (a disaccharide sugar), and other small saccharides—in other words, *sugars*. From a biochemical and physiological standpoint, these sugars are similar to sucrose, as all are convertible to *glucose* (blood sugar) in the body. To argue that soft drinks "do not contain sugar" because they are not sweetened with sucrose is misleading and not in the interest of public education about diet and health.

2. Your letter refers to my statement that the U.S. Department of Agriculture (USDA) changed its 2000 dietary guideline on sugar based on political pressure from sugar lobby organizations. As you well know, that statement is true as the USDA did change the sugar guideline as a result of efforts by sugar lobbying organizations. As to your suggestion that the change was motivated by the fact that the preponderance of scientific evidence does not support the recommendation to "limit" sugar intake, I think it is fair to say that the scientific evidence that relates sugar to health is incomplete and, therefore, subject to interpretation and a matter of reasoned opinion as much as it is of scientific "fact." Experts do not necessarily agree with the change in the dietary guideline, or the purported rationale for the change, nor do they have to on the basis of existing science (see #5 below).

3. Your letter contends that I have made an "inferred claim that sugar is physiologically addictive." You are misinformed about my views on the subject and incorrect about the claim you attribute to me, as I do not apply the word "addictive" to *any* food. Instead, I state that the *taste* for sugar is innate. Taste is not the same as addiction and I make every effort to make that distinction clear. *continued*

Figure 10.2 Letter from Marion Nestle to Venable Attorneys at Law

4. Your letter contends that I "clearly connote" that "sugar has been scientifically proven to be a prime contributor to heart disease, obesity and other diseases besides dental caries." You have not cited a single source or reference for the "connotation" you attribute to me. Your statement mischaracterizes the strength of my opinion about the role of sugars in elevating risk factors for chronic disease, but again I must point out that interpretation of research on sugar and health is a matter of reasoned opinion and experts do not always agree on such interpretation (see #5).

5. Your letter contends that "SAI [Sugar Association, Inc.] has provided me with truthful and non-misleading facts concerning these issues." Again I must point out that some experts disagree with the Sugar Association's opinion on these matters. For example, a paper in the March 2002 *Journal of the American Dietetic Association* (Vol. 102, pages 351–353) states that "whether sweetness comes from sucrose or HFCS [high fructose corn syrup], both are essentially disaccharides composed of one glucose and one fructose molecule," and that "Growing evidence is linking excessive intakes of added sugars with undesirable health risks of obesity leading to increased incidence of type 2 diabetes mellitus and its complications, especially cardiovascular disease." Thus, opinions may differ among experts even when based on the same set of scientific "facts."

In sum, I have never disseminated "distorted and damaging statements" about sugar. The First Amendment guarantees us both the right to air our opinions in public so as to stimulate debate in matters of public interest. The sense of fairness and academic integrity to which you appeal would seem to me to work both ways. Therefore, I ask that you immediately stop attributing unsupported false and misleading statements to me and cease threatening me with legal action—threats clearly designed to intimidate me into silence.

Yours sincerely,

Marion Nestle, Ph.D., MPH
Professor and Chair
New York University

Claiming the moral high ground seems questionable when support is from the tobacco and food industries and one then fights attempts to control their products, despite hundreds of thousands of deaths each year from smoking and poor diet. All in the name of freedom.

In June 2002, the Center for Consumer Freedom placed a full-page color ad in *U.S. News and World Report*. The ad stated:

You are too stupid . . . to make your own food choices. At least according to the food police and government bureaucrats who have proposed "fat taxes" on foods they don't want you to eat. . . . We think they are going too far. It's your food. It's your drink. It's your freedom.[46]

At about the same time this group ran radio advertisements with the same theme on stations in Washington, D.C. Their website (www .consumerfreedom.com) is where their attacking strategy is most evident. In responding to one of us (KB), they say:

"If children have healthy foods available, they'll eat healthy foods. If they have unhealthy foods available, they'll eat those. . . . Animals will do the same thing when put in a cage."

That was Kelly Brownell, mullah of the "Twinkie tax," in testimony before the U.S. Senate in late May. It's the latest silly rhetoric from one of the grand poobahs of the anticonsumer movement.[47]

Further, the Center for Consumer Freedom says:

Thanks to the relentless hounding by self-appointed "nannies"—those "food cops," health-care enforcers and vegetarian activists who "know what's best for us"—people are embarrassed to speak up in defense of adult beverages, high-calorie foods or their personal pleasure of smoking. Years of obscene and inflammatory rhetoric by the nanny culture have so demonized some products that the public is starting to equate any use with product abuse.[48]

Groups like the Center for Consumer Freedom will likely give the food industry a black eye and, contrary to their aim, might actually speed the policy changes they so oppose. This group fights on behalf of both tobacco and food industries, thus linking food to an industry with a terrible reputation. The nation accepts stern legal, regulatory, and legislative action with tobacco. With the Center for Consumer Freedom making the links between tobacco and food so evident, the public might become more open to similar measures with food.

An Industry Potentially Divided?

As we mentioned earlier, the food industry is not a uniform entity that sells nothing but unhealthy products. Segments of the industry sell very healthy foods. Even a given company selling mainly one product, like Kellogg with cereals, will have some products low in calories and high in nutrients and others the opposite. Changing the food environment to encourage healthy eating would be welcome news in some quarters and disaster in others.

Some industry groups have a dilemma, therefore. The GMA, for instance, represents a great many companies, including Coca-Cola, General Mills, Hershey, Kellogg, Mars, Nestle, PepsiCo, and Refined Sugars, Inc. But also on the list are Chiquita, Del Monte, Dole, and Ocean Spray. Such a group can survive only by favoring no food or company and by declaring there are no good or bad foods.

One might imagine controversies within the GMA about changing public policy. If snack foods and soft drinks are removed from schools, brands such as Coca-Cola, Pepsi, Hershey, and Mars might lose and the fruit companies might win. How would such conflict be resolved?

From actions thus far, it would appear that the snack food, soft drink, and fast-food constituents are prevailing. The GMA fiercely opposes favoring any type of food, banning certain foods from schools, taxing foods, and so on, even though some of their constituents would benefit. There are people within each of these industries who are very health-oriented and who would like to see change. We hope with time their voices will be heard.

Suing Big Food

A complex issue facing public health advocates is whether to support lawsuits against the food industry. The attorneys, fresh from making huge amounts on lawsuits against the tobacco companies, are on the attack. In July 2002, New York attorney Samuel Hirsch, representing fifty-six-year-old maintenance worker Caesar Barber and others, sued McDonald's, Wendy's, Kentucky Fried Chicken, and Burger King. In November 2002, Hirsch filed suit against McDonald's on behalf of obese teenagers. The suits claim that the fast-food restaurants contributed to or caused the obesity and subsequent health problems. The question is whether lawsuits against the major food companies are likely to be effective, but even more so, whether they will help or hinder public health efforts.

Prior to Hirsch filing these suits, several attorneys who were quite involved with tobacco litigation made a very public display of the possibility that food companies would be sued. John Banzhaf of George Washington University is the most prominent. By calling press conferences and issuing statements, he became the leading spokesperson for legal action against the food companies.[49]

These lawsuits will be a visible part of the obesity issue for years to come. How successful they will be and their effect on food company practices remains to be seen.

There is debate on the role legal action has played with tobacco. In a thorough analysis of legal action taken against tobacco companies, scientists Peter Jacobson and Kenneth Warner state:

On balance we conclude that litigation is a second-best solution. We see a distinct role for litigation as a complement to a broader, comprehensive approach to tobacco control policy making, rather than as an alternative to the traditional political apparatus of formulating and implementing public health policy. Our analysis suggests that, in general, public health goals are more directly achievable through the political process than through litigation, though situations such as those concerning tobacco control blur the bounds between litigation and the politics of public health. Litigation has stimulated a national debate over the role of smoking in society and may well move the policy agenda. But we conclude that a sustained legislative and regulatory presence ought to be the foundation of meaningful policy changes.[50]

Some legal actions have been successful against food companies, but not yet the large suits seeking to recover damages for the health effects of foods. Rather, the suits have targeted deceptive labeling and marketing practices. McDonald's was sued for having beef products in French fries, after claiming no such products were present. Other suits have been filed for companies using incorrect labels and making inappropriate nutrition claims about foods.

We support such targeted action. Consumers are often misled by the way foods are labeled and packaged and by claims companies make about their foods. The food industry should be held to a very high standard, and if legal action is necessary for this to occur, so be it.

The more thorny issue will be the impact of suits brought by attorneys to collect damages for health problems created by food. This seems a difficult case to make. With tobacco, one product (cigarettes) made by a handful of companies offered up a focused target. There is clear evidence the product is addictive and deadly, and "smoking gun" documents from the industry showed the companies knew the health implications of use of their product.

There are countless foods and thousands of companies selling them. Connecting specific health effects to a given product or company will be difficult. People do not eat just one food or the foods from just one company. The addiction issue with food is just now being studied. We suppose attorneys could calculate how many cheeseburgers, Big Macs, and chicken nuggets McDonald's has sold; estimate the amount of fat and calories ingested by the public as a consequence; and then guess at the effect on some disease such as cancer. However, this would be an extremely imprecise process.

Another key legal attack may be to claim that the food companies sell products that are harmful when "used as intended." Certainly the companies hope to sell as much of their food as possible but intended use is not stated or implied. The fast-food companies know that some customers are "heavy users,"[51] but whether this can be linked to health effects in an individual is not clear.

A key issue for public health is whether such legal forays will be helpful or harmful. There is potential in both directions. On the positive side, putting keen legal minds and their investigative teams to work may uncover evidence of wrongdoing. If companies have manipulated portion sizes knowing that intake of unhealthy food increases, used deceptive advertising, added caffeine to sugared beverages to make them addictive, or engaged in other deceitful acts, the public should know. Companies might be more reluctant to engage in deceptive practices in the future if the threat of discovery is high.

Another potential benefit is that the threat of mass lawsuits, regardless of legal merit, may help change the self-interests of the food industry. Until now, self-interest has argued for selling more food to as many people as possible. The threat of legal action, regulatory actions such as restricting advertising, and the cost of being demonized may encourage the industry to change some of their more troubling practices (such as advertising unhealthy foods to children).[52]

One negative effect of the lawsuits may be a backlash that finds the public sympathizing with the food companies, perhaps compromising other opportunities for change. Some attorneys who sued the tobacco companies made unspeakable amounts of money, precipitating a strong call for system reform. If attorneys suing the food companies are seen in a similar light, more sensible policy approaches might be tarnished by association. We believe that with food, as Jacobson and Warner concluded with tobacco, litigation is a second choice to be used if the political process is ineffective.

The attorneys suing the food industry say that public policy has failed, so we must default to litigation. Quite the contrary: the nation is only just now considering policy changes.

How the Industry Can Prove Its Sincerity

The food industry claims it is interested in public health, especially in children. They now have the opportunity to prove it. With this in mind, one of us (KB) wrote an Op-Ed article for *The Washington Post* with Dr. David Ludwig of Harvard Medical School and Children's Hospital Boston. An excerpt reads:

The time has come for the industry to demonstrate that it will be a trustworthy public health ally by adopting the following policies: (1) suspend all food advertising and marketing campaigns directed at children; (2) remove sugar-sweetened soft drinks and snack foods from vending machines in schools; (3) end sponsorship of scholastic activities and professional nutrition organizations linked to product promotion; and (4) refrain from political contributions that might influence national nutritional policy.[53]

There is even more the industry can do. An invaluable resource the food industry might make available is its marketing expertise. Ronald McDonald is one of the most effective advertising icons of all time. Coca-Cola, Pepsi, and other soft drinks are preeminent worldwide brands. The industry has perfected the use of cartoon characters, movie figures, and sports heroes. Their advertising brings life to animals and mythical figures. A colorful bird sells Froot Loops, a tiger sells Frosted Flakes, a rabbit peddles Trix, a friendly sea captain promotes Cap'n Crunch, and a leprechaun sells Lucky Charms. Creative genius underlies such campaigns, and marketing research is needed to mount campaigns effectively.

This talent, expertise, and experience, if harnessed for campaigns to promote healthy eating and activity, could be used to develop pro-nutrition campaigns.

It is incumbent on the industry to take action if they are to lay claim to public health as a priority. They cannot raise their flag on the high ground by making superficial efforts, boasting of them, and all the while aggressively marketing high-sugar, high-fat, high-calorie products, cultivating children as customers, selling problem foods in schools, and the like.

Back to the Crossroad

We began this chapter saying that the nation's leaders are at a crossroad. Decisions are made every day by elected and appointed leaders, those who convene panels to discuss nutrition policy, school administrators, and others in a position to address the obesity crisis.

The reflex action has been to invite the food industry into the war room. The language used to describe this inviting process is precisely what the food industry calls for—collaboration, inclusion, and involvement. There are advantages to this approach but also grave dangers. The dangers have been ignored, thus no protections are put in place to insure that conflicts of interest do not undermine methods to improve public health.

These conflicts are not hidden or secret. It is well known that the primary nutrition organization, the American Dietetic Association, receives money from the food industry at the same time it issues statements on what the nation should eat. Soft drinks and snack foods are peddled in schools, not through backroom payoffs but through contracts that are discussed in the press. Government and private groups issuing nutrition policy statements are not influenced in covert ways by the food industry—these groups invite the food industry to take part.

These situations scream *conflict of interest*, but the danger is being ignored. If government leaders were planning an antismoking strategy for the nation, would:

- People from Philip Morris and R.J. Reynolds be invited to serve on key panels that issue policy directives?
- The Secretary of Health and Human Services invite tobacco industry lobbying groups to meet with him and then urge them to "go on the offensive" against their critics?

One approach the nation might consider is to call a moratorium on input from the food industry, while offering it the chance to prove a commitment to public health. Taking the opposite turn leads to acceptance and even courting of food industry involvement, exemplified by Tommy Thompson's interactions with the food lobby. Leaders accept that the industry will be a trustworthy ally, that its interests can coexist with public health priorities, and that it will offer up its expertise to help improve diet. Maybe they are wrong.

There are several traps to avoid in dealing with this issue. The first trap is to create an "invite them or fight them" dichotomy. There are drawbacks to both approaches, so it is important to not push the debate in a way that the food industry must be declared either benevolent or evil. The industry does positive things and negative things as well. Recognizing and reinforcing the positive, while challenging and reversing the negative, is a more reasoned approach.

The second trap is for the nation to "back into" a position on food industry involvement based on political expediency and the pleasant-sounding language of coalition and collaboration. Informed, considered action is possible only after a full debate of the issues and clear awareness of the industry's behavior to date.

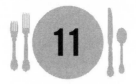

TAKING DECISIVE ACTION

First they ignore you. Then they laugh at you. Then they fight you. Then you win.

—M. K. GANDHI

This quote from Gandhi about social movements conveys the natural progression from the birth of an idea to broad social change. When we first proposed ideas for changing the food and activity environment, we and others were ignored. As we'll show below, laughing occurred next. Now the fight has been joined. The food industry and its lobbying groups, talk-show hosts, and Washington think tanks would not be fighting so hard if there were not credible ideas and movements to fight against.

Food issues may be less profound than Gandhi's struggle on behalf of an entire nation, but the changing diet and activity landscape has a major impact on the health and happiness of many millions of people. Issues of social justice arise because people in the lower social classes are most affected, exploitation of children is occurring, and the problem is extending to all corners of the world.

The environmental forces leading to poor diet and inactivity are overwhelming human biology. The human body has remarkable capacity to adapt to changing conditions, but there reaches a point where its resources are overmatched. Within a reasonable range of temperatures, the body adjusts and survives, but when temperatures are too extreme, the body succumbs.

The food environment has become too extreme for humans to adjust. Poor diet and physical inactivity, and the diseases they cause, are firmly entrenched in the American way of living. Persistent access to foods high in sugar, fat, and calories activates factors locked into the human genetic code, making weight gain in the population quite predictable. Physical activity is declining and cannot compensate.

U.S. and world health authorities have declared obesity an emergency. Words like *epidemic* and *crisis* are used to describe the severity of current conditions. Powerful forces are causing the problem, fueled in part by massive financial interests. Nothing short of bold, innovative action is likely to have an impact. A new committee here, another report there, the food companies making minor changes, and the President exhorting people once a year to exercise and eat better are helpful, but are no match for the toxic environment.

Bold action is possible when the population favors it or, in some cases, forces it, when leaders move slowly because of influence from special interests. America needs a social movement related to diet and activity. Such a movement is beginning. There are clear opportunities now to create the conditions for the movement to prosper.

The Necessary Elements for a Social Movement

Broad social movements take place when certain conditions come together. As discussed in Chapter 10, political scientists Rogan Kersh and James Morone have defined key elements for social health movements to take place.[1] Borrowing from their analysis and adding what we think are crucial elements particular to diet and obesity, we describe here what conditions must exist for the social movement to build.

A Crisis

There is clear awareness of the obesity crisis among health authorities. Report after report shows both awareness and alarm. Elected leaders are beginning to take notice, to the point where obesity legislation has been proposed in the U.S. Senate. A key question, then, is whether the public cares.

The public does appear to care—and in large numbers. More and more people recognize that obesity is a crisis and believe that policy action is indicated. In a population survey, Eric Oliver from Princeton and Taeku Lee from Harvard found that 86 percent of those surveyed believe that obesity is a serious health issue.[2]

The population awareness is influenced heavily by the media, and the media coverage of obesity is exploding. The International Food Information Council, which tracks media studies in major outlets, found that the number of articles on obesity went from less than 100 in the first quarter of 2000 to more than 1,000 from July to September 2002.[3]

Critical Mass of Health and Scientific Evidence

Having a strong body of scientific evidence is necessary to support calls for policy change. This evidence becomes persuasive currency in discussions with the media, the public, and elected leaders. Policy does not always move in directions suggested by science, but in the absence of science, it is difficult to justify calls for change.

Scientific evidence has been discussed throughout this book. When distilled to its basics, there is clear evidence that:

- Obesity is occurring in epidemic proportions.
- Obesity is a growing global crisis.
- Environmental factors are primarily responsible for the rapid increase in prevalence.
- Both poor diet and sedentary lifestyle are key contributors.
- Factors such as large portion sizes, economic incentives to eat more, and lack of access to healthy foods in poor areas are a few of the factors linked to increasing obesity.

The critical mass of science to support policy change is in place.

Victims

The injustice felt when victims suffer is often a key to mobilizing support for change. The entire population is affected by obesity, but when certain vulnerable groups are affected, something rings true in people's hearts.

This condition is certainly met with obesity. There are clear racial and economic disparities. Poor people have poorer diets, have many more challenges in being physically active, and, as a consequence, have high rates of obesity. With few healthy foods available in poor neighborhoods, dangerous streets, and more, poverty and obesity get linked in tragic ways.

The most salient victims are children. When companies with dangerous products (such as tobacco) prey on children or when children have a heavy burden of disease (as with obesity), the suffering touches us all. Even those who feel adults bring on their own problems will soften when thinking of children. Children are vulnerable and are a protected group in our culture. As the public becomes more aware of children as victims, the instinct to protect will be activated.

Emotion and Social Attitude Change

If there is any possibility for major social action and policy change, scientists cannot force it and health leaders cannot mandate it. The public must demand it. Grassroots calls for change can then join with efforts from the health community, elected officials, and business leaders. For such a movement to occur, people must care.

Caring occurs when something strikes an emotional nerve and we feel sad, bothered, outraged, or frustrated. Our heart is moved, and we are driven to act.

Emotions come from human experience, not statistics or numbers on health care costs. They come from seeing people suffer. As our mothers, fathers, grandparents, aunts, uncles, brothers, and sisters suffer strokes, lose limbs to diabetes, die from heart disease, and have painful deaths due to cancer, and we recognize that poor diet and inactivity are major reasons, we are touched as human beings. We want to see the suffering stop.

Few things mobilize us like suffering children. Watching them struggle with weight (and self-esteem), seeing them drawn to unhealthy food like insects to light, seeing how inactive they are, knowing how many years of life they will lose, and fully comprehending how their quality of life will suffer is heartbreaking.

In Chapter 1, we discussed Nicole Talbott, a high school student in California, who said:

Lunch for me is chips, soda, maybe a chocolate ice cream taco. Every day, just about the same thing. That's all I like to eat—the bad stuff.[4]

What lies in her future? Do we not owe her more? How have we allowed an environment to take shape that is so bad for Nicole and others like her? How can we let conditions stay this way?

Children need us; the nation can afford to fail them no longer. They need protection from the giant that looms over them. They need a giant of their own to defend them.

That giant is public opinion. As opinion changes and the food and activity environment is seen for what it is, the ground rules suddenly favor the good giant. A cascade of actions can occur based on public opinion, which is driven quite naturally by our emotions.

Political Leaders Willing to Resist Industry Influence

Political leaders must step forward as examples of courage. They can help sway public opinion, give voice to grassroots emotions, and initiate important policy changes. Here is a cause looking for high-profile leaders to become the banner bearers. It would not surprise us if such a person emerges from those who have been most passionate about advocacy for children.

There are many examples of political leaders yielding to industry pressure. As an example, Coca-Cola offered to build a bottling plant in Louisiana only if legislators agreed to reduce existing soft drink taxes. In 1993, the legislators voted to cut the tax in half by 1995 and repeal the tax entirely if Coca-Cola built a bottling plant worth $50 million or more. In 1997, Coca-Cola signed the contract. In addition to adding several hundred jobs, the plant was expected to generate $3 million each year in new taxes. Louisiana, however, lost $15 million in revenue from lowering soft drink taxes.[5]

As a few elected officials take the lead in protecting the nation from factors producing obesity, others will join the effort, thus providing a compelling social and political force to counteract the powerful presence of the food industry.

A Movement Taking Shape

There are many signs that obesity, poor diet, and physical inactivity have entered the national agenda, with public opinion shifting in ways that make policy change quite likely. Among the signs:

- Multiple reports have sounded the alarm that obesity is a national (and global) crisis. These reports are by respected individuals and groups, including the Centers for Disease Control and Prevention, National Institutes of Health, Surgeon General, Institute of Medicine, and the World Health Organization. These simply cannot be ignored.
- Legislation specifically on obesity has been introduced in the U.S. Senate.
- Public opinion polls are showing high levels of concern about obesity.
- Surprising numbers of people voice support for policies such as changing the food environment in schools.
- Media stories on obesity no longer focus on diets, but have shifted to health aspects of obesity, growing prevalence, the impact on children, the effects of the environment on the problem, and related issues.
- A number of local actions have occurred, including the ban on soft drinks by the Los Angeles Unified School District. These efforts embolden others to take action and show that the food industry is not invincible.

- The food industry is feeling the threat, suggesting the threat is very real. Through their spokespeople and lobbyists, the food companies are attacking their critics, trying to forestall shifting public opinion, and attempting to block proposals for policy change.

The historical parallels with the war on tobacco are fascinating. There was little support for policy changes when the first Surgeon General's Report on Smoking was released in 1964. Things changed as scientific evidence mounted, relentless antitobacco crusaders forged ahead, people saw victims (children and those affected by secondhand smoke), and awareness grew of an industry engaging in deceptive, dishonest practices. The public no longer trusted the tobacco industry, and the door opened for serious changes in policy. Aggressive actions such as banning smoking in public places and having extremely high taxes on cigarettes then became possible. A social movement had taken place.

Similar conditions are taking shape with diet and obesity. By the mid-1980s, the heath consequences of obesity were well established and were so great that pioneers who had sustained the field (Albert Stunkard, George Bray, Theodore VanItallie, George Blackburn, John Garrow, Per Bjorntorp, Jules Hirsch, and a few others) were joined by a new generation of scientists devoting their careers to studying obesity, including people now in key positions such as William Dietz at the Centers for Disease Control and Prevention and Susan Yanovski at the National Institutes of Health. With the integration of top-rate scientists in the nutrition and exercise fields, there is now a very active scientific community focusing on these issues.

During the 1980s, a few lone voices raised questions about the practices of the food industry, and while there were some victories (including food labeling requirements), calls for action at the national level were ignored. The subsequent growth in the number of scientific articles and media stories helped put obesity on the map. Public opinion began to change to the point that policy ideas, even those as radical as taxing food, are being debated in the mainstream (e.g., opinion polls now ask about these policies).

There are visible cases of the public demanding change (Seattle parents objecting to commercialism in schools—Chapter 6), public officials such as school principals kicking out the soft drink companies (North Community High School in Minneapolis ending soft drink contracts—Chapter 7), and editorials galore on how to deal with the obesity crisis. These signal significant changes in attitudes.

The academic world has also taken notice. Beyond those who have been studying obesity for years, new disciplines are turning their attention to this topic. Debates in law now occur on taxing foods, economists such as Tomas Philipson (Chapter 9) and political scientists such as Kersh and Morone (Chapter 10) are bringing new levels of expertise and analysis to the problem. Obesity is a phenomenon.

We stand now at a point in history where science and public opinion are converging and where the world realizes something dramatic must be done. Opinions about using public policy to prevent obesity are changing, and the time to make a difference is near.

The Need to Protect Children

Some of the first and most innovative approaches to obesity probably will take place with children. There are good reasons. Obesity is difficult to treat, so prevention is an obvious priority. The prevalence of obesity in children is growing even faster than that of adults, and it is easy to identify environmental contributors to poor diet and inactivity in children.

Eating and physical activity conditions for America's children are disastrous and growing worse. Children are being raised in a land of giant portions; compelling inducements to eat; schools peppered with soft drinks, snack foods, and other high-calorie items; commercialization running wild; and food companies doing their very best to attract even the youngest children as customers. This environment makes it very difficult to raise healthy children.

There is much to prevent. Obesity in children, not to mention the poor diet and inactivity that cause it, lead to very serious medical problems in both childhood and adult years. The quality of life and psychological matters such as self-esteem can be seriously affected. Improving diet and activity and preventing obesity in children must be made a national priority. An article in *USA Today* conveys how the food industry has locked on to the nation's children:

Ronald McDonald is re-acquainting himself with his most crucial customers, kids. . . . Nearly two years after McDonald's aired ads for its now extinct line of Arch Deluxe burgers that mockingly snubbed kids, the chain has come full circle. A slew of new promotions will be targeted at kids as young as two.

Clearly kids are king again at McDonald's. Over the past year, 89 percent of all kids 8 and under went to McDonald's at least once a month. "My goal for 1999 is to get that to 100," said R. J. Milano, vice president of marketing at McDonald's. "I'm going to own every kid transaction out there."[6]

Which Foods and Activities Should Change?

Supposing that changes in eating and physical activity would benefit the nation, the question turns to what should change. The activity part of the equation is much easier than dealing with food. Increased activity of any kind is likely to be beneficial. Finding the most cost-effective means of accomplishing this is more complicated, but clear progress is being made (see Chapter 4).

Food is fraught with much more controversy. Discussions inevitably lead to prospects of cutting back on things people enjoy, it is hard for nutrition experts to agree on the optimal diet, and the food industry fights aggressively to protect its interests. It is tempting to skirt the food controversy by focusing on physical activity. The food companies then become friendly and offer up money to help. Promoting physical activity is an important goal, but leaving food aside is ignoring the elephant in the center of the room.

Beginning in Chapter 1, we have discussed the difficult issue of declaring which foods in the nation's diet should increase or decrease. This issue arises repeatedly in any discussion of dietary change, from decisions of what should be allowed in school vending machines to how food prices might change to encourage healthy eating. We would like to reinforce several points.

First, the position championed by the food industry and supported by the American Dietetic Association is that there are no good or bad foods. This position has utility in some contexts but is out of step with a public health perspective on obesity. Certainly some foods are better than others when viewed in the context of the nation's diet.

At the risk of repeating what was said in Chapter 1, discussing whether a food such as bacon is good or bad leads nowhere. Most would probably agree that the nation would benefit if total bacon consumption went down and vegetable consumption increased. We could readily imagine the day when, without much objection (except from the affected food companies), policies could be put in place to encourage consumption of vegetables instead of bacon, oranges instead of French fries, and whole grains instead of potato chips.

It is beyond the scope of this book to create a list of foods that should be eaten more or less. It is the *concept* we argue for—that the nation *must* develop fair, sensible, but bold policies that will help people eat better. Groups of experts can create specific lists of foods when the time is right, but only when conflicts of interest can be removed from this process.

In such deliberations, many factors other than sugar, fat, and calories will require consideration. Two examples might be fiber and the calorie density of foods. Research shows that people feel satisfied with less food if the volume is high (even by just adding water) and that higher levels of fiber are associated with better control of body weight.[7] Discussions must begin now on how to classify foods in a rational way.

Balance in Viewing the Food Industry

In any vision of addressing the obesity crisis, the food industry is a central character. Villains to some and heroes to others, the food companies are an amazing story in business history. With some of the most successful advertising icons, slogans, and jingles of all time, the industry has been brilliant at selling its products and in rewarding its shareholders.

The food industry must be scrutinized as a possible contributing party if for no other reason than what people eat is a key determinant of how much they weigh. Opinions vary widely on the degree to which the industry has contributed. Widely varying opinions usually means the truth lies somewhere between extreme positions.

A History of Profound Changes

During the twentieth century, the food industry in America made a fundamental transition. Working to provide enough food to the population at a reasonable price was the early challenge, but then the landscape changed. Advances in agriculture technology produced enough food to feed the population and then to do so at very low cost. This afforded the population an opportunity it had not previously encountered—to eat food merely for pleasure and to consume more than the body needed to survive.

This opportunity was not anticipated by biology, and because the body can adjust to excess calorie intake by adding body fat, the upside potential for increasing food consumption in the population was enormous. Not being malicious but seeking to increase profits, the food industry found that by offering more food for less money and by engineering foods to taste good by changing sugar, fat, and flavors, people bought more and ate more, almost without limit.

Neither the food companies nor health experts would have noticed anything negative as this trend began. Obesity affected few people and the science establishing links between diet and health had not begun. Higher profits and happy consumers made legends of the companies and heroes of the people who ran them (such as Ray Kroc). The rush toward even higher profits, more efficient production, and increased consumption had a looming dark side, but it would take years before the nation noticed.

The nation finally realized there was a problem, but not until the 1990s was there much attention paid to obesity and the effects of poor diet on health and well-being. Not until now has there been the alarm the situation warrants. Waiting so long has left the nation with a massive problem that is supported by many features of day-to-day life in America.

Are They Heroes or Scoundrels?

We see both positive and negative features of the food industry's impact on the health and well-being of the nation. The price of food is very low in the United States, the number of choices tremendous, and food is widely available. These improve the nation's quality of life.

There have also been impressive health benefits attributable to the food industry. The low cost of producing food has made it easier for the country to address problems of hunger. Fortification of certain foods has helped remedy some common nutrition problems. Advances in handling, storage, and transportation make it easier to get foods such as fresh fruits and vegetables to a broader group of consumers. These are a few examples of the good that has come from developments in the food industry.

In this book, we have focused on poor diet and obesity, thus the possible negative impact of the food industry has been a focus. This is a story that must be told. The industry has vast resources to publicize its accomplishments, dwarfing those of the people and groups who feel the industry has done damage with some of its practices.

When the total story is told, the food industry is to be applauded for some activities and criticized for others. Negative practices in the industry do not negate the good it does, nor does the good justify ignoring the negative.

Embracing Positive Efforts

The food industry is developing or sponsoring a number of programs related to diet and activity. For the programs that are well-designed, effective, and free of commercial content, we salute the effort. An example is innovative programming by the International Food Information Council (IFIC), which is funded by the food industry.

IFIC has undertaken a number of worthwhile efforts, including the development of an excellent E-mail server list that informs subscribers about news items on diet, obesity, and physical activity (one can sub-scribe by sending an E-mail request to kelly@ific.org). The IFIC Foun-dation, in concert with a number of other groups, was instrumental in developing the ACTIVATE (Internet-based) program for the preven-tion of obesity in children, along with the website www.kidnetic.com (see Chapter 4). Designed to be engaging and attractive, this program should be helpful in increasing activity in children.

Other examples of progress are in changes in the foods themselves or in marketing healthy food in interesting ways. The McDonald's change in fat used to fry foods (now on hold) and the Frito-Lay health-ier snacks discussed in Chapter 10 are good examples, although we must consider the possibility that people will eat more of these foods and hence increase calorie intake. The fast-food restaurants have introduced healthier options. Grilled chicken sandwiches at all major chains, an array of salads at Wendy's, and yogurt with fruit at McDonald's are all positive changes. Tropicana has introduced a special Healthy Kids Orange Juice that is reformulated for children but is still 100 percent juice.

Less exciting but potentially still valuable are product-oriented pro-grams such as the "Better for You" snack options marketed by PepsiCo and its companies, such as Quaker and Frito-Lay. A nicely designed pro-gram called Sensible Snacking by PepsiCo has educational materials and a CD-ROM featuring Kenneth Cooper. It discusses nutrition, physical activity, and youth obesity and then emphasizes how a variety of Pep-siCo products can be used to improve one's snacking (Quaker Oatmeal and Granola bars, Tropicana juice, Rold Gold pretzels, and Frito-Lay's baked version of potato chips and Doritos).

As we have mentioned before, introducing healthier foods should not buy the food companies public relations immunity for promoting less healthy products and for exploitive practices such as marketing them to children. But their positive accomplishments also should not be overlooked.

Develop a Food Industry Code of Conduct

There will be slow, painful progress on the issue of obesity unless the food industry makes fundamental changes. One constructive step may be internal policing by the industry itself. If the industry can establish guidelines that represent strong, decisive action, and then develop a system whereby guidelines are actually followed, its credibility will increase and the chances of strict government controls on issues like advertising may diminish.

A code of conduct, principles of the trade, guidelines for business practices, or something similar might be developed to frame industry actions. It would be imperative for such an endeavor to tackle difficult issues such as advertising to children, use of children's television and movie characters for promotion, portion size control, product placements, health claims, and more.

The food industry may react to this proposal with utter disbelief, but bear with us for a minute. The tobacco industry once felt invulnerable and believed that with enough political influence, advertising, and public relations, critics would be overwhelmed, disgraced, or at least neutralized. They were wrong.

The food industry now stands at a critical juncture and may wish to benefit from lessons learned by tobacco. If the tobacco industry had instituted a monitoring process years ago in collaboration with health and public policy experts, the severe blows they have suffered might have been anticipated and some constructive, alternative plan developed.

Public opinion of the food industry is becoming more critical. The industry can respond by attacking the messengers, denying responsibility for contributing to the problem, and taking weak and tardy action, or by being vigilant of impending changes and acting in creative ways to change.

One reason a code of conduct might be helpful is that companies moving unilaterally in healthy directions may be at an initial strategic disadvantage. Introducing a few healthy foods is one thing, but a company ceasing advertising to children or selling only smaller portion sizes might suffer. If public opinion changes enough, such a company may achieve a public relations victory by becoming known as a leader, but otherwise the threat of strategic setbacks may deter companies from acting. Collective action would diminish this threat.

We admit some misgivings about proposing this course of action. If the guidelines permit actions not in the interest of public health or if by establishing guidelines the industry forestalls necessary action from the outside (e.g., federal guidelines for advertising to children), the effect may be counterproductive.

One possible safeguard would be to have the industry develop guidelines with meaningful input from a broad spectrum of people (including industry critics, parents, educators, etc.). This would decrease chances that guidelines would be weak, self-serving, and not credible. Outside boards, with objective individuals, could monitor progress, issue reports cards, and so on.

Broad Actions for the Nation

Earlier chapters in this book contain many specific suggestions for changes that might be made to improve the food and physical activity environment of the nation. Several broad actions may be important as well.

Coordination of Nutrition and Physical Activity Programs

A number of government agencies are involved with programs on nutrition and physical activity, but no agency, person, or group minds the entire store. The National Institutes of Health funds some research on nutrition, but so does the U.S. Department of Agriculture (USDA), the Centers for Disease Control and Prevention (CDC), the Department of Defense, and more. There does not exist a national nutrition strategic plan that organizes and directs these efforts.

As an example, we attempted to find a report, document, or book that would describe all subsidies relevant to food and agriculture. We wished to know, for example, how pork, beef, or poultry farmers/businesses were supported compared to support given to fruit and vegetable segments of the industry.

After much searching and many phone calls to people at the USDA and elsewhere, we made several discoveries. First, subsidies come in many forms. Price supports, purchase of surpluses, use of commodities in school lunch programs, and the subsidy of water for irrigation are but a few of the ways government intervenes with agriculture. Second, it appears these efforts are scattered and not done according to a strategic plan. To the extent there is an implicit plan, the goal is not to foster good nutrition but to help farmers and businesses. Third, we could not find a single document or person where we would find an all-encompassing view of the subsidy issue.

This subsidy story symbolizes what is true overall. The absence of a national plan leads to agencies and programs with conflicting aims. As one example, efforts to improve academic performance by the Department of Education may be undermined by USDA policies that permit unhealthy foods in schools.

The Homeland Security Department was created to coordinate the multiple agencies dealing with security issues and to prevent duplication of effort, lack of cooperation, communication problems, and inefficiency. Nutrition issues are on the agenda not only for the USDA, but various agencies of the Department of Health and Human Services (Centers for Disease Control and Prevention, National Institutes of Health, Office of the Surgeon General), the Federal Trade Commission, Food and Drug Administration, Federal Communications Commission, and even the Department of Education to begin the list.

Without broad oversight, there is contradiction and lack of decisive action. The amount of funding for obesity treatment versus prevention, for instance, has not been the product of deliberative action. Subsidies paid to the agriculture industry are not considered in the context of public health. Food advertising aimed at children is essentially unregulated, again without regard to the overall nutrition picture. And if anyone is alert to all the pieces, it is the food industry.

This said, there is a risk that centralizing nutrition programs will increase opportunities for commercial interests to exploit the system, as there would be fewer people to target with lobbying and fewer elected leaders to court. Central nutrition oversight should be done with the aim of maximizing impact on public health, and buffers must be created between the decision-making process and the food and agriculture industries.

Encourage Practices Known to Affect Obesity

With all that is known about obesity, there is relatively little agreement yet on specific actions to be taken for its prevention. There are, however, several actions around which consensus is building. It may be worthwhile addressing these immediately.[8]

Encourage Breast-Feeding. Studies from around the world have shown lower rates of obesity in breast-fed than in formula-fed children.[9] Different reasons have been proposed. One is that the child, rather than the feeder, dictates how much is consumed during breast-feeding, perhaps leading to food intake dictated by hunger rather than external cues. In addition, breast-fed children also seem willing to try a greater variety of foods, perhaps because breast milk is more variable in taste than is formula. This may be helpful in establishing preferences for foods such as vegetables. It also appears that women who breast-feed are more likely to lose the weight gained during their pregnancy.[10]

Reduce Television Viewing and Other Sedentary Activities. We noted in Chapters 2 and 5 how television viewing is associated with increased obesity, less physical activity, and poorer measures of health. Promoting less time with the television has been proposed as one means for addressing the obesity crisis, especially in children.[11] Ridding bedrooms of televisions, not watching television at meal times, and reducing time spent with video games and the computer may also be logical goals to pursue.

Promote Physical Activity. As we discussed in detail in Chapter 4, there is consensus that declining activity is contributing to obesity and that increasing activity in the population is an important goal. There is little opposition to this goal, so the task is to find ways to accomplish the goal and to create a funding base to make and then sustain broad changes. There is good evidence that increasing activity will help with weight control and improve health in other ways, so promoting activity should be an enterprise undertaken immediately.

Reverse the Distorted Economics of Food

This issue has been discussed many times throughout this book, particularly in Chapter 9, but is so fundamental to promoting change at the national level that we mention it once more. Economics have a powerful impact on behavior, and current economic conditions are structured in ways that promote obesity and unhealthy eating. It will be difficult to make significant progress on the national diet and obesity crisis without addressing economic factors.

Curbing Food Commercialism in Public and Community Institutions

A number of cities have agreed to purchase police cars with ads painted on them, perhaps with logos of companies such as McDonald's.[12] The exposure of these ads, not to mention credibility, would be significant. This is just the latest example of commercialism gone awry. Sports stadiums, football bowl games, and countless other enterprises have commercial sponsors. How often do we hear that some product is the "official sponsor" of some event? Unless the sponsors are wasting money, we can assume these have an impact on consumer behavior.

In August 2001, the most visited museum in the world, the National Air and Space Museum of the Smithsonian Institution, began a ten-year, $16 million contract with McDonald's. The museum agreed to feature McDonald's foods in the cafeteria, creating what may be the busiest McDonald's in the United States, but also foods from two companies owned by McDonald's, Donatos Pizzeria and Boston Market.[13] McDonald's made a $5 million gift to the museum.

Another surprising location for unhealthy food is hospitals. In a survey of sixteen hospitals listed in *U.S. News and World Report*'s "Honor Roll," 38 percent had regional or national fast-food franchises, four were contracting with two franchises at the same time, and one had closed a fast-food franchise but opened a hospital restaurant with similar foods.[14]

Said to be one of the city's busiest, there is a McDonald's in the Children's Hospital of Philadelphia. On its window during a visit one of us (KB) made there to lecture in 2001 was a large picture of the "New

Cheddar Bacon Sausage McMuffin." Between two halves of an English muffin, starting from the bottom, were cheese, sausage, egg, cheese, and bacon. It is hard to imagine a better way to deliver fat and calories.

The commercialism, particularly with food, seems to have no bounds. Will we someday encounter "Philadelphia, an Official McDonald's City," "Welcome to Wichita: Pepsi Proud," "CBS Snickers Nightly News," "The Kit-Kat Statue of Liberty," or the "Fritos Electoral College"? Forgive the sarcasm, but there appear to be no boundaries, and at some point the nation must say enough is enough.

Expect More of Celebrities

There is a long, star-studded list of popular people endorsing food products. There are the obvious ones, including Michael Jordan, Shaquille O'Neal, Kobe Bryant, and Britney Spears, but endorsements of other kinds are becoming more common. In 2001, for instance, Coca-Cola paid Warner Brothers $150 million for the global marketing rights for the first Harry Potter movie. Pleas to J. K. Rowling, the author of the Harry Potter books, to stop the use of her characters to promote soft drinks to children were unsuccessful.

It is time to expect more of celebrities. These individuals would never lend their names, faces, and impact to selling cigarettes. This would be a public relations disaster, not to mention they might have reservations about helping sell such products. This is precisely what should happen with endorsements of unhealthy foods. Highly visible people, perhaps through pro bono work, could have a very positive impact by helping promote healthy foods and physical activity.

Mobilize Parents to Demand More for Their Children

Raising a child to eat a healthy diet and be physically active has become a terribly difficult task. Parents and children deserve more help from the nation. Parents fighting for their children can be a powerful, compelling voice for making both local and national changes. If parents can be organized and mobilized to lobby on behalf of their children, they will be heard.

A first step may be to show parents the full extent of how the food companies entice children, not only through advertising, product placements on TV and in movies, and celebrity endorsements, but through connections with schools. Made alert to subtle ties between food companies and their schools, parents may demand change. For instance, Betty Crocker, owned by General Mills, is a "proud sponsor of the National PTA."[15] The Betty Crocker website claims the National PTA as a "partner" and links to the National PTA website for "helpful parenting resources." We assume the PTA has been paid or receives resources of some kind to allow its name to be used in this way.

Parents can protest with school officials and school boards, organize boycotts of companies they feel are exploitative, or demand other actions that will be in the best interests of their children.

Resist Feeling the Task Is Too Daunting

Feeling defeated before you start is a sure way to fail. Changing the environment is a daunting task, to be sure, but progress is clearly possible.

During the past forty years, antismoking advocates pressed ahead when faced with daunting challenges. Smoking was as much a part of America as unhealthy food is now. Massively powerful companies fought progress in a relentless, sometimes vicious manner. Because of bold action by the early pioneers, a significant public health victory became possible.

As individuals and as a nation, we must not be seduced by pessimism. It can happen easily. We cannot undo all advances in technology or give up agricultural advances that feed the world. But we can produce small victories that then multiply and quite possibly produce some major victories with time.

We have no doubt the environment can change. It *is* changing, in fact, just more slowly than needed to address an epidemic. Finally, the crisis has been recognized, and there is now the opportunity, awareness, and growing public will to act.

Change will occur. If the nation stands idle and permits the food environment to grow continually worse, watching from a distance as physical activity becomes less and less likely, we will get what we deserve—a worsening epidemic, a massive burden of disease, and shameful conditions for children. Being courageous and innovative, standing tall in the face of pressure from the food industry, and taking decisive action is what the nation needs, what our children deserve, and what appears to be in our future.

Gandhi's Prediction

We end this book by returning to the quote from Gandhi: "First they ignore you. Then they laugh at you. Then they fight you. Then you win." Gandhi was referring to social movements related to political freedom, and "they" were powerful government forces seeking to maintain a status quo that suppressed individual liberties and blocked democratic rule.

These stages appear to fit the movement that has been occurring on diet and obesity. Early writings, dating back a decade and more, were ignored. Then the laughing began. For instance, in response to our question about how different Ronald McDonald was from Joe Camel, the *Boston Globe* said in a 1998 editorial:

Brownell . . . isn't satisfied with trying to persuade you to eat less junk food. He wants Big Brother to make you eat less junk food. Ben and Jerry will be transformed from kindly Vermont hippies to foul peddlers of heart disease.[16]

The fighting came next, was focused mainly on the idea of a "fat tax," and continues today. The fighting came from different sources, including the press.

First, public health groups will determine that hamburgers cause cancer and heart disease. The trial lawyers will begin class actions on behalf of adults who blame their illness on . . . special sauce.

—*WALL STREET JOURNAL* EDITORIAL[17]

And from the shadow groups funded by industry money:

If enough smokers get behind the fat tax idea to encourage government nannies and the other "good for you" social engineers to energize themselves, maybe, just maybe, other mainstream Americans will wake up to the fact that the slippery slope is real and not just an argument.

—NATIONAL SMOKERS ALLIANCE[18]

The vigilantes and the nannies are ganging up on the quintessential American meal—a cheeseburger, side of fries, and a large soda. Vegetarian activists want to tax meat to reduce consumption. A Yale University professor is generating support for a "twinkie tax" on high-calorie foods like French fries. . . .

—CENTER FOR CONSUMER FREEDOM[19]

There has also been concerted fighting from the food industry groups such as the Snack Food Association, National Soft Drink Association, Sugar Association, and Grocery Manufacturers of America. The fighting is organized and strong, and comes from the food industry, its lobbying groups, trade associations, some people in the press, and media figures such as Rush Limbaugh. What is striking, however, is the perception in these circles that danger lies ahead and the fact that the ideas we have proposed are now part of public discourse.

The media has softened to public policy proposals related to obesity. There were early signs in the late 1990s. One example was the last issue of *U.S. News and World Report* in 1997. The cover story was entitled "16 Silver Bullets: Smart Ideas to Fix the World." One of the sixteen ideas was our concept of taxing foods as part of a broad strategy to improve the nation's diet:

This would be unabashed social engineering, but so is virtually everything the government does about public health dangers, such as air pollution or drunk driving, that pose smaller threats to most people's life expectancy.

—U.S. NEWS AND WORLD REPORT, 1997[20]

Other examples:

Is it really such a crazy idea? It's too bad Brownell isn't more popular.
—THE NEW REPUBLIC, 1998[21]

A Weighty Case Against Big Macs
—ELLEN GOODMAN, BOSTON GLOBE, 2002[22]

From the medical literature:

More radical solutions should be considered: taxing soft drinks and fast foods; subsidizing nutritious foods, like fruits and vegetables; labeling of the contents of fast food; and prohibiting marketing and advertising to children.
—THE LANCET, 2002[23]

And from anonymous messages received from the public:

I couldn't agree with you more regarding the typical American diet. It is a sad state of affairs when it is cheaper to buy a box of Little Debbie cupcakes than a bag of apples.

By taking the actions you suggest, we would be helping people to give up unhealthful eating habits, in much the same way that laws against cigarette advertising and smoking have created a shift in attitudes toward smoking.

And from health professionals:

Coming from New Zealand it was even more profound for me to observe first hand the "toxic environment" of the U.S., particularly since New Zealand is obviously following the lead of the U.S.—they call it progress.
—NUTRITION PROFESSOR FROM NEW ZEALAND

Believe us, there is opposition as well. We have described this in many places throughout the book. Only a few years ago, the opposition overwhelmed the support and it was easy to be discouraged, but the balance is becoming more even. The quote that follows is beginning to typify what experts are saying, and what experts say can influence public opinion:

The prevalence of obesity is increasing globally, with nearly half a billion of the world's population now considered to be overweight or obese. The obesity epidemic is related both to dietary factors and to an increasingly sedentary lifestyle. . . . Of particular concern is the fact that obesity is increasing among children and adolescents. National health policy makers must take action to deal with the obesity problem. Prevention should be the primary target.

—STEPHAN ROSSNER, OBESITY EXPERT FROM SWEDEN [24]

A very tangible sign of change is that for the first time in U.S. history, Congress in 2002 began consideration of comprehensive legislation dealing specifically with obesity. Sponsored by Senators Bill Frist from Tennessee, Jeff Bingaman from New Mexico, and Christopher Dodd from Connecticut, this legislation is impressive more for its existence than substance but does represent an encouraging first step. One of us (KB) was invited for Senate testimony for initial hearings on the bill. Knowing that this testimony would include recommendations of the sort suggested in this book, Senate leaders specifically invited this input.

There has been a change in public attitude in the past several years, joined by attitude changes in the media, the scientific community, and government leaders. From not caring about obesity and blaming the problem on those who had it, there is now recognition that prevalence is alarming, that a health crisis looms, and that the food and activity environment must change.

Change will continue to occur. We expect that:

- The prevalence of obesity will continue to rise, intensifying national and global alarm.
- The toxic food and activity environment will be listed more frequently as the top cause.
- Government leaders will be forced to act.
- Acceptance of public policy measures as a means of preventing obesity will continue to grow.

Now that we have progressed through the ignoring, laughing, and fighting stages, it is our passionate hope that Gandhi's prediction that "then you win" will come true. The nation and her people are who must win. Future generations of children must win by being raised in a different food and activity environment. Helping children avoid poor diet and sedentary living, along with the obesity, diabetes, heart disease, and cancer that follow, would be a wonderful gift we could bestow on those who follow us.

Reaching this goal of "winning" will require even more passionate and committed people to promote change at local and national levels, a few courageous and visible leaders to propose bold action, and the country to follow through, even if it means tangling with formidable forces. We see these changes occurring now, as part of the growing social movement we mentioned earlier. It is our ambition to help stimulate this movement and to provide a blueprint of actions that might be taken now and in the future.

There is broad willingness to hear new ideas for dealing with the world's obesity crisis, if not yet to embrace them. Hearing the ideas is a good first step. Embracing them may not be far behind.

Perhaps then, the nation can win.

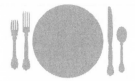

SUMMARY OF
RECOMMENDED ACTIONS

This book offers many proposals for addressing the diet and inactivity that contribute so much to disease and disability and undermine the nation's effort to be healthy, happy, and productive. This is our summary of the action points of this book.

Chapters 1 and 2 (Thinking Differently)

- Appreciate that a changing environment has caused the world's obesity epidemic and that the environment is the logical place to intervene.
- Recognize that personal resources (responsibility) can be overwhelmed when the environment is toxic, that our culture already places heavy emphasis on personal responsibility, and that further emphasis is likely to have limited impact on the obesity epidemic.
- Move beyond the old "no good foods or bad foods" stance to a public health perspective in which we identify types of foods the nation should consume less or consume more.
- Recognize that treating obesity is very difficult and can be costly; thus, prevention must be a national priority.

- Appreciate that investing in children is likely to produce the first victories in the fight against poor diet and inactivity.
- Pledge to the nation's children that we will provide them a healthy environment.
- Resist the temptation to blame parents and instead offer them a healthy environment in which to raise their children.

Chapter 3 (Global Priorities)

- Recognize that overnutrition now rivals hunger as the world's leading nutrition issue.
- Learn from successes in countries such as Finland and Mauritius about large-scale efforts to change diet and activity.
- Support research to better understand the nutrition and activity transitions that are occurring around the world.
- Work with international and national health and government officials to develop creative programs for preventing obesity.
- Establish a culture around the world where promoting unhealthy food is unacceptable.

Chapter 4 (Physical Activity)

- Develop a national strategic plan to increase physical activity.
- Earmark transportation funding to increase activity (bike paths and walking paths, buses with bike racks, traffic calming, etc.).
- Design activity-friendly communities.
- Build exercise facilities knowing they will be used.
- Promote walking and biking to school and enhance physical education.
- Offer incentives for physical activity and strive to decrease sedentary behavior.
- Promote activity through work sites and physician practices.

Chapter 5 (Commercialization of Childhood)

- Object to thinking of children as market objects.
- Protest to companies such as Disney and Nickelodeon for offering up their characters to sell unhealthy foods.

- Encourage celebrities not to promote unhealthy food and to help promote healthy eating and physical activity.
- Encourage television and movie executives to stop using food product placements in programming aimed at children.
- Encourage legislators to prohibit marketing of products to children.
- Level the playing field so healthy foods are promoted at least as much as unhealthy foods.
- As occurred with the Fairness Doctrine and tobacco, mandate equal time for pro-nutrition and activity messages to counter those for unhealthy foods.
- Create a "superfund" to promote healthy eating, perhaps from assessments placed on food advertisements or small taxes on the sale of unhealthy foods.
- Enforce the Children's Television Act.
- Promote media literacy among children (advertising inoculation).

Chapters 6 and 7 (Food and Soft Drinks in Schools)

- Show how healthy eating and activity are connected with academic performance.
- Permit commercial television (such as Channel One) in the schools only if it is free of advertising for unhealthy foods.
- Rid children's books and educational materials of references to unhealthy foods and cease connection with brand-name food products.
- If food is to be used as academic incentive, use healthy foods.
- Have nonfood or healthy food fund-raisers.
- Do not allow food company logos or advertisements on school property, including buses.
- Improve school lunch programs and use the cafeteria as a learning laboratory.
- Find alternatives to snack foods, soft drinks, and fast foods in schools with the goal of eliminating unhealthy foods entirely.
- Support programs that teach children about nutrition and activity.

- Make schools commercial-free zones and use zoning laws to prohibit establishments with unhealthy foods from operating near schools.
- Have only healthy foods and beverages in vending machines. If this is not possible, use the pricing of selections to encourage purchase of healthy items.
- Require schools to be open and clear about industry contracts and connections.
- Challenge industry claims that they are helping education.

Chapter 8 (Portions)

- Help make the public, health professionals, and government leaders aware that larger portion sizes lead to greater eating and that people do not appear to compensate for the additional calories at later meals.
- Educate people, beginning with children, on appropriate serving sizes.
- Encourage food companies to show reasonable portions in advertisements and to avoid suggestions about eating large amounts.
- Require food labeling at restaurants.
- Require food packaging to have the number of USDA servings in a container accompany weight or volume figures on the front of containers.

Chapter 9 (Economic Issues)

- Help make the public aware of the powerful economic forces that contribute to obesity, noting how the fundamental imbalance of incentives to eat unhealthy vs. healthy foods (low cost, convenience, accessibility, and taste for unhealthy choices) by itself would predict an epidemic of obesity.
- Increase awareness of social inequities (e.g., conditions that predispose the poor to obesity) and increase access to healthy foods and opportunities to be active for those living in poverty.

- Engage federal food programs as allies in the fight against obesity. These are the National School Lunch Program, Food Stamp Program, Head Start, and WIC.
- Consider changing the price structure of food, first by lowering the cost of healthy foods and perhaps by increasing the cost of unhealthy foods.
- Think of food taxes not as a means of punishing people for "bad" choices but rather for raising revenue for programs aimed at improving the nation's diet.
- Sensitize consumers to financial inducements to buy large amounts of unhealthy foods.

Chapters 10 and 11 (Interacting with the Food Industry and Conclusions)

- Celebrate positive changes the industry makes in its products and the support it provides for programs aimed at improving diet and activity.
- Make transparent the impact of the industry on national nutrition policy.
- Increase awareness of industry tactics in dealing with being challenged; reinforce the reasonable tactics and fight against those that will impede progress.
- Challenge the industry for connections with tobacco and for funding provided to shadow groups like the Center for Consumer Freedom that fight efforts to curtail smoking or to change practices of the food industry.
- Encourage political leaders to be bold and innovative in addressing the obesity crisis and to remove political barriers to taking action.
- Curb food commercialism in public and community institutions (museums, hospitals, ads on police cars, etc.).
- Promote activities known to help with body weight (breast-feeding, decreased television watching).
- Mobilize parents to demand a healthy environment for their children.

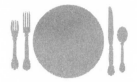

NOTES

Chapter 1

1. Centers for Disease Control and Prevention. Obesity and overweight: A public health epidemic. CDC website. Available at www.cdc.gov/nccdphp/dnpa/obesity/epidemic.htm. Accessed Jul. 21, 2002.

2. World Health Organization. *Obesity: Preventing and Managing the Global Epidemic.* Geneva, Switzerland: World Health Organization, 1998.

3. Sturm R. The effects of obesity, smoking, and problem drinking on chronic medical problems and health care costs. *Health Affairs,* 2002;21:245–253; Sturm R, Wells KB. Does obesity contribute as much to morbidity as poverty or smoking? *Public Health,* 2001;115:229–295.

4. Ebbeling CB, Pawlak DB, Ludwig DS. Childhood obesity: public health crisis, commonsense cure. *Lancet,* 2002;360:473–482.

5. Krebs-Smith SM. Progress in improving diet to reduce cancer risk. *Cancer,* 1998;83:1425–1432.

6. Booth FW, Chakravathy MV, Gordon SE, Spangenburg EE. Waging war on physical inactivity: using modern molecular ammunition against an ancient enemy. *Journal of Applied Physiology,* 2002;93:3–30.

7. Booth SL, Sallis JF, Ritenbaugh C, Hill JO, Birch LL, Frank LD, Glanz K, Himmelgreen DA, Mudd M, Popkin BM, Rickard KA, St Jeor S, Hays NP. Environmental and societal factors affect food choice and physical activity: rationale, influences, and leverage points. *Nutrition Reviews,* 2001;59:S21–39.

8. Nestle M. *Food Politics: How the Food Industry Influences Nutrition and Health.* Berkeley, CA: University of California Press, 2002.

9. *Advertising Age.* Leading national advertisers. Jun. 28, 2002. Available at www.adage.com/news.cms?newsId =35204. Accessed Nov. 24, 2002.

10. Siener K, Rothman D, Farrar J. Soft drink logos on baby bottles: do they influence what is fed to children? *Journal of Dentistry for Children,*1997;64:55–60.

11. Brownell KD. Get slim with higher taxes (Editorial). *New York Times,* December 1994, A29.

12. Schlosser E. *Fast Food Nation: The Dark Side of the All American Meal.* Boston: Houghton Mifflin, 2001.

13. McDonald's corporate website. Available at www.mcdonalds.com/corporate/press/corporate/index.html. Accessed April 1, 2003. Text from McDonald's press release, December 9, 1996. Available at www.mcspot light.org/media/press/prnews_9dec96.html. Accessed Sep. 2, 2002.

14. Egan T. In bid to improve nutrition, schools expel soda and chips. *New York Times,* May 20, 2002, A1.

15. Ebbeling CB, Pawlak DB, Ludwig DS. Childhood obesity: public health crisis, commonsense cure. *Lancet,* 2002;360:473–482.

16. Pollan M. *The Botany of Desire.* New York: Random House, 2001; Lappe FM, Lappe A. *Hope's Edge: The Next Diet for a Small Planet.* New York: Tarcher/Putnam, 2002; Scott JC. *Seeing Like a State: How Certain Schemes to Improve the Human Condition Have Failed.* New Haven: Yale University Press, 1998; Nestle M. *Food Politics: How the Food Industry Influences Nutrition and Health.* Berkeley, CA: University of California Press,

2002; Sims LS. *The Politics of Fat: Food and Nutrition Policy in America.* Armonk, New York: M.E. Sharpe, 1988; Fowler C, Mooney P. *Shattering: Food, Politics, and the Loss of Genetic Diversity.* Tucson: University of Arizona Press, 1996.

17. Tillotson JE. Food brands: Friend or foe? *Nutrition Today*, 2002;37:78–80.

18. Wadden TA, Brownell KD, Foster GD. Obesity: confronting a global epidemic. *Journal of Consulting and Clinical Psychology*, 2002;70:510–525.

19. McDonald's press release, Dec. 9, 1996. Available at www.mcspotlight.org/media/press/prnews_9dec96 .html. Accessed Sep. 2, 2002.

20. McDonald's corporate website. Available at www.mcdonalds.com/corporate/info/history/history2/ index.html. Accessed Sep. 2, 2002.

21. Heckman JJ. The importance of starting early. Presentation to the National Head Start Conference, Washington, DC, Jun. 26, 2002.

22. Heckman J, Lochner L, Smith J, Taber C. The effects of government policy on human capital investment and wage inequality. *Chicago Policy Review*, 1997;1:1–40.

23. Karoly LA, Greenwood PW, Everingham SS, Hoube J, Kilburn MR, Rydell CP, Sanders M, Chiesa J. *Investing in Our Children: What We Know and Don't Know About the Costs and Benefits of Early Childhood Interventions.* Washington, DC: Rand Corporation, 1998.

24. Department of Health and Human Services. *The Surgeon General's Call to Action Prevent and Decrease Overweight and Obesity.* Washington, DC: U.S. Government Printing Office, 2001.

25. Institute of Medicine. *Weighing the Options: Criteria for Evaluating Weight Management Programs.* Washington, DC: National Academy Press, 1995.

26. Puhl R, Brownell KD. Bias, discrimination, and obesity. *Obesity Research*, 2001;9:788–805.

27. For more information on weight bias, stigma, and discrimination, see the website of The Rudd Institute (www.RuddInstitute.org).

28. Nestle M. *Food Politics: How the Food Industry Influences Nutrition and Health.* Berkeley, CA: University of California Press, 2002; Sims LS. *The Politics of Fat: Food and Nutrition Policy in America.* Armonk, New York: M.E. Sharpe, 1988.

29. Grocery Manufacturers of American (GMA). Top administration officials brief GMA board. GMA website. Available at www.gmabrands.com/news/docs/NewsRelease.cfm?DocID=1028&. Accessed Nov. 17, 2002.

30. Freeland-Graves J, Nitzke S. Position of the American Dietetic Association: total diet approach to communicating food and nutrition information. *Journal of the American Dietetic Association*, 2002;102:100–108.

31. Brownell KD. *The LEARN Program for Weight Management 2000.* Dallas: American Health Publishing Co., 2000.

32. National Soft Drink Association website. Available at www.nsda.org/softdrinks/CSDHealth/Index.html. Accessed Nov. 18, 2002.

33. Grocery Manufacturers of America website. Available at www.gmabrands.com/nutrition/solutions.htm. Accessed Nov. 18, 2002.

34. National Confectioners Association website. Available at www.candyusa.org/Publications/chbrochure.pdf. Accessed Nov. 18, 2002.

35. National Confectioners Association website. Available at www.candyusa.org/Press/Health/overweight .shtml. Accessed Nov. 18, 2002.

Chapter 2

1. Quoted in Amos J. Obesity is changing human shape. *BBC News, World Edition*, Sep. 9, 2002.

2. Squires S. Into our stomachs and out of our minds. *The Washington Post*, Jul. 28, 2002, p. B03.

3. World Health Organization. *Obesity: Preventing and Managing the Global Epidemic.* Geneva, Switzerland: World Health Organization, 1998; James WPT. A world view of the obesity problem. In CG Fairburn & KD Brownell (Eds) *Eating Disorders and Obesity: A Comprehensive Handbook.* New York: Guilford Publications, 2002, pp. 411–416; Popkin BM. The nutrition transition and obesity in the developing world. *Journal of Nutrition*, 2001;131:871S–873S; Brownell KD. The environment and obesity. In CG Fairburn & KD Brownell (Eds) *Eating Disorders and Obesity: A Comprehensive Handbook* (2nd Ed). New York: Guilford Press, pp. 433–438.

4. There is an excellent special issue of the journal *Public Health Nutrition* (2002, Vol. 5, issue 1A) on nutrition transitions around the world. The contents can be accessed through the website of Dr. Barry Popkin at the University of North Carolina (www.nutrans.org). Click on Bellagio Conference papers.

5. Bhatnagar D, Anand IS, Durrington PN, Patel DJ, Wander GS, Mackness MI, Creed F, Tomenson B, Chandrashekhar Y, Winterbotham M. Coronary risk factors in people from the Indian subcontinent living in West London and their siblings in India. *Lancet*, 1995;345:405–409.

6. Ravussin E, Valencia ME, Esparza J, Bennett PH, Schulz LO. Effects of a traditional lifestyle on obesity in Pima Indians. *Diabetes Care*, 1994;17:1067–1074; Lindsay RS, Cook V, Hanson RL, Salbe AD, Tataranni A, Knowler WC. Early excess weight gain of children in the Pima Indian population. *Pediatrics*, 2002;109:E33.

7. Doblhammer G, Vaupel JW. Lifespan depends on month of birth. *Proceedings of the National Academy of Sciences*, 2001;98:2934–2939.

8. Stunkard AJ, Sorensen TI, Hanis C, Teasdale TW, Chakraborty R, Schull WJ, Schulsinger F. An adoption study of human obesity. *New England Journal of Medicine*, 1986;314:193–198; Stunkard AJ, Harris JR, Pedersen NL, McClearn GE. The body-mass index of twins who have been reared apart. *New England Journal of Medicine*, 1990;322:1483–1487.

9. Barsh GS, Farooqi IS, O'Rahilly S. Genetics of body weight regulation. *Nature*, 2000;404:644–651; Bouchard C. Genetic influences on body weight. In CG Fairburn & KD Brownell (Eds) *Eating Disorders and Obesity: A Comprehensive Handbook* (2nd Ed). New York: Guilford Press, pp. 16–21; Leibel RL. Genetic influences on body weight. In CG Fairburn & KD Brownell (Eds) *Eating Disorders and Obesity: A Comprehensive Handbook* (2nd Ed). New York: Guilford Press, pp. 26–31.

10. Levin BE. The obesity epidemic: metabolic imprinting on genetically susceptible neural circuits. *Obesity Research*, 2000;8:342–347.

11. Bray GA. *Contemporary Diagnosis and Management of Obesity*. Newtown, PA: Handbooks in Health Care, 1998.

12. Quote from Pinel JPJ, Assanand S, Lehman DR. Hunger, eating, and health. *American Psychologist*, 2000;55:1105–1116, p. 1105; Peters JC, Wyatt HR, Donahoo WT, Hill JO. From instinct to intellect: the challenge of maintaining healthy weight in the modern world. *Obesity Reviews*, 2002;3:69–74, p. 69.

13. Tordoff MG. Obesity by choice: the powerful influence of nutrient availability on nutrient intake. *American Journal of Physiology: Regulatory, Integrative and Comparative Physiology*, 2001;282:R1536–1539.

14. Ramirez I, Tordoff MG, Friedman MI. Dietary obesity and hyperphagia; what causes them? *Physiology and Behavior*, 1989;45:163–168.

15. Sclafani A. Personal communication via electronic mail to authors (KDB), Aug. 6, 2002.

16. Rolls BJ. Sensory-specific satiety. *Nutrition Reviews*, 1986;44:93–101.

17. Rolls BJ. The role of energy density in the overconsumption of fat. *Journal of Nutrition*, 2000;130 (2S Suppl):268S–271S; Rolls BJ. *The Volumetrics Weight Control Plan: Feel Full on Fewer Calories*. New York: HarperCollins, 2000.

18. Hill JO, Peters JC. Environmental contributions to the obesity epidemic. *Science*, 1998;280:1371–1374.

19. Institute of Medicine. *Weighing the Options: Criteria for Evaluating Weight Management Programs*. Washington, DC: National Academy Press, 1995.

20. Hietmann BL, Lissner L, Osler M. Do we eat less fat, or just report so? *International Journal of Obesity*, 2000:24:435–442.

21. Nestle M. *Food Politics: How the Food Industry Influences Nutrition and Health*. Berkeley, CA: University of California Press, 2002.

22. Ibid.

23. Frito-Lay (PepsiCo) website. Available at www.pepsico.com/press/20020118f.shtml. Accessed Aug. 21, 2002.

24. Jacobson MF. Liquid candy: how soft drinks are harming Americans' health. Report from Center for Science in the Public Interest, 1998. Available at www.cspinet.org/sodapop/liquid_candy.htm. Accessed Aug. 30, 2002; Ludwig DS. The glycemic index: physiological mechanisms related to obesity, diabetes, and cardiovascular disease. *JAMA*, 2002;287:2414–2423; Fulmer M. Food firms hope you can never have enough of a sweeter thing. *Los Angeles Times*, Apr. 28, 2002.

25. Howard BV, Wylie-Rosett J. Sugar and cardiovascular disease. A statement for healthcare professionals from the Committee on Nutrition of the Council on Nutrition, Physical Activity, and Metabolism of the American Heart Association. *Circulation*, 2002;106:523–527.

26. Guthrie JF, Morton JF. Food sources of added sweeteners in the diets of Americans. *Journal of the American Dietetic Association*, 2000;100:43–51.

27. Institute of Medicine Food and Nutrition Board, National Academy of Sciences. *Dietary Reference Intakes for Energy, Carbohydrates, Fiber, Fat, Protein and Amino Acids (Macronutrients)*. Washington, DC: National Academy Press, 2002.

28. Fulmer M. Food firms hope you can never have enough of a sweeter thing. *Los Angeles Times*, Apr. 28, 2002.

29. Bray GA. Diobesity: A global problem. *International Journal of Obesity*, 2002;26 (Suppl 1):S63; Bray GA. The fluoride hypothesis and diobesity: how to prevent diabetes by preventing obesity. In A Halperin, G Mederios-Neto, C Bouchard (Eds) *Progress in Obesity Research VII*. London: John Libbey & Co., 2003.

30. Heinz Company website. Available at www.heinz.com/jsp/di/q22002/q220023.jsp. Accessed Aug. 19, 2002.

31. Sherwood NE, Jeffery RW, French SA, Hannan PJ, Murray DM. Predictors of weight gain in the Pound of Prevention Study. *International Journal of Obesity & Related Metabolic Disorders*, 2000;24:395–403.

32. French SA, Jeffery RW, Forster JL, McGovern PG, Kelder SH, Baxter JE. Predictors of weight change over two years among a population of working adults: the Healthy Worker Project. *International Journal of Obesity & Related Metabolic Disorders*, 1994:18:145–154.

33. Rissanen A, Hakala P, Lissner L, Mattlar CE, Koskenvuo M, Ronnemaa T. Acquired preference especially for dietary fat and obesity: a study of weight-discordant monozygotic twin pairs. *International Journal of Obesity & Related Metabolic Disorders*, 2002;26:973–977.

34. Astrup A, Ryan L, Grunwald GK, Storgaard M, Saris W, Melanson E, Hill JO. The role of dietary fat in body fatness: evidence from a preliminary meta-analysis of ad libitum low-fat dietary intervention studies. *British Journal of Nutrition*, 2000;83 (Suppl 1):S25–32.

35. Hill JO, Melanson EL, Wyatt HT. Dietary fat intake and regulation of energy balance: implications for obesity. *Journal of Nutrition*, 2000:130 (2S Suppl):284S–288S, p. 284S.

36. Taubes G. What if it's all been a big fat lie? *New York Times Magazine*, July 7, 2002.

37. Squires S. Experts declare story low on saturated facts. *The Washington Post*, Aug. 27, 2002, p. HE01.

38. Astrup A. Dietary fat is a major player in obesity—but not the only one. *Obesity Reviews*, 2002;3:57–58; Willett WC. Dietary fat plays a major role in obesity: no. *Obesity Reviews*, 2002;3:59–68.

39. Quatromoni PA, Copenhafer DL, D'Agostino RB, Millen BE. Dietary patterns predict the development of overweight in women: the Framingham Nutrition Studies. *Journal of the American Dietetic Association*, 2002;102:1240–1246.

40. Wurtman RJ, Wurtman JJ. Brain serotonin, carbohydrate-craving, obesity and depression. *Advances in Experimental Medicine & Biology*, 1996;398:35–41; Wurtman JJ. *Carbohydrate Craver's Diet*. Boston: Houghton Mifflin, 1983.

41. Fernstrom JD. Tryptophan, serotonin and carbohydrate appetite: will the real carbohydrate craver please stand up! *Journal of Nutrition*, 1988;118:1417–1419.

42. Colantuoni C, Schwenker J, McCarthy J, Rada P, Ladenheim B, Cadet J-L, Schwartz GJ, Moran TH, Hoebel BG. Excessive sugar intake alters binding to dopamine and mu-opioid receptors in the brain. *NeuroReport*, 2001;12:3549–3552; Colantuoni C, Rada P, McCarthy J, Patten C, Avena NM, Chadeayne A, Hoebel BG. Evidence that intermittent, excessive sugar intake causes endogenous opioid dependence. *Obesity Research*, 2002;10:478–488; Hoebel BG, Rada PV, Mark GP, Pothos EN. Neural systems for reinforcement and inhibition of behavior: Relevance to eating, addiction, and depression. In D Kahneman, E Diener, N Schwarz (Eds) *Well-being: Foundations of Hedonic Psychology*. New York: Russell Sage Foundation, 1999, pp. 558–572.

43. Colantuoni C, Rada P, McCarthy J, Patten C, Avena NM, Chadeayne A, Hoebel BG. Evidence that intermittent, excessive sugar intake causes endogenous opioid dependence. *Obesity Research*, 2002;10:478–488.

44. Drewnowski A, Krahn DD, Demitrack MA, Nairn K, Gosnell BA. Naloxone, an opiate blocker, reduces the consumption of sweet high-fat foods in obese and lean female binge eaters. *American Journal of Clinical Nutrition*, 1995;61:1206–1212; Drewnowski A. Metabolic determinants of binge eating. *Addictive Behaviors*, 1995;20:733–745.

45. Drewnowski quoted in Roan S. The sugar habit. *Los Angeles Times*, Nov. 11, 2002.

46. Philipson T. The world-wide growth in obesity: an economic research agenda. *Health Economics*, 2001;10:1–7.

47. Dietz WH, Gortmaker SL. Do we fatten our children at the TV set? television viewing and obesity in children and adolescents. *Pediatrics*, 1985;75:807–812; Gortmaker SL, Must A, Sobol AM, Peterson K, Colditz GA, Dietz WH. Television viewing as a cause of increasing obesity among children in the United States, 1986–1990. *Archives of Pediatric and Adolescent Medicine*, 1996;150:356–362.

48. Dennison BA, Erb TA, Jenkins PL. Television viewing and television in bedroom associated with overweight risk among low-income preschool children. *Pediatrics*, 2002;109:1028–1035; Hu FB, Leitzmann MF, Stampfer MJ, Colditz GA, Willett WC, Rimm EB. Physical activity and television watching in relation to risk for type 2 diabetes mellitus in men. *Archives of Internal Medicine*, 2001;161:1542–1548; Borzekowski DL, Robinson TN. The 30-second effect: an experiment revealing the impact of television commercials on food preferences of preschoolers. *Journal of the American Dietetic Association*, 2001;101:42–46; Andersen RE, Crespo CJ, Bartlett SJ, Cheskin LJ, Pratt M. Relationship of physical activity and television watching with body weight and level of fatness among children: results from the third National Health and Nutrition Examination Survey. *JAMA*, 1998;279:938–942.

49. Fung TT, Hu FB, Yu J, Chu NF, Spiegelman D, Tofler GH, Willett WC, Rimm EB. Leisure-time physical activity, television watching, and plasma biomarkers of obesity and cardiovascular disease risk. *American Journal of Epidemiology*, 2000;152:1171–1178; Kronenberg F, Pereira MA, Schmitz MK, Arnett DK, Evenson KR, Crapo RO, Jensen RL, Burke GL, Sholinsky P, Ellison RC, Hunt SC. Influence of leisure time physical activity and television watching on atherosclerosis risk factors in the NHLBI Family Heart Study. *Atherosclerosis*, 2000;153:433–443.

50. Dietz WH. The obesity epidemic in young children. Reduce television viewing and promote playing. *BMJ*, 2001;322:313–314; Robinson TN. Reducing children's television viewing to prevent obesity: a randomized controlled trial. *JAMA*, 1999;282:1561–1567; Robinson TN. Television viewing and childhood obesity. *Pediatric Clinics of North America*, 2001;48:1017–1025.

51. Certain LK, Kahn RS. Prevalence, correlates, and trajectory of television viewing among infants and toddlers. *Pediatrics*, 2002:109;634–642.

52. Dennison BA, Erb TA, Jenkins PL. Television viewing and television in bedroom associated with overweight risk among low-income preschool children. *Pediatrics*, 2002;109:1028–1035; Saelens BE, Sallis JF, Nader PR, Broyles SL, Berry CC, Taras HL. Home environmental influences on children's television watching from early to middle childhood. *Journal of Developmental & Behavioral Pediatrics*, 2002;23:127–132.

53. Coon KA, Goldberg J, Rogers BL, Tucker KL. Relationships between use of television during meals and children's food consumption patterns. *Pediatrics*, 2001;107:E7; Dennison BA, Erb TA, Jenkins PL. Is family dinnertime undone by TV? *Obesity Research*, 2001;9:92S.

54. Klesges R, Shelton M, Klesges L. Effects of television on metabolic rate: potential implications for childhood obesity. *Pediatrics*, 1993;9:281–286.

55. National Restaurant Association website. Available at www.restaurant.org/faq.cfm#population. Accessed Aug. 19, 2002.

56. French SA, Harnack L, Jeffery RW. Fast food restaurant use among women in the Pound of Prevention Study: dietary, behavioral, and demographic correlates. *International Journal of Obesity & Related Metabolic Disorders*, 2000;24:1353–1359; Jeffery RW, French SA. Epidemic obesity in the Untied States: are fast foods and television viewing contributing? *American Journal of Public Health*, 1998;88:277–280; Zoumas-Morse C, Rock CL, Sobo EJ, Neuhouser ML. Children's patterns of macronutrient intake and associations with restaurant and home eating. *Journal of the American Dietetic Association*, 2001;101:923–925.

57. Gillman MW, Rifas-Shiman SL, Frazier AL, Rockett HR, Camargo CA Jr, Field AE, Berkey CS, Colditz GA. Family dinner and diet quality among older children and adolescents. *Archives of Family Medicine*, 2000;9:235–240.

58. National Restaurant Association website. Available at www.restaurant.org/faq.cfm#population. Accessed Aug. 19, 2002.

59. Schwartz MB, Hrabosky JI, Brownell KD. Nutrition analysis of children's meals at fast food and family restaurants. Paper submitted for publication.

60. French SA, Story M, Neumark-Sztainer D, Fulkerson JA, Hannan P. Fast food restaurant use among adolescents: associations with nutrient intake, food choices and behavioral and psychosocial variables. *International Journal of Obesity & Related Metabolic Disorders*, 2001;25:1823–1833.

61. When you're here, you're thirsty. *Harper's Magazine*, Oct. 2002, 14.

62. Press release "College Students Snack to Satisfy Hunger" from the National Snack Food Association. Available at www.sfa.org/press.html. Accessed Nov. 19, 2002.

63. Zizza C, Siega-Riz AM, Popkin BM. Significant increase in young adults' snacking between 1977–1978 and 1994–1996 represents a cause for concern! *Preventive Medicine*, 2001;32:303–310; Jahns L, Siega-Riz AM, Popkin BM. The increasing prevalence of snacking among U.S. children between 1977 to 1996. *Journal of Pediatrics*, 2001;138:493–498.

64. Marmonier C, Chapelot D, Fantino M, Louis-Sylvestre J. Snacks consumed in a nonhungry state have poor satiating efficiency; influence of snack composition on substrate utilization and hunger. *American Journal of Clinical Nutrition*, 2002;76:518–528.

65. Food Commission. Children's food: ten junk products for every healthy one. *Food Magazine*, April, 2000. Available at http://ourworld.compuserve.com/homepages/foodcomm/00d.htm. Accessed Aug. 27, 2002.

66. International Federation of Competitive Overeating website. Available at www.ifoce.com. Accessed Aug. 26, 2002.

67. Quoted in Duenwald M. Good health is linked to grocer. *New York Times*, Nov. 12, 2002.

68. Centers for Disease Control and Prevention. Obesity and overweight: a public health epidemic. CDC website. Available at www.cdc.gov/nccdphp/dnpa/obesity/epidemic.htm. Accessed Jul. 21, 2002; World Health Organization. *Obesity: Preventing and Managing the Global Epidemic.* Geneva, Switzerland: World Health Organization, 1998.

69. Centers for Disease Control and Prevention website. Body mass index calculator. Available at www.cdc.gov/nccdphp/dnpa/bmi. Accessed Aug. 23, 2002.

70. Flegal KM, Carroll MD, Ogden CL, Johnson CL. Prevalence and trends in obesity among U.S. adults, 1999–2000. *JAMA*, 288:1723–1727; Freedman DS, Khan LK, Serdula MK, Galuska DA, Dietz WH. Trends and correlates of class 3 obesity in the United States from 1990 through 2000. *JAMA*, 2002;288:1758–1761.

71. Kumanyika SK. Obesity in minority populations. In CG Fairburn & KD Brownell (Eds) *Eating Disorders and Obesity: A Comprehensive Handbook* (2nd Ed). New York: Guilford Press, 2002, pp. 439–444; Kumanyika SK, Krebs-Smith SM. Preventive nutrition issues in ethnic and socioeconomic groups in the United States. In

A Bendich & RK Deckelbaum (Eds) *Primary and Secondary Preventive Nutrition*. Totowa, NJ: Humana Press, 2000, pp. 325–356.

72. Ogden CL, Flegal KM, Carroll MD, Johnson CL. Prevalence and trends in overweight among U.S. children and adolescents, 1999–2000. *JAMA*, 2002;288:1728–1732; Goran, MI. Metabolic precursors and effects of obesity in children: a decade of progress, 1990–1999. *American Journal of Clinical Nutrition*, 2001;73:158–171; Filozof C, Gonzalez C, Sereday M, Mazza C, Braguinsky J. Obesity prevalence and trends in Latin-American countries. *Obesity Reviews*, 2001;2:99–106; Chinn S, Hughes JM, Rona RJ. Trends in growth and obesity in ethnic groups in Britain. *Archives of Disease in Childhood*, 1998;78:513–517; Acton KJ, Burrows NR, Moore K, Querec L, Geiss LS, Engelgau MM. Trends in diabetes prevalence among American Indian and Alaska Native children, adolescents, and young adults. *American Journal of Public Health*, 2002;92:1485–1490; Reaven P, Nader PR, Berry C, Hoy T. Cardiovascular disease insulin risk in Mexican-American and Anglo-American children and mothers. *Pediatrics*, 1998;101:E12.

73. Kumanyika SK. Obesity treatment in minorities. In TA Wadden & AJ Stunkard (Eds) *Handbook of Obesity Treatment*. New York: Guilford Press, 2001.

74. Crawford D, Jeffery RW, French SA. Can anyone successfully control their weight? Findings of a three year community-based study of men and women. *International Journal of Obesity & Related Metabolic Disorders*, 2000;24:1107–1110.

75. Table adapted from information on American Obesity Association website. Available at www.obesity.org/subs/fastfacts/Health_Effects.shtml. Accessed Aug. 23, 2002.

76. National Heart, Lung, and Blood Institute. NHLBI clinical guidelines on the identification, evaluation, and treatment of overweight and obesity in adults: the evidence report. *Obesity Research*, 1998:6 (Suppl 2):51S–209S; National Task Force on the Treatment and Prevention of Obesity. Overweight, obesity, and health risk. *Archives of Internal Medicine*, 2000:160:898–904; Must A, Spadano J, Coakley EH, Field AE, Colditz G, Dietz WH. The disease burden associated with overweight and obesity. *JAMA*, 1999;282:1523–1529.

77. Manson JE, Willett WC, Stampfer MJ, Colditz GA, Hunter DJ, Hankinson SE, Hennekens CH, Speizer FE. Body weight and mortality among women. *New England Journal of Medicine*, 1995;333:677–685.

78. Kenchaiah S, Evans JC, Levy D, Wilson PWF, Benjamin EJ, Larson MG, Kannel WB, Vasan RS. Obesity and the risk for heart failure. *New England Journal of Medicine*, 2002;347:305–313; Haney DQ. New culprit found in heart attacks: Doctors urged to test for hidden inflammation. Associated Press, Aug. 4, 2002; Jonsson S, Hedblad B, Engstrom G, Nilsson P, Bergland G, Janzon L. Influence of obesity on cardiovascular risk. Twenty-three-year follow-up of 22,025 men from an urban Swedish population. *International Journal of Obesity*, 2002:26:1046–1053; March of Dimes study on obesity and pregnancy complications. Available at www.marchofdimes.com. Accessed Nov. 17, 2002.

79. Lakka H-M, Laaksonen DE, Lakka TA, Niskanen LK, Kumpusalo E, Tuomilehto J, Salonen JT. The metabolic syndrome and total and cardiovascular disease mortality in middle-aged men. *JAMA*, 2002;288:2709–2716.

80. Fontaine KR, Barofsky I. Obesity and health-related quality of life. *Obesity Reviews*, 2001;2:173–182; Kushner RF, Foster GD. Obesity and quality of life. *Nutrition*, 2000;16:947–952; Burns CM, Tijhuis MA, Seidell JC. The relationship between quality of life and perceived body weight and dieting history in Dutch men and women. *International Journal of Obesity & Related Metabolic Disorders*, 2001;25:1386–1392.

81. Thompson D, Wolf AM. The medical-care cost burden of obesity. *Obesity Reviews*, 2001:2:189–197; Allison DB, Zannolli R, Narayan KM. The direct health care costs of obesity in the United States. *American Journal of Public Health*, 1999;89:1194–1199.

82. Sturm R. The effects of obesity, smoking, and problem drinking on chronic medical problems and health care costs. *Health Affairs*, 2002;21:245–253; Sturm R, Wells KB. Does obesity contribute as much to morbidity as poverty or smoking? *Public Health*, 2001;115:229–295.

83. Ebbeling CB, Pawlak DB, Ludwig DS. Childhood obesity: public health crisis, commonsense cure. *Lancet*, 2002;360:473–482; Dietz WH, Gortmaker SL. Preventing obesity in children and adolescents. *Annual Review of Public Health*, 2001:22:337–353; Strauss RS, Pollock HA. Epidemic increase in childhood overweight, 1986–1998. *JAMA*, 2001;286:2845–2848. Ogden CL, Flegal KM, Carroll MD, Johnson CL. Prevalence and trends in overweight among U.S. children and adolescents, 1999–2000. *JAMA*, 2002;288:1728–1732.

84. Ebbeling CB, Pawlak DB, Ludwig DS. Childhood obesity: public health crisis, commonsense cure. *Lancet*, 2002;360:473–482; Wang Y, Montiero CM, Popkin BM. Trends of obesity and underweight in older children and adolescents in the United States, Brazil, China, and Russia. *American Journal of Clinical Nutrition*, 2002;75:971–977.

85. Guo SS, Wu W, Chumlea WC, Roche AF. Predicting overweight and obesity in childhood from body mass index values in childhood and adolescence. *American Journal of Clinical Nutrition*, 2002:76:653–658; Whitaker RC, Wright JA, Pepe MS, Seidel KD, Dietz WH. Predicting obesity in young adulthood from childhood and parental obesity. *New England Journal of Medicine*, 1997;337:869–873; Freedman DS, Khan LK, Dietz WH,

Srinivasan SR, Berenson GS. Relationship of childhood obesity to coronary heart disease risk factors in adulthood: the Bogalusa Heart Study. *Pediatrics*, 2001;108:712–718.

86. Ebbeling CB, Pawlak DB, Ludwig DS. Childhood obesity: public health crisis, commonsense cure. *Lancet*, 2002;360:473–482.

87. Sinha R, Fisch G, Teague B, Tamborlane WV, Banyas B, Allen K, Savoye M, Rieger V, Taksali S, Barbetta G, Sherwin RS, Caprio S. Prevalence of impaired glucose tolerance among children and adolescents with marked obesity. *New England Journal of Medicine*, 2002;346:802–810.

88. Tounian P, Aggoun Y, Dubern B, Varille V, Guy-Grand B, Sidi D, Girardet JP, Bonnet D. Presence of increased stiffness of the common carotid artery and endothelial dysfunction in severely obese children: a prospective study. *Lancet*, 2001:358:1400–1404; Dean H, Flett B. Natural history of Type 2 diabetes diagnosed in childhood; long-term follow-up in young adult years. Paper presented at the annual meeting of the American Diabetes Association, San Francisco, June, 2002.

89. French SA, Story M, Perry CL. Self-esteem and obesity in children and adolescence: a literature review. *Obesity Research*, 1995;3:479–490.

90. Wang G, Dietz WH. Economic burden of obesity in youths aged 6–17 years: 1979–1999. *Pediatrics*, 2002;109. Available at www.pediatrics.org/cgi/content/full/109/5/e81. Accessed Aug. 25, 2002.

91. Nolte R, Franckowiak SC, Crespo CJ, Andersen RE. U.S. military weight standards: What percentage of U.S. young adults meet the current standards? *American Journal of Medicine*, 2002:113:486–490.

92. Siener K, Rothman D, Farrar J. Soft drink logos on baby bottles: do they influence what is fed to children? *Journal of Dentistry for Children*, 1997;64:55–60.

93. Davison KK, Birch LL. Obesigenic families: parents' physical activity and dietary intake patterns predict girls' risk of overweight. *International Journal of Obesity*, 2002;26:1186–1193; Davison KK, Birch LL. Child and parent characteristics as predictors of change in girls' body mass index. *International Journal of Obesity & Related Metabolic Disorders*, 2001;25:1834–1842; Kalakanis LE, Goldfield GS, Paluch RA, Epstein LH. Parental activity as a determinant of activity level and patterns of activity in obese children. *Research Quarterly for Exercise & Sport*, 2001;72:202–209.

94. Bray GA. Diobesity: A global problem. *International Journal of Obesity*, 2002;26 (Suppl 1):S63; Bray GA. The fluoride hypothesis and diobesity: how to prevent diabetes by preventing obesity. In A Halperin, G Mederios-Neto, C Bouchard (Eds) *Progress in Obesity Research VII*. London: John Libbey & Co., 2003.

Chapter 3

1. Nordic Business Report. Finns are becoming fatter—report. Nordic Business Report via Comtex. November 12, 2001; Swiss Radio International. Tubby Swiss urged to slim down. Nov. 11, 2002; Latimer W. Obesity in Canadians a big problems—say local health officials. *Strathroy Age Dispatch*, July 22, 2002; Reuters News Service (Singapore). Experts chew the fat over Asian obesity guidelines. July 10, 2002; *New Zealand Herald*. Obesity epidemic in New Zealand, Health Minister says. *New Zealand Herald*, July 18, 2002; Vietnam News Agency (Hanoi). Viet Nam faces both obesity and malnutrition problems. July 29, 2002; Kazmi A. Survey reveals unhealthy lifestyle. *Gulf News* (UAE). July 18, 2002; Zhelev V. Bulgarians are Europe's most overweight or obese citizens, experts say. Associated Press, Sofia, Bulgaria, July 22, 2002; *Straits Times* (Singapore). One in four Malaysians is overweight from overeating. *Straits Times*, August 20, 2002; ABC Radio Australia News. French Polynesia launches campaign to fight obesity. Nov. 14, 2002; Reuters (Shanghai). China's little emperors getting bigger. Reuters, June 2, 2002; Lorenzi R. Italy moves to tackle obesity epidemic. Reuters health, Florence, Italy, July 2, 2002; Montgomery D. Fitness czar for a lazy Scotland. *The Daily Herald* (UK), June 7, 2002; Belgian News (Brussels). Obesity epidemic in Belgium. *Belgian News*, June 5, 2002; *Pacific Business News*. Tonga obesity rate 60 percent. Sep. 23, 2002.

2. James WPT. A world view of the obesity problem. In CG Fairburn & KD Brownell (Eds) *Eating Disorders and Obesity: A Comprehensive Handbook*. New York: Guilford Publications, 2002, pp. 411–416.

3. Quotes in Winslow R, Landers P. Rising global obesity reflects changes in diet and lifestyle. *Wall Street Journal*, July 1, 2002.

4. World Health Organization. *Obesity: Preventing and Managing the Global Epidemic*. Geneva, Switzerland: World Health Organization, 1998.

5. Ross E. WHO gets aggressive on obesity. Associated Press (Geneva). May 15, 2002.

6. Friedrich MJ. Epidemic of obesity expands its spread to developing countries. *JAMA*, 2002;287:1382–1386.

7. Winslow R, Landers P. Rising global obesity reflects changes in diet and lifestyle. *Wall Street Journal*, July 1, 2002.

8. Popkin BM. An overview on the nutrition transition and its health implications: the Bellagio meeting. *Public Health Nutrition*, 2002;5:93–103; Popkin BM. The nutrition transition and obesity in the developing world.

Journal of Nutrition, 2001;131:871S–873S; Drewnowski A, Popkin BM. The nutrition transition: new trends in the global diet. *Nutrition Reviews*, 1997;55:31–43.

9. Popkin BM. The nutrition transition and obesity in the developing world. *Journal of Nutrition*, 2001;131:871S–873S.

10. Brownell KD, Ludwig DS. Fighting obesity and the food lobby. *Washington Post*, June 9, 2002.

11. McDonald's corporate website. Available at www.mcdonalds.com/corporate/info/history/history5/index .html. Accessed Sep. 2, 2002.

12. Coca-Cola corporate website. Available at www.coca-cola.com/golocal/index.html. Accessed Aug. 1, 2002.

13. Mars, Inc. website. Available at http://gcv.mms.com. Accessed Aug. 13, 2002.

14. Text from McDonald's press release, December 9, 1996. Available at www.mcspotlight.org/media/press/ prnews_9dec96.html. Accessed Sep. 2, 2002.

15. Cowing E. Why India has no beef with McDonald's. *The Scotsman*, December. 8, 2000, p. 4.

16. McDonald's corporate website. Available at www.mcdonalds.com/corporate/index.html. Accessed Aug. 1, 2002.

17. Watson J. China's Big Mac attack. *Foreign Affairs*, 2000;79:120.

18. Harding L. Real lives: Give me a Big Mac, but hold the beef. *Guardian Features Pages*, Dec. 28, 2000, p. 4.

19. KFC corporate website. Available at www.kfc.com/about/kfcfacts.htm. Accessed Aug. 28, 2002.

20. Cowing E. Why India has no beef with McDonald's. *The Scotsman*, Dec. 8, 2000, p. 4.

21. Ibid.

22. Ringham E. New economy finds room for the West. *Minneapolis Star Tribune*, June 21, 2001, p. 23A.

23. Watson J. China's Big Mac attack. *Foreign Affairs*, 2000;79:120.

24. *The Hindu*. Fast food yes, but no trouble please. FT Asia Africa Intelligence Wire. Oct. 17, 2001.

25. Iritani E. Ruling the roost in China: KFC has developed a new secret recipe—measured expansion, cagey marketing, and cheerful service—and the customers are flocking in. *Los Angeles Times*, Sept. 10, 2001, A1.

26. Jitpleecheep S. Chinese outlet joins delivery bandwagon. *Bangkok Post*, Feb. 23, 2001.

27. Dunkin' Donuts website. Available at www.dunkindonuts.com/aboutus/funfacts.jsp. Accessed Sep. 2, 2002.

28. Herrmann A. Happy meals in an unhappy world. *Chicago Sun-Times*, Oct. 18, 2000, p. 57.

29. Ibid.

30. Watson J. China's Big Mac attack. *Foreign Affairs*, 2000;79:120.

31. Fisher M. Meal deals in world hotspots. *Toronto Sun* (Editorial), Oct. 19, 2001, p. 16.

32. Herrmann A. Happy meals in an unhappy world. *Chicago Sun-Times*, Oct. 18, 2000, p. 57.

33. Greenway H. Arches not so golden to some in India. *Boston Globe* (Op-Ed), June 4, 2001, p. A11.

34. Fisher M. Meal deals in world hotspots. *Toronto Sun* (Editorial), Oct. 19, 2001, p. 16.

35. Reuters. Mexican artist leads anti-McDonald's campaign. Reuters, Aug, 19, 2002. Available at www.mcspotlight.org/media/press/campaigns/reuters190802.html. Accessed Sep. 2, 2002.

36. Wall M. KFC into India: a case study of resistance to globalization discourse. In R Andersen & L Strate (Eds) *Critical Studies in Media Commercialism*. Oxford: Oxford University Press, 2000, pp. 291–309.

37. Schlosser E. *Fast Food Nation: The Dark Side of the All American Meal.* Boston: Houghton Mifflin, 2001, p. 244.

38. See the special issue of the journal *Public Health Nutrition* (2002, Vol. 5, issue 1A) on nutrition transitions around the world. The contents can be accessed through the website of Dr. Barry Popkin at the University of North Carolina (www.nutrans.org). Click on Bellagio Conference papers; Doak C. Large-scale interventions and programmes addressing nutrition-related chronic diseases and obesity: examples from fourteen countries. *Public Health Nutrition*, 2002;5:275–277.

39. Uusitalo U, Feskens EJ, Tuomilehto J, Dowse G, Haw U, Fareed D, Hemraj F, Gareeboo H, Alberti KG, Zimmet P. Fall in total cholesterol concentration over five years in association with changes in fatty acid composition of cooking oil in Mauritius: cross sectional survey. *BMJ*, 1996;313:1044–1046.

40. Puska P, Pietinen P, Uusitalo U. Influencing public nutrition for noncommunicable disease prevention: from community intervention to national programme—experiences from Finland. *Public Health Nutrition*, 2002;5:245–251.

41. Coitinho D, Monteiro CA, Popkin BM. What Brazil is doing to promote healthy diets and active lifestyles. *Public Health Nutrition*, 2002;5:263–267.

42. Zhai F, Fu D, Du S, Ge K, Chen C, Popkin BM. What is China doing in policy-making to push back the negative aspects of the nutrition transition? *Public Health Nutrition*, 2002;5:269–273.

43. Swinburn B, Egger G, Raza F. Dissecting obesogenic environments: the development and application of a framework for identifying and prioritizing environmental interventions for obesity. *Preventive Medicine*, 1999;29:563–570.

Chapter 4

1. Testimony of Keith Laughlin, President of the Rails-to-Trails Conservancy before the subcommittee on Highways and Transit of the House Committee on Transportation and Infrastructure, U.S. House of Representatives, July 22, 2002, Available at www.railstrails.org/whatwedo/policy/testimony0725.htm. Accessed Sep. 19, 2002.

2. Blair SN, Booth M, Gyarfas I, Iwane H, Marti B, Matsudo V, Morrow MS, Noakes T, Shephard R. Development of public policy and physical activity initiatives internationally. *Sports Medicine*, 2000; 154:904–911.

3. McGinnis JM, Foege WH. Actual causes of death in the United States. *JAMA*, 1993;270:207–212; Hahn RA, Teutsch SM, Rothenberg RB, Marks JS. Excess deaths from nine chronic diseases in the United States, 1986. *JAMA*, 1990;264:2654–2659.

4. Morgan JE. *University Oars: Being a Critical Enquiry into the After-Health of the Men Who Rowed in the Oxford and Cambridge Boat Race from the Year 1829–1869, Based on the Personal Experience of the Rowers Themselves.* London: Macmillan, 1873.

5. U.S. Department of Health and Human Services (1996). *Physical Activity and Health: Report of the Surgeon General.* Atlanta, GA: U.S. Department of Health and Human Services, Centers for Disease Control, National Center for Chronic Disease Prevention and Health Promotion; Pate RR, Pratt M, Blair SN, Haskell WL, Macera CA, Bouchard C, Buchner D, Ettinger W, Heath GW, King AC, Kriska A, Leon AS, Marcus BH, Morris J, Paffenbarger RS Jr., Patrick K, Rippe JM, Sallis J, Wilmore JH. Physical activity and public health: A recommendation from the Centers for Disease Control and the American College of Sports Medicine, *JAMA*, 1995;273:402–407.

6. Mokdad A, Bowman B, Ford E, Vinicor F, Marks J, Koplan J. The continuing epidemics of obesity and diabetes in the United States. *JAMA*, 2001;286:1195–1200; Serdula M, Mokdad A, Williamson D, Galuska D, Mendlein J, Health G. Prevalence of attempting weight loss and strategies for controlling weight. *JAMA*, 1999;282: 1353–1358.

7. Duncan G. Couch potatoes may overestimate their activity. *Preventive Medicine*, 2001;33:18–26.

8. Centers for Disease Control and Prevention website, section on physical activity. Available at www.cdc.gov/nccdphp/dnpa/physicalactivity.htm. Accessed Aug. 31, 2002; U.S. Department of Health and Human Services. *Physical Activity and Health: Report of the Surgeon General.* Atlanta, GA: U.S. Department of Health and Human Services, Centers for Disease Control, National Center for Chronic Disease Prevention and Health Promotion, 1996; Pate RR, Freedson PS, Sallis JF, Taylor WC, Sinard SG, Trost SG, Dowda M. Compliance with physical activity guidelines: prevalence in a population of children and youth. *Annals of Epidemiology*, 2002;12:303–308; Trost SG, Pate RR, Sallis JF, Freedson PS, Taylor WC, Dowda M, Sirard J. Age and gender differences in objectively measured physical activity in youth. *Medicine and Science in Sports and Exercise*, 2002;34:350–355; Gordon-Larsen P, McMurray R, Popkin B. Adolescent physical activity and inactivity vary by ethnicity: The National Longitudinal Study of Adolescent Health. *Journal of Pediatrics*, 1999;135:301–306; Angle M. Teens slack off on exercise, but older folks keep up—Over 55 group works out the most, study says. *USA Today*, Aug. 6, 2001, 4D; Kim SYS, Glynn NW, Kriska AM, Baron BA, Kronsberg SS, Daniels SR, Crawford PB, Sabry ZI, Liu K. Decline in physical activity in black girls and white girls during adolescence. *JAMA*, 2002;347:709–715.

9. Centers for Disease Control and Prevention, National Center for Chronic Disease Prevention and Health Promotion. Kids Walk to School Program. Available at http://rtc.railtrails.org/whatwedo/policy/saferoutes.asp. Accessed Aug. 31, 2002; Rails-to-Trails Conservancy. Safe Routes to School Program. Available at http://rtc.railtrails.org/whatwedo/policy/saferoutes.asp. Accessed Aug. 31, 2002.

10. Blair SN, Kampert JB, Kohl HW 3rd, Barlow CE, Macera CA, Paffenbarger RS Jr, Gibbons LW. Influences of cardiorespiratory fitness and other precursors on cardiovascular disease and all-cause mortality in men and women. *JAMA*, 1996;276:205–210; Pate RR, Pratt M, Blair SN, Haskell WL, Macera CA, Bouchard C, Buchner D, Ettinger W, Heath GW, King AC, Kriska A, Leon AS, Marcus BH, Morris J, Paffenbarger RS Jr., Patrick K, Rippe JM, Sallis J, Wilmore JH. Physical activity and public health: A recommendation from the Centers for Disease Control and the American College of Sports Medicine, *JAMA*, 1995:273:402–407; Myers J, Prakash M, Froelicher V, Do D, Partington S, Atwood JE. Exercise capacity and mortality among men referred for exercise testing. *New England Journal of Medicine*, 2002;346:793–801; Rockhill B, Willett WC, Manson JE, Leitzmann MF, Stampfer MJ, Hunter DJ, Colditz GA. Physical activity and mortality: a prospective study among women. *American Journal of Public Health*, 2001;91:578–583; Lee IM, Paffenbarger RS. Physical activity and stroke incidence. *Stroke*, 1998;29:2049–2054; Irwin ML, Ainsworth BE, Mayer-Davis EJ, Addy CL, Pate RR, Durstine JL. Physical activity and the metabolic syndrome in a tri-ethnic sample of women. *Obesity Research*, 2002;10:1030–1037; Feskanich D, Willett W, Colditz G. Walking and leisure-time activity and risk of hip fracture in postmenopausal women. *JAMA*, 2002; 288:2300–2306.

11. Manson JE, Greenland P, LaCroix AZ, Stefanick M, Mouton CP, Oberman A, Perri MG, Sheps DS, Pettinger MB, Siscovick DS. Walking compared with vigorous exercise for the prevention of cardiovascular events in women. *New England Journal of Medicine*, 2002;347:716–725.

12. U.S. Department of Health and Human Services. *Physical Activity and Health: Report of the Surgeon General*. Atlanta, GA: U.S. Department of Health and Human Services, Centers for Disease Control, National Center for Chronic Disease Prevention and Health Promotion, 1996.

13. Sinha R, Fisch G, Teague B, Tamborlane WV, Banyas B, Allen K, Savoye M, Rieger V, Taksali S, Barbetta G, Sherwin RS, Caprio S. Prevalence of impaired glucose tolerance among children and adolescents with marked obesity. *New England Journal of Medicine*, 2002;346:802–810; Ebbeling CB, Pawlak DB, Ludwig DS. Childhood obesity: public health crisis, commonsense cure. *Lancet*, 2002;360:473–482.

14. U.S. Department of Health and Human Services. *Physical Activity and Health: Report of the Surgeon General*. Atlanta, GA: U.S. Department of Health and Human Services, Centers for Disease Control, National Center for Chronic Disease Prevention and Health Promotion, 1996; Hansen C, Stevens L, Coast J. Exercise duration and mood state: How much is enough to feel better? *Health Psychology*, 2001;20:267–275.

15. Baker CW, Brownell KD. Physical activity and maintenance of weight loss: Physiological and psychological mechanisms. In C Bouchard (Ed) *Physical Activity and Obesity*. Champaign, IL: Human Kinetics Press, 2000, pp. 311–328; King GA, Fitzhugh EC, Bassett DR Jr, McLaughlin JE, Strath SJ, Swartz AM, Thompson DL. Relationship of leisure-time physical activity and occupational activity to the prevalence of obesity. *International Journal of Obesity*, 2001;25:606–612.

16. Sorensen TIA. Is physical inactivity the cause or the consequence of obesity? Paper presented at the 9th International Congress on Obesity, Sao Paulo, Brazil. *International Journal of Obesity and Related Metabolic Disorders*, 2002:26 (Suppl 1):S64.

17. DiPietro L, Kohl HW, Barlow CE, Blair SN. Improvements in cardiorespiratory fitness attenuate age-related weight gain in healthy men and women: The Aerobics Center Longitudinal Study. *International Journal of Obesity*, 1998;22:55–62; Berkey CS, Rockett HR, Field AE, Gillman MW, Frazier AL, Camargo CA, Jr., Colditz GA. Activity, dietary intake, and weight changes in a longitudinal study of preadolescent and adolescent boys and girls. *Pediatrics*, 2000;105:E56; Sherwood NE, Jeffery RW, French SA, Hannan PJ, Murray DM. Predictors of weight gain in the Pound of Prevention study. *International Journal of Obesity and Related Metabolic Disorders*, 2000;24:395–403.

18. Andersen RE, Wadden TA, Bartlett SJ, Zemel B, Verde TJ, Franckowiak SC. Effect of lifestyle activity vs. structured aerobic exercise in obese women. *JAMA*, 1999;281:335–340; Wing RR, Hill JO. Successful weight loss maintenance. *Annual Review of Nutrition*, 2001;21:323–341; Jakicic J, Winters C, Lang W, Wing R. Effects of intermittent exercise and use of home exercise equipment on adherence, weight loss, and fitness in overweight women. *JAMA*, 1999;282:1554–1560.

19. McGuire MT, Wing RR, Klem ML, Lang W, Hill JO. What predicts weight regain in a group of successful weight losers? *Journal of Consulting & Clinical Psychology*, 1999;67:177–185.

20. Blair SN, Kampert JB, Kohl HW 3rd, Barlow CE, Macera CA, Paffenbarger RS Jr, Gibbons LW. Influences of cardiorespiratory fitness and other precursors on cardiovascular disease and all-cause mortality in men and women. *JAMA*, 1996;276:205–210; Wei M, Kampert JB, Barlow CE, Nichaman MZ, Gibbons LW, Paffenbarger RS Jr, Blair SN. Relationship between low cardiorespiratory fitness and mortality in normal-weight, overweight, and obese men. *JAMA*, 1999;282:1547–1553.

21. U.S. Department of Health and Human Services. *Physical Activity and Health: Report of the Surgeon General*. Atlanta, GA: U.S. Department of Health and Human Services, Centers for Disease Control, National Center for Chronic Disease Prevention and Health Promotion, 1996; Prentice AM. Obesity—the inevitable penalty of civilization? *British Medical Bulletin*, 1997;53:229–237.

22. Flint, A. Suburban sprawl seen as health hazard, discourages daily exercise, scientist says. *Boston Globe*, Oct. 8, 2001,B2; Pierce N. Modern schools often illustrate "dumb growth": State rules on the site size and rehab push systems toward school sprawl. *Charlotte Observer*, Sep. 3, 2001; Website of Citistates Group. Available at http://citistates.com. Accessed Nov. 18, 2002.

23. Koplan JP, Dietz WH. Caloric imbalance and public health policy. *JAMA*, 1999;282:1579–1581.

24. Surface Transportation Policy Project. Report entitled *Mean Streets 2000: a transportation and quality of life campaign report*. Available at www.transact.org. Accessed Sep. 15, 2002.

25. Bell AC, Ge K, Popkin BM. The road to obesity or the path to prevention: motorized transportation and obesity in China. *Obesity Research*, 2002;10:277–283.

26. Berrigan D, Troiano RP. The association between urban form and physical activity in U.S. adults. *American Journal of Preventive Medicine*, 2002;23(Suppl):74–79.

27. Robinson TN, Hammer LD, Killen JD, Kraemer HC, Wilson DM, Hayward C, Taylor CB. Does television viewing increase obesity and reduce physical activity? Cross-sectional and longitudinal analyses among adolescent girls. *Pediatrics*, 1993;91:273–280; Andersen RE, Crespo CJ, Bartlett SJ, Cheskin LJ, Pratt M. Relationship of physical activity and television watching with body weight and level of fatness among children:

results from the third National Health and Nutrition Examination Survey. *JAMA*, 1998;279:938–942; Hu FB, Leitzmann MF, Stampfer MJ, Colditz GA, Willett WC, Rimm EB. Physical activity and television watching in relation to risk for type 2 diabetes mellitus in men. *Archives of Internal Medicine*, 2001;161:1542–1548.

28. Salzer J. State may let districts make rules on PE class; Board of Education votes to leave decision on grades 6–8 to each system. *Atlanta Journal and Constitution*, May 12, 2000, 1E.

29. Centers for Disease Control and Prevention. Youth risk behavior surveillance–United States, 1999. *Morbidity and Mortality Weekly Report 2000*, 1999;49:1–94; Secretary of Health and Human Services and Secretary of Education. Promoting better health for young people through physical activity and sports: A report to the President. Fall, 2000. Available online: www.cdc.gov/nccdphp/dash/presphysactrpt. Accessed Sep. 9, 2001; Kilborn P. No work for a bicycle thief: children pedal around less. *New York Times*, Jun. 7, 1999, A1; Strauss R, Rodzilsky D, Burack G, Cokin M. Psychosocial correlates of physical activity in healthy children. *Archives of Pediatric and Adolescent Medicine*, 2001;155:897–902; Trost SG, Pate RR, Ward DS, Saunders R, Riner W. Determinants of physical activity in active and low-active sixth grade African American youth. *Journal of School Health*, 1999;69:29–34.

30. Davies GA. Talking school sport: government physical education requirements "too low." *The Daily Telegraph*, Jul. 17, 2002.

31. Sallis JF, Conway TL, Prochaska JJ, McKenzie TL, Marshall SJ, Brown M. The association of school environments with youth physical activity. *American Journal of Public Health*, 2001;91:618–620.

32. American Heart Association. Children's need for physical activity: Fact sheet. Available online: www.americanheart.org/Health/Lifestyle?Physical_Activity?ChildFac.html. Accessed Mar. 22, 2001.

33. National Association for Sport and Physical Education. Shape of the Nation Report. Available online: http://fyi.cnn.com/2001/fyi/teachers.ednews/10/10/fitness.ed.ap/index.html. Accessed Oct. 12, 2001.

34. National Association of State Boards of Education (NASBE). Policy Update, Feb. 1997;5.

35. Simons-Morton BG, Taylor WC, Snider SA, Huang IW. The physical activity of fifth-grade students during physical education classes. *American Journal of Public Health*, 1993;83:262–264.

36. Sallis JF, Conway TL, Prochaska JJ, McKenzie TL, Marshall SJ, Brown M. The association of school environments with youth physical activity. *American Journal of Public Health*, 2001;91:618–620; U.S. Department of Health and Human Services Prevention Report. Available at www.cdc.gov/nccdphp/dnpa/physicalactivity.htm. Accessed Oct. 24, 2002.

37. Sallis JF, Bauman A, Pratt M. Environmental and policy interventions to promote physical activity. *American Journal of Preventive Medicine*, 1998;15:379–397; Pate RR, Trost SG, Mullis R, Sallis JF, Wechsler H, Brown DR. Community interventions to promote proper nutrition and physical activity among youth. *Preventive Medicine*, 2000;31:S138–S149; King AC. Community and public health approaches to the promotion of physical activity. *Medicine and Science in Sports and Exercise*, 1994;26:1405–1412.

38. U.S. Department of Health and Human Services Prevention Report. Available at www.cdc.gov/nccdphp/dnpa/physicalactivity.htm. Accessed Oct. 24, 2002.

39. Colorado on the Move project website. Available at www.coloradoonthemove.com. Accessed Sep. 2, 2002.

40. Pronk N. Presentation to joint meeting of Kaiser Permanente and the Centers for Disease Control and Prevention, Denver, June 28, 2002. Information on the 10,000 Steps program available at www.healthpartners.com/Menu/0,1791,1630,00.html. Accessed Sep. 2, 2002; Lindberg R. Active living: on the road with the 10,000 Steps program. *Journal of the American Dietetic Association*, 2000;100:878–879.

41. The Elevator Escalator Safety Foundation. Available at www.eesf.org/fact.htm. Accessed Sep. 15, 2002.

42. Brownell KD, Stunkard AJ, Albaum JM. Evaluation and modification of exercise patterns in the natural environment. *American Journal of Psychiatry*, 1980;137:1540–1545.

43. Blamey A, Mutrie N, Aitchison T. Health promotion by encouraged use of stairs. *BMJ*, 1995;311:289–290.

44. Andersen RE, Franckowiak SC, Snyder J, Bartlett SJ, Fontaine KR. Can inexpensive signs encourage the use of stairs? Results from a community intervention. *Annals of Internal Medicine*, 1998;129:363–369; Andersen RE, Franckowiak SC, Zuzak KB, Cummings ES, Crespo CJ. Community intervention to encourage stair use among African American commuters. *Medicine and Science in Sports and Exercise*. 2000;32 (suppl):S38.

45. Boutelle KN, Jeffery RW, Murray DM, Schmitz KH. Using signs, artwork, and music to promote stair use in a public building. *American Journal of Public Health*, 2001;91:2004–2006.

46. Coleman KJ, Gonzalez EC. Promoting stair use in a U.S.–Mexico border community. *American Journal of Public Health*, 2001;91:2007–2009.

47. O'Regan E. Oh boy, girls are left trailing when it comes to exercise. *Irish Independent*, Aug. 8, 2001. Available online: www.unison.ie.irish_independent/stories.php3?ca-9&si=489698&issue_id=5023&printer=1. Accessed Jan. 7, 2002.

48. *Philippine Daily News*. Thai elementary school launches weight loss program for students. Aug. 8, 2001.

49. Smithers R. Teachers seek school car ban: Quarter mile exclusion zone would improve health and help children gain independence. CDC Physical Activity E-mail Roster. Jul. 27, 1999.

50. Lantin B. Health and well-being: Ways to keep children on the hop concentrating on fun, not sport, encourages youngsters to get active. *Daily Telegraph* (London), Mar. 2, 2000, 24.

51. *National Post*. Huge study tests fitness of Nova Scotia kids. Sep. 20, 2001.

52. McKenzie TL, Stone EJ, Feldman HA, Epping JN, Yang M, Strikmiller PK, Lytle LA, Parcel GS. Effects of the CATCH physical education intervention: teacher type and lesson location. *American Journal of Preventive Medicine*, 2001;21:101–109; Nader PR, Stone EJ, Lytle LA, Perry CL, Osganian SK, Kelder S, Webber LS, Elder JP, Montgomery D, Feldman HA, Wu M, Johnson C, Parcel GS, Luepker RV. Three-year maintenance of improved diet and physical activity: the CATCH cohort. Child and Adolescent Trial for Cardiovascular Health. *Archives of Pediatrics & Adolescent Medicine*, 1999;153:695–704; Sallis JF, McKenzie TL, Alcaraz JE, Kolody B, Faucette N, Hovell MF. The effects of a two-year physical education program (SPARK) on physical activity and fitness in elementary school students. Sports, Play and Active Recreation for Kids. *American Journal of Public Health*, 1997;87:1328–1334.

53. Sallis J, McKenzie T, Kolody B, Lewis M, Marshall S, Rosengard P. Effects of health-related physical education on academic achievement: Project SPARK. *Research Quarterly for Exercise and Sport*, 1999;70:127–134; Daley A, Ryan J. Academic performance and participation in physical activity by secondary school adolescents. *Perceptual and Motor Skills*, 2000;91:531–534.

54. Hillman CH, Weiss EP, Hagberg JM, Hatfield BD. The relationship of age and cardiovascular fitness to cognitive and motor processes. *Psychophysiology*, 2002;39:303–312.

55. U.S. Department of Health and Human Services. Physical activity and health: A report of the Surgeon General. Atlanta, GA: U.S. Department of Health and Human Services, Centers for Disease Control and Prevention, National Center for Chronic Disease Prevention and Health Promotion, 1996; Escobedo L, Marcus S, Holtzman D, Giovino G. Sports participation, age at smoking initiation, and the risk of smoking among U.S. high school students. *JAMA*, 1993;269:1391–1395; Zill N, Nord C, Loomis L. Adolescent time use, risky behavior, and outcomes: An analysis of national data. Rockville, MD: Westat, 1995; Secretary of Health and Human Services and Secretary of Education. Promoting better health for young people through physical activity and sports: A report to the President. Available online: www.cdc.gov/nccdphp/dash/presphysactrpt. Fall, 2000. Accessed Sep. 1, 2001. Pate R, Health G, Dowda M, Trost S. Associations between physical activity and other health behaviors in a representative sample of U.S. adolescents. *American Journal of Public Health*, 1996;86:1577–1581.

56. International Food Information Council website. Available at www.ific.org. Accessed Oct. 23, 2002.

57. King A. Community and public health approaches to the promotion of physical activity. *Medicine and Science in Sports and Exercise*, 1994;26:1405–1412; Sallis J, Bauman A, Pratt M. Environmental and policy interventions to promote physical activity. *American Journal of Preventive Medicine*, 1998;15:379–397.

58. Department of Health and Human Services, Centers for Disease Control and Prevention. Kidswalk-to-School: A Guide to Promote Walking to School. Available at www.cdc.gov/nccdphp/dnpa/kidswalk/resources.htm. Accessed Sep. 23, 2002.

59. Canadian Association for the Advancement of Women and Sport and Physical Activity. On-the-move walking clubs. Aug. 16, 2001. Available online: www.caaws.ca/Whats_New/aug01/on-the-move.htm. Accessed Sep. 1, 2001.

60. Available online: www.bikesbelong.org. Accessed Jul. 10, 2000.

61. Olken R. Bikes Belong Coalition awards second grant to Los Angeles County Bicycle Coalition. Aug. 2, 2000. Available online: www.bikesbelong.org. Accessed Aug. 16, 2000.

62. National Walkable Community Teleconference. Available online: www.lgc.org/clc. Jun. 11, 1999. Accessed May 24, 1999.

63. Jilla S. Cycling can add two years to your life, so it's about time you got out of your car. *Sunday Times* (UK), Aug. 5, 2001, 38.

64. King A. Community and public health approaches to the promotion of physical activity. *Medicine and Science in Sports and Exercise*, 1994;26:1405–1412.

65. Troped PJ, Saunders RP, Pate RR, Reininger B, Ureda JR, Thompson SJ. Associations between self-reported and objective physical environmental factors and use of a community rail-trail. *Preventive Medicine*, 2001;32:191–200; Brownson RC, Housemann RA, Brown DR, Jackson-Thompson J, Kind AC, Malone BR, Sallis JF. Promoting physical activity in rural communities: walking trail access, use, and effects. *American Journal of Preventive Medicine*, 2000;18:235–241.

66. Testimony of Keith Laughlin, President of the Rails-to-Trails Conservancy before the subcommittee on Highways and Transit of the House Committee on Transportation and Infrastructure, U.S. House of Representatives, Jul. 22, 2002. Available at www.railstrails.org/whatwedo/policy/testimony0725.htm. Accessed Sep. 19, 2002.

67. Centers for Disease Control and Prevention website on resources and programs for increasing physical activity. Available at www.cdc.gov/nccdphp/dnpa/physicalactivity.htm. Accessed Oct. 24, 2002.

68. Webster B. Children on bicycles learn to beat the school-run blues. *The London Times*, June 17, 2002.

69. Wyatt K. Health officials say only a quarter of U.S. children regularly walk or bike to school. Associated Press, Aug. 15, 2002.

70. Sustrans website. Available at www.sustrans.org.uk/webcode/home.asp. Accessed Nov. 18, 2002; National Cycle Network in Devon website. Available at www.devon.gov.uk/tourism/ncn. Accessed Nov. 18, 2002; Walters J. Joanna Walters braves tempest and hungry horses on Britain's new rural cycle paths. *The Observer*, Aug. 4, 2002.

71. Reger B, Cooper L, Booth-Butterfield S, Smith H, Bauman A, Wootan M, Middlestadt S, Marcus B, Greer F. Wheeling Walks: a community campaign using paid media to encourage walking among sedentary older adults. *Preventive Medicine*, 2002;35:285–292; Hellmich N. A city sold on fitness: Wheeling dealing with lots of new ad-inspired walkers. *USA Today*, Aug. 29, 2001.

72. Indy in Motion website from Indianapolis. Available at www.mchd.com/iim_launch.htm. Accessed Nov. 18, 2002; Hagen P. Kick into motion: A new program uses walking in parks and free fitness classes to tackle obesity. *Indianapolis Star*, Oct. 25, 2002.

73. Dunn AL, Marcus BH, Kampert JB, Garcia ME, Kohl HW 3rd, Blair SN. Comparison of lifestyle and structured interventions to increase physical activity and cardiorespiratory fitness: a randomized trial. *JAMA*, 1999;281:327–334; Sevick MA, Dunn AL, Morrow MS, Marcus BH, Chen GJ, Blair SN. Cost-effectiveness of lifestyle and structured exercise interventions in sedentary adults: results of project ACTIVE. *American Journal of Preventive Medicine*, 2000;19:1–8.

74. Associated Press. Fit workers have fewer injuries. *Holland Sentinel*. Jul. 13, 2001. Available online: www.hollandsentinel.com/stories/071101/bus_0711010035.shtml. Accessed Sep. 9, 2001.

75. Website of the Sisters Together: Move more, eat better program. Available at www.niddk.nih.gov/health/nutri/sisters/sisters.htm. Accessed Oct. 27, 2002.

76. Gortmaker SL, Peterson K, Wiecha J, Sobol AM, Dixit S, Fox MK, Laird N. Reducing obesity via a school-based interdisciplinary intervention among youth: Planet Health. *Archives of Pediatrics & Adolescent Medicine*, 1999;153:409–418; Planet Health program website, done through the Harvard School of Public health. Available at www.hsph.harvard.edu/prc/planet.html. Accessed Oct. 30, 2002.

77. Haines A, McMichael T, Anderson R, Houghton J. Fossil fuels, transport, and public health. *BMJ*, 2000;321:1168–1169.

78. Secretary of Health and Human Services and Secretary of Education (Fall 2000). Promoting better health for young people through physical activity and sports: A report to the President. Available online: www.cdc.gov/nccdphp/dash/presphysactrpt. Accessed Sep. 1, 2001.

79. *Nation's Health*. From the American Public Health Association. Obesity rates increasing among youth: Daily physical education, activity crucial for youth. Feb. 2001, 1.

80. Press conference held by President Bush, June 20, 2002. Available at www.whitehouse.gov/news/releases/2002/06/20020620-2.html. Accessed Oct. 30, 2002.

81. Blair SN, Booth M, Gyarfas I, Iwane H, Marti B, Matsudo V, Morrow MS, Noakes T, Shephard R. Development of public policy and physical activity initiatives internationally. *Sports Medicine*, 2000; 154:904–911; U.S. Department of Health and Human Services. *Physical Activity and Health: Report of the Surgeon General*. Atlanta, GA: U.S. Department of Health and Human Services, Centers for Disease Control, National Center for Chronic Disease Prevention and Health Promotion, 1996; Brownson RC, Baker EA, Housemann RA, Brennan LK, Bacak SJ. Environmental and policy determinants of physical activity in the United States. *American Journal of Public Health*, 2001;91:1995–2003.

82. Website of the Surface Transportation Policy Project. Available at www.transact.org. Accessed Oct. 27, 2002; Speech of Barbara McCann, Campaign Director of the Surface Transportation Policy Project before Congressional Health Fair for the U.S. House of Representatives, June, 2002.

83. Brownson RC, Housemann RA, Brown DR, Jackson-Thompson J, Kind AC, Malone BR, Sallis JF. Promoting physical activity in rural communities: walking trail access, use, and effects. *American Journal of Preventive Medicine*, 2000;18:235–241; Tudor-Locke C, Ainsworth BE, Popkin BM. Active commuting to school: an overlooked source of children's physical activity? *Sports Medicine*, 2001;31:309–313; King AC, Castro C, Wilcox S, Eyler AA, Sallis JF, Brownson RC. Personal and environmental factors associated with physical inactivity among different racial-ethnic groups of U.S. middle-aged and older-aged women. *Health Psychology*, 2000;19:354–364.

84. American Academy of Pediatrics. Physical fitness and activity in schools (Policy Statement). *Pediatrics*, 2000;105:1156–1157.

85. Desmon S. Pupils often skip gym in Arundel middle schools. County calls it elective; state says it's required. *Baltimore Sun*, Mar. 1, 2001,1B.

86. Hartocollis A. Study faults gym program in city schools. *New York Times*, Mar. 3, 2001, B1.

87. Centers for Disease Control. Guidelines for school and community programs to promote lifelong physical activity among young people. *Morbidity and Mortality Weekly Report*, 1997;46:1–36.

88. P.E.4Life website. Available at www.pe4life.org. Accessed Apr. 12, 2003.

89. McMurray RG, Harrell JS, Bangdiwala SI, Bradley CB, Deng S, Levine A. A school-based intervention can reduce body fat and blood pressure in young adolescents. *Journal of Adolescent Health*, 2002;31:125–132.
90. Epstein LH, Paluch RA, Consalvi A, Riordan K, Scholl T. Effects of manipulating sedentary behavior on physical activity and food intake. *Journal of Pediatrics*, 2002;140:334–339; Saelens BE. The rate of sedentary activities determines the reinforcing value of physical activity. *Health Psychology*, 1999;18:655–659.
91. Dietz WH. The obesity epidemic in young children. Reduce television viewing and promote playing. *BMJ*, 2001;322:313–314; Robinson TN. Reducing children's television viewing to prevent obesity: a randomized controlled trial. *JAMA*, 1999;282:1561–1567.
92. Shephard RJ. Work site fitness and exercise programs: A review of methodology and health impact. *American Journal of Health Promotion*, 1996;10:436–452.
93. PACE Project website. Available at www.paceproject.org. Accessed Sep. 8, 2002. This site contains information about PACE, along with published papers on the topic; The Writing Group for the Activity Counseling Trial Research Group. Effects of physical activity counseling in primary care: the Activity Counseling Trial; a randomized controlled trial. *JAMA*, 2001;286:677–687; Wee CC. Physical activity counseling in primary care: the challenge of effecting behavior change. *JAMA*, 2001;286:677–687; Goldstein MG, Pinto BM, Marcus BH, Lynn H, Jette AM, McDermott S, DePue JD, Milan FB, Dube C, Tennstedt S, Rakowski W. Physician-based physical activity counseling for middle-aged and older adults: a randomized trial. *Annals of Behavioral Medicine*, 2001;21:40–47.

Chapter 5

1. Willett W. The food pushers (review of M. Nestle's book *Food Politics*). *Science*, 2002;297:198–199.
2. (a) M&M's (b) Kit Kat (c) Coca-Cola (d) Lucky Charms (e) Lay's potato chips (f) Folgers (g) Trix (h) Life (i) McDonald's (j) Burger King (k) Campbell Soup (l) Frosted Flakes (m) Cocoa Puffs (n) Skittles (o) Mountain Dew (p) KFC (q) Sprite (r) Rice Krispies (s) Pork (t) McDonald's
3. *Advertising Age*. The Advertising Century. Available at www.adage.com/century. Accessed Nov. 13, 2002.
4. Horovitz B. McDonald's going after the small fry. *USA Today*, Oct. 8, 1998, 3B.
5. Food Commission. Advertising to children: UK the worst in Europe. *Food Magazine*, 1997, Jan/Mar.
6. Avery R, Mathios A, Shanahan J, Bisogni C. Food and nutrition messages communicated through prime-time television. *Journal of Public Policy & Marketing*, 1997;16:217–233; Zuckerman D, Zuckerman S. Television's impact on children. *Pediatrics*, 1985;75: 233–240; Roberts D, Foehr U, Rideout V, Brodie M. Kids and media at the new millennium: A comprehensive national analysis of children's media use. Menlo Park, California: The Henry J. Kaiser Family Foundation Report, 1999; Committee on Public Education. Children, adolescents, and television. *Pediatrics*, 2001;107: 423–426.
7. Self Regulatory Guidelines for Children's Advertising. Available at www.bbb.org/advertising/childad.asp. Accessed Dec. 20, 2001.
8. Jackson D. Black families need to live with less TV. *Boston Globe*, Aug. 24, 2001, A25.
9. Certain LK, Kahn RS. Prevalence, correlates, and trajectory of television viewing among infants and toddlers. *Pediatrics*, 2002;109:634–642.
10. Consoli J. Television: clutter climbs higher. *Mediaweek*, A/S/M Communications, Inc., Apr. 12, 1999.
11. Television Bureau of Advertising (1998). TV Basics. Available at www.tvb.org/tvfacts/index.html. Accessed Oct. 15, 1999.
12. Nestle M, Jacobson MF. Halting the obesity epidemic: A public health policy approach. *Public Health Reports*, 2000;115:12–24.
13. Food Commission. Advertising to children: UK the worst in Europe. *Food Magazine*, 1997, Jan./Mar.
14. Television Bureau of Advertising. TV Basics. Available at www.tvb.org/tvfacts/index.html. Accessed Dec. 15, 2001.
15. Kunkle D, Roberts D. Young minds and marketplace values: Issues in children's advertising. *Journal of Social Issues*, 1991;47: 57–72.
16. McNeal J. *Kids as Customers: A Handbook of Marketing to Children*. Lexington, MA: Lexington Books, 1992; Del Vecchio G. *Creating Ever-Cool: A Marketer's Guide to a Kid's Heart*. Gretna, LA: Pelican, 1997; Acuff DS, Reiher RH. *What Kids Buy and Why: The Psychology of Marketing to Kids*. New York: Free Press, 1997.
17. Center for Media Education. Marketing to children harmful: Experts urge candidate to lead nation in setting limits. Press Release. Available online: www.cme.org/press/001018pr.html. Accessed Aug. 2, 2001.
18. Vaeth E. Fast-food restaurants aim ad dollars at kiddie market. *Atlanta Business Chronicle*, Oct. 20, 1997.
19. Campbell K, Davis-Packard K. How ads get kids to say, "I want it!" *Christian Science Monitor*, Sep. 18, 2000, 1.

20. Consumer's Union. Selling America's kids: Commercial pressures on kids of the '90s. Consumer's Union Educational Services Department, Yonkers, NY, quote from p. 1. Available at www.igc.org/consunion/other/sellingkids.summary.htm. Accessed Sep. 22, 2001.

21. Taras HL, Gage M. Advertised foods on children's television. *Archives of Pediatrics and Adolescent Medicine*, 1995;149:649–652; Horgen KB, Choate M, Brownell KD. Food advertising: targeting children in a toxic environment. In DG Singer & JL Singer (Eds) *Handbook of Children and the Media*. Thousand Oaks, CA: Sage, pp. 447–462; Center for Media Education (1998). The Campaign for Kids' TV: Children and Television. www.cme.org. Accessed Oct. 1, 1999; Williams JO, Achterberg C, Sylvester GP. Targeting marketing of food products to ethnic minority youths. In CL Williams & SYS Kimm (Eds) Prevention and treatment of childhood obesity. *Annals of the New York Academy of Sciences*, 1993;699:107–114; Cotunga N. TV ads on Saturday morning children's programming: What's new? *Journal of Nutrition Education*, 1998;20:125–127.

22. Gussow J. It even makes milk a dessert: A report on the counternutritional messages of children's television advertising. *Clinical Pediatrics*, 1973;12:68–71.

23. Kotz K, Story M. Food advertisements during children's Saturday morning television programming: Are they consistent with dietary recommendations? *Journal of the American Dietetic Association*, 1994;94: 1296–1300; Wallack L, Dorfman L. Health messages on television commercials. *American Journal of Health Promotion*, 1992;6:190–196.

24. McCollum C. Fast food chains get jump on holiday season with movie promotions. *San Jose Mercury News*, Nov. 22, 1998. Available online: http://web.lexis-nexis.com/universe/docu...zV&_md5=9a30829469b08 bcafc57eb0c55d26eaf. Accessed Aug. 15, 2001.

25. Keebler Corporation Chips Deluxe: Everything about our best-selling cookie is magical! 1997 Annual Report.

26. Bell R. Advertising. Judgment: Justice Bell's Verdict, Section 7. Jun. 19, 1997. Available at www.mcspot light.org/case/trial/verdict/verdict_jud2b.html. Accessed Nov. 17, 2002; Jacobson M. Center for Science in the Public Interest. Liquid candy: How soft drinks are harming Americans' health. Available at www.cspi net.org/sodapop/liquid_candy.htm. Accessed Aug. 6, 2001.

27. Lewis C, Lewis M. The impact of television commercials on health-related beliefs and behaviors of children. *Pediatrics*, 1974;53:431–435; Martin M. Children's understanding of the intent of advertising: A meta-analysis. *Journal of Public Policy and Marketing*, 1997;16:205–224; Kunkle D, Roberts D. Young minds and marketplace values: Issues in children's advertising. *Journal of Social Issues*, 1991;47:57–72.

28. Kunkel D. Children and television advertising. In DG Singer & J L Singer (Eds) *The Handbook of Children and Media*. Thousand Oaks, CA: Sage, 2001, pp. 375–393.

29. Donahue T, Meyer T, Henke L. Black and white children's perceptions of television commercials. *Journal of Marketing*, 1978;42:34–40.

30. Leiber L. Commercial and character slogan recall by children aged 9–11 years: Budweiser versus Bugs Bunny. Center on Alcohol Advertising, Trauma Foundation, 1996.

31. Fischer P, Schwartz M, Richards J, Goldstein A, Rojas T. Brand logo recognition by children aged 3 to 6 years. Mickey Mouse and Old Joe Camel. *Journal of the American Medical Association*, 1991;266:3145–3148.

32. Dibb S. Advertising: Witnesses (Statement of advertising researcher, witness for defense). Nov. 1994. Available at www.mcspotlight.org/cgi-bin/zv/people/witnesses/advertising/dibb_sue.html. Accessed Nov. 17, 2002.

33. Gorn GJ, Goldberg ME. The impact of television advertising on children from low-income families. *Journal of Consumer Research*, 1997;4:86–88; Borzekowski DL, Robinson TN. The 30-second effect: An experiment revealing the impact of television commercials on food preferences in preschoolers. *Journal of the American Dietetic Association*, 2001;101:42–46.

34. Grube JW, Wallack L. Television beer advertising and drinking knowledge, beliefs, and intentions among school children. *American Journal of Public Health*, 1994;84:254–259.

35. Signorelli N, Staples J. Television and children's conception of nutrition. *Health Communication*, 1997;9:289–301.

36. Galst JP, White MA. The unhealthy persuader: The reinforcing value of television and children's purchase-influencing attempts at the supermarket. *Child Development*, 1996;47:1089–1096.

37. Goldberg ME, Gorn GJ, Gibson W. TV messages for snack and breakfast foods: Do they influence children's preferences? *Journal of Consumer Research*, 1978;5:73–81.

38. Taras HL, Sallis JF, Patterson TL, Nader PR, Nelson JA. Television's influence on children's diet and physical activity. *Journal of Developmental & Behavioral Pediatrics*, 1989;10:176–180.

39. Coon KA, Goldberg J, Rogers BL, Tucker KL. Relationships between use of television during meals and children's food consumption patterns. *Pediatrics*, 2001;107:E7; Dennison BA, Erb TA, Jenkins PL. Is family dinnertime undone by TV? *Obesity Research*, 2001;9:92S.

40. Carruth BR, Goldberg DL, Skinner JD. Do parents and peers mediate the influence of television advertising on food-related purchases? *Journal of Adolescent Research*, 1991;6:253–271.

41. Atkin CK. Television advertising and socialization to consumer role. In D Pearl, L Bouthilet, J Lazar (Eds) *Television and Behavior: Ten Years of Scientific Progress and Implications for the Eighties.* Rockville, MD: National Institute of Mental Health, 1982, pp. 191–200; Liebert RM, Sprafkin JN, *The Early Window: Effects of Television on Children and Youth* (3rd Ed). New York: Pergamon, 1988; Horgen KB, Choate M, Brownell KD. Food advertising: targeting children in a toxic environment. In DG Singer & JL Singer (Eds) *Handbook of Children and the Media.* Thousand Oaks, CA: Sage, pp. 447–462.

42. American Academy of Pediatrics, Committee on Communications. Children, adolescents, and advertising. *Pediatrics*, 1995;95:295–297. Available at www.aap.org/policy/00656.html. Accessed Aug. 18, 2002.

43. Dennison BA, Erb TA, Jenkins PL. Television viewing and television in bedroom associated with overweight risk among low-income preschool children. *Pediatrics*, 2002:109:1028–1035.

44. Miller SH. Feeding fast-food's frenzy: McDonald's latest item joins a crowded field of trinketlike toys. *Indianapolis Star*, May 22, 1999, B01.

45. The supermarket surveyed was the Super Stop & Shop in Branford, Connecticut. Fourteen-year-old Kristy Brownell and ten-year-old Greg Nobile identified TV and movie characters. Survey completed in September, 2002.

46. General Mills website. Available at www.generalmills.com/careeropportunities/ourcareers_promotion.asp. Accessed Aug. 12, 2002.

47. Talaski K. Kellogg, Disney unite for breakfast: co-branded products to promote characters on a daily basis. *Detroit News*, Sep.6, 2001. Available online: http://detnews.com/2001/business/0109/07/b01-286526.htm. Accessed Aug. 13, 2002.

48. Netactive website. Success story: Disney Interactive, General Mills, & EarthLink. Available online: www.netactive.com. Accessed Aug. 15, 2002.

49. Frito-Lay (PepsiCo) press release. The Walt Disney Company and Frito-Lay form multi-year strategic alliance. Oct. 10, 2002. Available at www.pepsico.com/news/fritolay/2002/20021010f.shtml. Accessed Dec. 19, 2002.

50. Entertainment Resources & Marketing Association website. Available at www.erma.org/nav/frame.html. Accessed Nov. 18, 2002.

51. Feature This! corporate website. Available at www.featurethis.com/celeb_endrs.html. Accessed Nov. 17, 2002.

52. Memo from Rogers & Cowan, Inc., June 19, 1980. Available at www.library.ucsf.edu/tobacco/mangini/html/cc/022/otherpages/2.html. Accessed Nov. 18, 2002.

53. Bates J. Summer Sneaks: Attack of the Killer Tot Meals. May 11, 1997.

54. Natale R. The surreal thing: Use of computer graphics in product placement. *Los Angeles Magazine*, Sept., 1999.

55. Website for *Kidscreen* magazine. Available at www.kidscreen.com. Accessed Nov. 15, 2002.

56. Kid Power Xchange website. Available at www.kidpowerx.com/index.htm. Accessed Nov. 15, 2002.

57. Article from *Selling to Kids* magazine. Available at www.findarticles.com/cf_dls/m0FVE/1_6/69482549/p1/article.jhtml. Accessed Nov. 15, 2002.

58. Kids and your bottom line. *Restaurant Hospitality*, 2000;84:49.

59. Leo Burnett website. Available at www.leoburnett.com/content/contacts/recruiting/chicago.html. Accessed Nov. 16, 2002.

60. Horovitz B. McDonald's rediscovers its future with kids. *USA Today*, Apr. 18, 1997.

61. American Academy of Pediatrics, Committee on Communications. Children, adolescents, and advertising. *Pediatrics*, 1995;95:295–297. Available at www.aap.org/policy/00656.html. Accessed Aug. 18, 2002.

62. Stop Commercial Exploitation of Children website. Available at www.commercialexploitation.com. Accessed Aug. 22, 2002.

63. Center for Media Education (1998). The Campaign for Kids' TV: Children and Television. Available at www.cme.org. Accessed Oct. 1, 1999.

64. The "Save Harry" website of the Center for Science in the Public Interest. Available at http://saveharry.com. Accessed Nov. 16, 2002.

65. The Lancet. Selling to—and selling out—children. *Lancet*, 2002;360:959; McLellan F. Marketing and advertising: Harmful to children's health. *Lancet*, 2002;360:1001.

66. Children's Advertising Review Unit. Available at www.caru.org. Accessed Nov. 16, 2002.

67. Gotting P. Junk food meeting to discuss ban on TV ads. *The Sydney Morning Herald*, Jun. 20, 2002.

68. Shanahan M. Under fire, state dilutes anti-soda ads. *Portland Press Herald*, Nov. 16, 2002.

69. Examples of writing and testimony of Guy Johnson on behalf of the National Soft Drink Association. Available at www.nsda.org/softdrinks/CSDHealth/guyjohnson.html and www.cga.state.ct.us/2002/jfr/s/2002SB-00584-R00PH-JFR.htm. Accessed Nov. 16, 2002.

70. Quote from Guy Johnson testifying before the New York State Assembly. Available at www.consumerfreedom.com/headline_detail.cfm?HEADLINE_ID=1405. Accessed Nov. 16, 2002.

71. Shanahan, op. cit.

72. Advertising Research Resource Center. Available online at www.advertising.utexas.edu/research/biblio/FTC.html. Accessed Oct. 19, 2001.

73. Federal Trade Commission (May 1994). Enforcement Policy Statement on Food Advertising. Available at www.ftc.gov/bcp/policystmt/ad-food.htm. Accessed Oct. 19, 2001.

74. Pearson L, Lewis K. Preventive intervention to improve children's discrimination of the persuasive tactics in televised advertising. *Journal of Pediatric Psychology*, 1998:13:163–170.

75. Goldberg ME, Gorn GJ, Gibson W. TV messages for snack and breakfast foods: Do they influence children's preferences? *Journal of Consumer Research*, 1978;5:73–81.

76. Galst JP. Television food commercials and pro-nutritional public services announcements as determinants of young children's snack choices. *Child Development*, 1980;51:935–938.

77. Gorn GJ, Goldberg ME. Behavioral evidence of the effects of televised food messages on children. *Journal of Consumer Research*, 1982;9:200–205.

78. Robinson T. Reducing children's television viewing to prevent obesity. *Journal of the American Medical Association*, 1999;282:1561–1567.

79. Taras HL, Sallis JF, Nader PR, Nelson J. Children's television viewing habits and the family environment. *American Journal of Diseases of Children*, 1990;144:357–359.

80. Hogan M, Bar-on M, Beard L, Corrigan S, Gedissman A, Palumbo F, Rich M, Shifrin D, Roberts M, Villani S, Holroyd J, Sherry NS, Strasburger V. Media education. *Pediatrics*, 1999;104:341–343.

81. Faith M, Berman N, Heo M, Pietrobelli A, Gallagher D, Epstein L, Eiden M, Allison D. Effects of contingent television on physical activity and television viewing in obese children. *Pediatrics*, 2001:107:1043–1048.

82. Smart-Mouth.org website of the Center for Science in the Public Interest. Available at www.cspinet.org/smartmouth. Accessed Nov. 16, 2002.

83. Government of Quebec website. Available at http://publicationsduquebec.gouv.qc.ca/fr/cgi/frameset .cgi?url=/documents/lr/P_40_1/P40_1_A.html. Accessed Aug. 22, 2002.

84. Website of Stop Commercial Exploitation of Children. Available at www.commercialexploitation.com/scholastic_victory.htm. Accessed Nov. 16, 2002.

85. Valkenburg P. Media and youth consumerism. *Journal of Adolescent Health*, 2000;27 (Suppl.2):52–56.

86. Roper poll covered in "Selling to kids: reading, writing, buying" from *Consumer Reports*, September 1998, p. 46; Lake, Snell, Perry, and Associates. *Television in the digital age: A report to the Project on Media Ownership and the Benton Foundation*, December, 1998.

87. Department of Health and Human Services. *The Surgeon General's Call to Action: Prevent and Decrease Overweight and Obesity*. Washington, DC: U.S. Government Printing Office, 2001.

88. Oliver JE, Lee T. Public opinion and the politics of America's obesity epidemic. Paper submitted to the *American Journal of Political Science*. Available at http://ksgnotes1.harvard.edu/Research/wpaper.nsf/rwp/RWP02-017/$File/rwp02_017_lee.pdf. Accessed Nov. 16, 2002; Olson BH. Paper for presentation at the annual Experimental Biology meeting. Contact is Dr. Beth Olson at Michigan State University.

89. American Academy of Pediatrics, Committee on Communications. Children, adolescents, and advertising. *Pediatrics*, 1995;95:295–297. Available at www.aap.org/policy/00656.html. Accessed Aug. 18, 2002; Center for Media Education, Institute for Public Representation. *A Report on Station Compliance with the Children's Television Act*. Washington, DC: Georgetown University Law Center, 1992.

90. Singer DG, Singer JL (Eds) *Handbook of Children and the Media*. Thousand Oaks, CA: Sage, 2001.

91. Portions of this chapter were adapted from an earlier work by the authors (Horgen KB, Choate M, Brownell KD. Food advertising: targeting children in a toxic environment. In DG Singer & JL Singer (Eds) *Handbook of Children and the Media*. Thousand Oaks, CA: Sage, pp. 447–462).

Chapter 6

1. Manning S. Students for sale: how corporations are buying their way into America's classrooms. *The Nation*, Sep. 27, 1999.

2. Levine J. Food industry marketing in elementary schools: Implications for school health professionals. *Journal of School Health*, 1999;69:290–291.

3. Sullivan W. Schools sell fries to pay for books. *Yale Daily News*, Oct. 17, 2002. Available at www.yaledailynews.com/article.asp?AID=20193. Accessed Nov. 18, 2002.

4. Carter RC. The impact of public schools on childhood obesity. *JAMA*, 2002;288:2180; Story M. School-based approaches for preventing and treating obesity. *International Journal of Obesity*, 1999:23:S43–S51.

5. Study conducted between 12/1/02 and 1/18/02 on The Status of Vending Machines, Schools and Physical Activity in KY Schools. Conducted by the University of Kentucky Cooperative Extension, Lexington Fayette County Health Department, and the Kentucky Dept. of Public Health.

6. French SA, Fulkerson JA, Story M. School food policies and practices: A statewide survey of secondary school principals. *Journal of the American Dietetic Association*, in press.

7. Nutrition Program Facts, National School Lunch Program, Food and Nutrition Service, U.S. Department of Agriculture. Available at www.fns.usda.gov/cnd/Lunch. Accessed Nov. 20, 2002.

8. Background on the National School Lunch Program. Physicians Committee on Responsible Medicine. Available at www.healthyschoollunches.org/background.html. Accessed Nov. 20, 2002.

9. U.S. Department of Agriculture. Foods Sold in Competition with USDA School Meal Programs: A Report to Congress. Jan, 21, 2002. Available at www.fns.usda.gov/cnd/Lunch/CompetitiveFoods/report_congress .htm. Accessed Nov. 22, 2002.

10. French SA, Story M, Fulkerson JA, Gerlach AF. Food environment in secondary schools: A la carte, vending machines, food policies, and practices. *American Journal of Public Health*, in press; Kubik MY, Lytle LA, Hannan PJ, Perry CL, Story M. The association of the school food environment with dietary behaviors of young adolescents. *American Journal of Public Health*, in press; Widley MB, Pampalone SZ, Pelletier RL, Zive MM, Elder JP, Sallis JF. Fat and sugar levels are high in snacks purchased from student stores in middle schools. *Journal of the American Dietetic Association*, 2000;100:319–322.

11. Kubik MY, Lytle LA, Hannan PJ, Perry CL, Story M. The association of the school food environment with dietary behaviors of young adolescents. *American Journal of Public Health*, in press.

12. Rohde M. Cafeteria style: Nicolet students line up for fast food. *Milwaukee Journal Sentinel*, Sep. 16, 1998.

13. Consumer's Union. Selling America's kids: Commercial pressures on kids of the 90s. Summary. Available online: www.consumersunion.org/other/sellingkids/summary.htm. Accessed Jan. 11, 2002.

14. Primedia Inc. home page. Channel One network. Available online: www.primediainc.com. Accessed Aug. 7, 2002.

15. Coeyman, M. Follow the customer: New media ventures may help marketers target a market. *Restaurant Business*, 1995;94:36.

16. Brand J, Greenberg B. Commercials in the classroom: The impact of Channel One advertising. *Journal of Advertising Research*, 1994;34:18–23.

17. Schlafly R. Channel One comes under fire. Jun. 1999. Available at www.eagleforum.org/column/1999/june99/99-06-02.html. Accessed Aug. 7, 2001.

18. Richards J, Wartella E, Morton C, Thompson L. The growing commercialization of schools: Issues and practices. *Annals of the American Academy of Political and Social Science*, 1998;557:148–163.

19. Turn off Channel One. Editorial. *Seattle Times*, Mar. 8, 2000. Available at http://archives.seattletimes .nwsource.co...chaned&date=20000318&query=Channel percent2bOne. Accessed Aug. 17, 2001.

20. Adbusters. Watch or go to jail: Students locked up after refusing to watch Channel One. Available at http://adbusters.org/magazine/34/jail.html. Accessed Jan. 7, 2002.

21. Channel One still plays to captive audiences, but some schools are stopping the music. *Education Reporter*, Dec. 1998. Available at www.eagleforum.org/educate/1998/dec98/channel1.html. Accessed Aug. 7, 2001.

22. Obligation, Inc. Press releases about Channel One, 1998. Nov. 24, 1998. Available at www.obligation .org/ch198/html. Accessed Aug. 7, 2001.

23. Trotter A. Report blasts "hidden" public costs of Channel One news program. *Education Week on the Web*. Apr. 8, 1998. Available at wysiwyg://139/http://www.edweek.com/ew/vol-17/30chan.h17. Accessed Aug. 7, 2001.

24. Zernike K. Coke to dilute push in schools for its products. *New York Times*, Mar. 14, 2001, A1.

25. *Mathematics: Applications and Connections, Course 1*. New York: Glencoe/McGraw-Hill, 1999.

26. Manning S. Classrooms for sale. *New York Times*, Mar. 24, 1999; Hayes CL. New report examines commercialism in schools. *New York Times*, Sep. 14, 2000; Fisher M. Easy cash eroding their principles. *The Washington Post*, Feb. 27, 2001, B1.

27. *Education Reporter*. Study says commercialism rampant in public schools. *Education Reporter*, Nov. 2000. Available at www.eagleforum.org/educate/2000/nov00/commercialism.shtml. Accessed Aug. 7, 2001.

28. Consumers Union. Captive kids: A report on commercial pressures on kids at schools. Available at www.consumersunion.org/other/captivekids/prologue.htm. Accessed Nov. 22, 2002.

29. Consumer's Union. Selling America's kids: Commercial pressures on kids of the 90s. In *School Promotion*, p. 2. Available at www.consumersunion.org/other/sellingkids/inschoolpromo.htm. Accessed Jan. 11, 2002.

30. Ibid.

31. Molnar A, Morales J. Commercialism@school.com. Center for the Analysis of Commercialism in Education, Sep., 2000. Available at www.uwm.edu/Dept/CACE/documents/cace-oo-02.htm. Accessed Aug. 7, 2001.

32. Dunkin' Donuts website. Available at http://stores.dunkindonuts.com/newyork. Accessed Sep. 2, 2002.

33. Vorman J. Schools say NO to sodas. Oct. 21, 1998. Available at www.bus.utexas.edu/~west/wwwboard/messages/84.html. Accessed Aug. 3, 2001.

34. Commercialism in the schools. Available at wysiwyg://navrt.6/http://www.commercialfree.org/commercialismtext.html. Accessed Aug. 6, 2001.

35. *Education Reporter.* Study says commercialism rampant in public schools. *Education Reporter,* Nov. 2000, 178. Available at www.eagleforum.org/educate/2000/nov00/commercialism.shtml. Accessed Aug. 7, 2001.

36. Sandham J. From walls to roofs, schools sell ad space. *Education Week,* Jun. 4, 1997. Available at www.edweek.org/ew/ewstory.cfm?slug=36ads.h16&keywords=roofs. Accessed Nov. 18, 2002.

37. Rothstein R. Schools' chosen cure for money ills: a sugar pill. *New York Times,* Aug. 21, 2002.

38. National PTA website, position statement on commercialization in the classroom. Available at www.pta.org/ptawashington/issues/commercial.asp. Accessed Aug. 21, 2002.

39. Rothstein R. Schools' chosen cure for money ills: a sugar pill. *New York Times,* Aug. 21, 2002.

40. 60 *Federal Register* 31188 (1995) (codified at 7CFR 210, 220).

41. Cullen KW, Eagan J, Baranowski T, Owens E, deMoor C. Effects of a la carte and snack bar foods at school on children's lunchtime intake of fruits and vegetables. *Journal of the American Dietetic Association,* 2000;100:1482–1486.

42. Healthy school nutrition environments. U.S. Department of Agriculture website. Available at www.fns.usda.gov/cnd/healthyeating/default.htm. Accessed Nov. 18, 2002.

43. Wechsler H, Brener ND, Kuester S, Miller C. Food service and foods and beverages available at school: results from the School Health Policies and Programs Study 2000. *Journal of School Health,* 2001;71:313–324.

44. Physicians Committee for Responsible Medicine. School lunch report card. Fall, 2002. Available at www.pcrm.org/news/health020828lunchreport.html. Accessed Nov. 24, 2002.

45. Figlio DN, Winicki J. Food for thought: The effects of school accountability plans on school nutrition. Working paper 9319, National Bureau of Economic Research. Available at www.nber.org/papers/w9319.

46. Associated Press. Study finds junk food can raise test scores. Nov. 20, 2002.

47. Perry CL, Bishop DB, Taylor G, Murray DM, Mays RW, Dudovitz BS, Smyth M, Story M. Changing fruit and vegetable consumption among children: the 5 A Day Power Plus program in St. Paul, Minnesota. *American Journal of Public Health,* 1998;88:603–609; Walsh CM, Dannhauser A, Joubert G. The impact of a nutrition education programme on the anthropometric nutritional status of low-income children in South Africa. *Public Health Nutrition,* 2002;5:3–9; Story M, Lytle LA, Birnbaum AS, Perry CL. Peer-led, school-based nutrition education for young adolescents: feasibility and process evaluation of the TEENS study. *Journal of School Health,* 2002;72:121–127; Williams CL, Bollella MC, Strobino BA, Spark A, Nicklas TA, Tolosi LB, Pittman BP. "Healthy-start": outcome of an intervention to promote a heart healthy diet in preschool children. *Journal of the American College of Nutrition,* 2002;21:62–71.

48. Sahota P, Rudolf MC, Dixey R, Hill AJ, Barth JH, Cade J. Randomised controlled trial of primary school-based intervention to reduce risk factors for obesity. *BMJ,* 2001;323:1029–1032.

49. Toh CM, Cutter J, Chew SK. School-based intervention has reduced obesity in Singapore. *BMJ,* 2002;324:427.

50. Borja ME, Bordi PL, Lambert CU. New lower-fat dessert recipes for the school lunch program are well accepted by children. *Journal of the American Dietetic Association.* 1996;96:908–910.

51. Wechsler H, Basch CE, Zybert P, Shea S. Promoting the selection of low-fat milk in elementary school cafeterias in an inner-city Latino community: evaluation of an intervention. *American Journal of Public Health,* 1998;88:427–433.

52. Nader PR, Stone EJ, Lytle LA, Perry CL, Osganian SK, Kelder S, Webber LS, Elder JP, Montgomery D, Feldman HA, Wu M, Johnson C, Parcel GS, Luepker RV. Three-year maintenance of improved diet and physical activity: the CATCH cohort. Child and Adolescent Trial for Cardiovascular Health. *Archives of Pediatrics & Adolescent Medicine,* 1999;153:695–704.

53. French SA, Story M, Fulkerson JA, Gerlach AF. Food environment in secondary schools: A la carte, vending machines, food policies, and practices. *American Journal of Public Health,* in press.

54. French SA, Jeffery RW, Story M, Breitlow KK, Baxter JS, Hanna P, Snyder MP. Pricing and promotion effects on low-fat vending snack purchases: the CHIPS study. *American Journal of Public Health,* 2001;91:112–117; French SA, Jeffery RW, Story M, Hannan P, Snyder MP. A pricing strategy to promote low-fat snack choices through vending machines. *American Journal of Public Health,* 1997;87:849–851; Hannan P, French SA, Story M, Fulkerson JA. A pricing strategy to promote sales of lower fat foods in high school cafeterias: acceptability and sensitivity analysis. *American Journal of Health Promotion,* 2002;17:1–6.

55. Schulte B. More nutritious, less delicious. *The Washington Post,* Jun. 27, 2002.

56. American School Food Service Association website. Available at www.asfsa.org. Accessed Nov. 20, 2002.

57. Oleck J. Go ahead, make my lunch; restaurants vying for school meal market. *Restaurant Business Magazine,* 1994;93:54.

58. Morse J. Flunking lunch. *Time,* Dec. 2, 2002.

59. Ibid.

60. Wechsler H, Brener ND, Kuester S, Miller C. Food service and foods and beverages available at school: results from the School Health Policies and Programs Study 2000. *Journal of School Health*, 2001;71:313–324.

61. Candy out, granola in. *Down East*, Nov. 2001, citing from the *Bangor Daily News*, p. 21.

62. Brownell KD, Ludwig DS. Fighting obesity and the food lobby (Editorial). *The Washington Post*, Jun. 17, 2002.

63. Manning S. Students for sale: how corporations are buying their way into America's classrooms. *The Nation*, Sep. 27, 1999; Consumers Union. Selling America's kids: Commercial pressures on kids of the 90s. Available at www.consumersunion.org/other/sellingkids/index.htm. Accessed Nov. 22, 2002; Brody J. Schools teach 3C's: Candy, cookies, chips. *New York Times*, Sep. 24, 2002; Consumers Union. Captive kids: A report on commercial pressures on kids at schools. Available at www.consumersunion.org/other/captivekids/prologue.htm. Accessed Nov. 22, 2002.

64. Consumer Alert Web page. Available at www.consumeralert.org. Accessed Nov. 22, 2002.

65. Manning S. Classrooms for sale. *New York Times*, Opinion Page, Mar. 24, 1999.

66. Quoted in report by the Consumers Union. Captive kids: A report on commercial pressures on kids at schools. Available at www.consumersunion.org/other/captivekids/prologue.htm. Accessed Nov. 22, 2002.

67. Nakamura D. U.S. schools hooked on junk food proceeds. *The Washington Post*, Feb. 27, 2001.

68. Henry T. Coca-Cola rethinks school contracts. *USA Today*, Jun. 19, 2001.

69. Lord M. Schools without soda? Coca-Cola revamps its sales and marketing. *U.S. News and World Report*, Mar. 26, 2001.

70. Senate considers free fruits, veggies for schools. *CNN.com/education*, Sep. 7, 2001. Available at http://fyi.cnn.com/2001/fyi/teachers.ednews/09/07/school.veggies.ap. Accessed Sep. 12, 2001.

71. *Education Reporter*. Study says commercialism rampant in public schools. *Education Reporter*, Nov., 2000, 178. Available at www.eagleforum.org/educate/2000/nov00/commercialism.shtml. Accessed Aug 7, 2002.

72. Nakamura D. U.S. schools hooked on junk food proceeds. *The Washington Post*, Feb. 27, 2001.

73. Marketing to students. *Education Reporter*, Jan. 2000, 168. Available at www.eagleforum.org/educate/2000/jan00/marketing.htm. Accessed Aug. 7, 2001.

74. Ibid.

75. Perry CL, Bishop DB, Taylor G, Murray DM, Mays RW, Dudovitz BS, Smyth M, Story M. Changing fruit and vegetable consumption among children: the 5A Day Power Plus program in St. Paul, Minnesota. *American Journal of Public Health*, 1998;88:603–609.

76. White Dog Café in Philadelphia. Website available at www.whitedog.com. Accessed Nov. 18, 2002.

77. Buehrle S. Henry battles junk food in school: Bill would set limits on snack machines. *Cincinnati Enquirer*, Mar. 13, 2002.

78. Information on Nutrition Friendly Schools program. Department of Nutrition, Pennsylvania State University. Available at http://nutrition.hhdev.psu.edu/projectpa/html/PromoHSNE.html. Accessed Nov. 18, 2002.

79. Uhlman M. Reading, writing, and 100 percent juice. *Philadelphia Inquirer*, May 18, 2002.

80. Health Promoting Schools website. Available at www.sofweb.vic.edu.au/hps/abouthps.htm. Accessed Nov. 19, 2002; the *Journal of School Health* published a number of articles on the Health Promoting Schools program in Australia in 2000 (Vol. 70, No. 6); Nader P. Health Promoting Schools: Why not in the United States? *Journal of School Health*, 2000;70:247.

81. Stuhldreher WL, Koehler AN, Harrison MK, Deel H. The West Virginia standards for school nutrition. *Journal of Child Nutrition & Management*, 1998;22:79–86.

82. U.S. Department of Health and Human Services. *Healthy People 2010: Understanding and Improving Health* (2nd Ed). Washington, DC: U.S. Department of Health and Human Services, 2000.

83. Competitive Food Service. 7CFR, 210.2 and 210.12; 220.2 and 220.12. *Federal Register*, Jan.1, 1986.

84. Centers for Disease Control and Prevention. Guidelines for school health programs to promote lifelong healthy eating. *Journal of School Health*, 1997;67:9–26.

85. Consumers Union. Captive kids: A report on commercial pressures on kids at schools. Available at www.consumersunion.org/other/captivekids/prologue.htm. Accessed Nov. 22, 2002.

86. Hungry Red Planet nutrition program, Health Media Lab. Available at www.hungryredplanet.com/html/contact2.html. Accessed Nov. 26, 2002.

87. Recommendations for competitive food standards in California schools. National Consensus Panel on School Nutrition. California Center for Public Health Advocacy, March 2002. Available at www.publichealthadvocacy.org/school_food_standards/school_food_standards.html. Accessed Nov. 20, 2002.

88. Nestle M. *Food Politics: How the Food Industry Influences Nutrition and Health*. Berkeley, CA: University of California Press, 2002; Sims LS. *The Politics of Fat: Food and Nutrition Policy in America*. Armonk, New York: M.E. Sharpe, 1988.

89. Anonymous. Vending machines—Are they worth it? *Journal of Physical Education, Recreation, and Dance*, May/June 2001. Available at wysiwyg://240/http://www.ahealthyme.com/article/bellhowell/100884063. Accessed Aug. 3, 2001.

90. Consumers Union. Captive kids: A report on commercial pressures on kids at schools. Available at www.consumersunion.org/other/captivekids/recommendations.htm. Accessed Nov. 22, 2002.

91. Jacobson MF, Brownell KD. Small taxes on soft drinks and snack foods to promote health. *American Journal of Public Health*, 2000;90: 854–857.

92. Dunsmore D. Cola vending machines: Rich contracts that may not be so "sweet." *Teacher Newsmagazine*, Mar. 2001;13. Available online: www.bctf.bc.ca/ezine/archive/2001-03/support/15Richcontracts.html. Accessed Aug. 3, 20001.

93. Healthy school nutrition environments. U.S. Department of Agriculture website. Available at www.fns.usda .gov/cnd/healthyeating/default.htm. Accessed Nov. 18, 2002.

Chapter 7

1. National Soft Drink Association. Business partnerships between beverage companies and schools. Available online: www.nsda.org/Issues/Partnerships/index.html. Accessed Aug. 6, 2002.

2. Beck J. Teen suspended from school for wearing Pepsi T-shirt on Coke Day. *Chicago Tribune*, April 1, 1998, Available online: www.flipside.org/vol1/apr98/pc4-16.htm. Accessed Aug. 3, 2001.

3. Nestle M. Soft drink "pouring rights": marketing empty calories to children. *Public Health Reports*, 2000;115:308–319; Fried EJ, Nestle M. The growing political movement against soft drinks in schools. *JAMA*, 2002;288:2181.

4. Wechsler H, Brener ND, Kuester S, Miller C. Food service and foods and beverages available at school: results from the School Health Policies and Programs Study, 2000. *Journal of School Health*, 2001;71:313–324.

5. Rothstein R. Schools' chosen cure for money ills: a sugar pill. *New York Times*, Aug. 21, 2002

6. National Soft Drink Association. The value we bring. Available at www.nsda.org/Issues/Partnerships/value.html. Accessed Aug. 6, 2002.

7. National Soft Drink Association. Business partnerships between beverage companies and schools. Available at www.nsda.org/Issues/Partnerships/index.html. Accessed Aug. 6, 2002.

8. French SA, Fulkerson JA, Story M. School food policies and practices: A statewide survey of secondary school principals. *Journal of the American Dietetic Association*, in press.

9. Study conducted between 12/1/02 and 1/18/02 on The Status of Vending Machines, Schools and Physical Activity in KY Schools. Conducted by the University of Kentucky Cooperative Extension, Lexington Fayette County Health Department, and the Kentucky Dept. of Public Health.

10. Zoldan D. Soft drink makers are shelling out to promote drinks in local schools. *Naples News*, Oct. 11, 1998. Available at www.naplesnews.com/today/marco/a89013k.htm. Accessed Aug. 3, 2001.

11. DeGette C. To insure revenue, Coke is it: schools urged to boost sales. *Denver Post*, Nov. 22, 1998, B1.

12. Fisher M. Easy cash eroding their principles. *The Washington Post*, Feb. 27, 2001, B1.

13. Slobogin K. Soft-drink issue bubbles in schools, Congress: Lawmakers mull capping campus soda sales. Apr. 30, 2001. Available at www.cnn.com/2001/fyi/news/04/30/school.junk.food. Accessed Aug. 3, 2001.

14. Hays C. Today's lesson: Soda rights: Consultant helps schools sell themselves to vendors. *New York Times*, May 21, 1999, C1.

15. Kaufman M. Fighting the cola wars in schools. *The Washington Post*, Mar. 23, 1999, Z12. Available at www.washingtonpost.com/wp-srv/national/colawars032399.htm. Accessed Aug. 3, 2001.

16. National Soft Drink Association website. www.nsda.org/softdrinks/CSDHealth/Nutrition/NutritionPR/Consumption43.html. Accessed Aug 6, 2002.

17. American Dietetic Association. Fact Sheet on Straight Facts on Beverage Choices. Available at www.nsda.org/softdrinks/CSDHealth/901 percent20Soft percent20drink percent20sheet.pdf. Accessed Aug. 6, 2002.

18. Johnson G. Facts about soft drinks and nutrition. From National Soft Drink Association website. Available online: www.nsda.org/softdrinks/CSDHealth/guyjohnson.html. Accessed Aug. 6, 2002.

19. Nestle M. *Food Politics: How the Food Industry Influences Nutrition and Health*. Berkeley, CA: University of California Press, 2002.

20. Jacobson M. Center for Science in the Public Interest. Liquid candy: How soft drinks are harming Americans' health. www.cspinet.org/sodapop/liquid_candy.htm. Accessed Aug. 6, 2001.

21. Troiano RP, Briefel RR, Carroll MD, Bialostosky K. Energy and fat intakes of children and adolescents in the United States: Data from the National Health and Nutrition Examination Surveys. *American Journal of Clinical Nutrition*, 2000;72:1343S–1353S.

22. Cullen KW, Ash DM, Warneke C, de Moor C. Intake of soft drinks, fruit-flavored beverages, and fruits and vegetables by children in grades 4–6. *American Journal of Public Health*, 2002;92:1475–1478.

23. Jacobson M. Center for Science in the Public Interest. Liquid candy: How soft drinks are harming Americans' health. Available at www.cspinet.org/sodapop/liquid_candy.htm. Accessed Aug. 6, 2001.

24. DiMeglio DP, Mattes RD. Liquid versus solid carbohydrate: effects of food intake and body weight. *International Journal of Obesity and Related Metabolic Disorders*, 2000;24:794–800.

25. Rolls BJ, Kim S, Fedoroff IC. Effects of drinks sweetened with sucrose or aspartame on hunger, thirst and food intake in men. *Physiology & Behavior*, 1990;48:19–26.

26. Raben A, Vasilaras TH, Møller AC, Astrup A. Sucrose compared with artificial sweeteners: different effects on ad libitum food intake and body weight after 10 weeks of supplementation in overweight subjects. *American Journal of Clinical Nutrition*, 2002;76:721–729.

27. National Soft Drink Association website. Studies show soft drink consumption by school-aged children is not linked to obesity, poor diet quality or lack of exercise Available online: www.nsda.org/softdrinks/CSD Health/Nutrition/NutritionPR/Consumption43.html. Accessed Aug. 6, 2002.

28. Ebbeling CB, Pawlak DB, Ludwig DS. Childhood obesity: public health crisis, commonsense cure. *Lancet*, 2002;360:473–482.

29. Ludwig DS, Peterson KE, Gortmaker SL. Relation between consumption of sugar-sweetened drinks and childhood obesity: A prospective, observational analysis. *Lancet*, 2001;357:505–508.

30. Harnack L, Stang J, Story M. Soft drink consumption among U.S. children and adolescents: Nutritional consequences. *Journal of the American Dietetic Association*, 1999:99:436–441.

31. Ballew C. Beverage choices affect adequacy of children's nutrient intakes. *JAMA*, 2001;285:524.

32. Pereira MA, Jacobs DR, VanHorn L, Slattery ML, Kartashov AI, Ludwig DS. Dietary consumption, obesity, and the insulin resistance syndrome in young adults: the CARDIA study. *JAMA*, 2002;287:2081–2089.

33. Cullen KW, Ash DM, Warneke C, de Moor C. Intake of soft drinks, fruit-flavored beverages, and fruits and vegetables by children in grades 4–6. *American Journal of Public Health*, 2002;92:1475–1478.

34. Pereira MA, Jacobs DR, VanHorn L, Slattery ML, Kartashov AI, Ludwig DS. Dietary consumption, obesity, and the insulin resistance syndrome in young adults: the CARDIA study. *JAMA*, 2002;287:2081–2089.

35. Lin YC, Lyle RM, McCabe LD, McCabe GP, Weaver CM, Teegarden D. Dairy calcium is related to changes in body composition during a two-year exercise intervention in young women. *Journal of the American College of Nutrition*, 2000;19:754–760; Zemel MB. Regulation of adiposity and obesity risk by dietary calcium: mechanisms and implications. *Journal of the American College of Nutrition*, 2002;21:146S–151S; Heaney RP, Davies KM, Barger-Lux MJ. Calcium and weight: clinical studies. *Journal of the American College of Nutrition*, 2002;21:152S–155S.

36. Zemel MB. Mechanisms of dairy modulation of adiposity. *Journal of Nutrition*, 2003;133:252S–256S.

37. *FDA Consumer*. Coffee and Cola—the good news and the bad news. Sep. 2000;34:5.

38. Wyshak G. Teenaged girls, carbonated beverage consumption, and bone fractures. *Archives of Pediatrics and Adolescent Medicine*, 2000;154:610.

39. Al-Dlaigan YH, Shaw L, Smith A. Dental erosion in a group of British 14-year-old school children. Part II: Influence of dietary intake. *British Dental Journal*, 2001;190:258–261.

40. Meskin LH. Outrageous II. *Journal of the American Dental Association*, 2001;132:10.

41. Maihofer MG. "Pouring wrongs": MDA discourages pop deals. *Journal of Michigan Dental Association*, 2000;82:10.

42. *Curriculum Administrator*. Dentists and parents complain about the selling of soft drinks in Toledo schools, Feb. 2001;37:13.

43. Spruill WT. PDA establishes position statement on cola contracts in schools. *Penn Dental Journal*, 2000;65:29–32.

44. American Dental Association. ADA weighs in on school vending machines. From ADA website. Available at www.ada.org/public/media/newsrel/0202/nr-05.html. Accessed Aug. 7, 2002.

45. Guthrie JF, Morton JF. Food sources of added sweeteners in the diets of Americans. *Journal of the American Dietetic Association*, 2000;100:43–51.

46. Discussion following testimony of Lisa Katic of the Grocery Manufacturers of America (GMA) to the Senate Committee on Health, Education, Labor, and Pensions, May 21, 2002. Available at www.fdch.com. Accessed Jul. 11, 2002

47. Brownell KD, Woolston S, Horgen KB. Beverage machine options in 10 Connecticut high schools. Paper in preparation.

48. Soft drinks won't get hard sell in Crested Butte and Gunnison Schools. *Denver Post*, Jul. 7, 1999, B6.

49. Snyder S. School board scuttles deal with Coke. *Philadelphia Inquirer*, Feb. 8, 2000, B1.

50. Davila E. Pepsi contract plan goes flat for local school board. *Santa Fe New Mexican*, Apr. 19, 2000, B1.

51. Murphy K. Madison schools reject Coke contract. *Milwaukee Journal Sentinel*, Aug. 30, 2000, 2B.

52. Slobogin K. Soft-drink issue bubbles in schools, Congress: Lawmakers mull capping campus soda sales. Apr. 30, 2001. Available at www.cnn.com/2001/fyi/news/04/30/school.junk.food. Accessed Aug. 3, 2001.

53. Nichols R. A baby step toward a Coke-free school zone. *Philadelphia Inquirer,* Oct. 27, 1999.

54. Commercialization in our schools: Positive trends in recent commercialization studies. OSSTF/FEESO. www.osstf.on.ca/www/abosstf/ampa01.commercialization/postivetrends.html. Accessed Aug 3, 2001.

55. Anonymous. Vending machines—Are they worth it? *Journal of Physical Education, Recreation, and Dance,* May/June 2001. Available at wysiwyg://240/http://www.ahealthyme.com/article/bellhowell/100884063. Accessed Aug. 3, 2001.

56. Winter G. Some states fight junk food sales in schools. *New York Times,* Sep. 9, 2001, A1.

57. News-Journal Wire Services. Coke to alter marketing strategy in U.S. Schools. Available at Wysiwyg://60/http://www.news-journalonline.com/2001/March/14/AREA4.htm. Accessed Aug. 6, 2001.

58. Lord M. School without soda? Coca-Cola revamps its sales and marketing. *U.S. News & World Report,* Mar. 26, 2001. Available at www.usnews.com/utils/search. Accessed Nov. 25, 2001.

59. McKay B. Coke finds its exclusive school contracts aren't so easily given up. *Wall Street Journal,* Jun. 26, 2001, B1.

60. Henry T. Coca-Cola rethinks school contracts. *USA Today,* Jun. 19, 2001. Available at wysiwyg://199/ http://www.usatoday.com/news/nation/2001-03-13-coke.htm. Accessed Aug. 3., 2001.

61. McKay B. Coke finds its exclusive school contracts aren't so easily given up. *Wall Street Journal,* Jun. 26, 2001, B1.

62. Zernike K. Coke to dilute push in schools for its products. *New York Times,* Mar. 14, 2001, A1.

63. Bachmann T. Coke's counter move. *Beverage Industry,* Jan., 2001;92:6.

64. Slobogin K. Soft-drink issue bubbles in schools, Congress: Lawmakers mull capping campus soda sales. Apr. 30, 2001. Available at www.cnn.com/2001/fyi/news/04/30/school.junk.food. Accessed Aug. 3, 2001.

65. McKay B. Coke finds its exclusive school contracts aren't so easily given up. *Wall Street Journal,* Jun. 26, 2001, B1.

66. Moore NY. Schools can undo healthy choices at home. *St. Paul Pioneer Press,* Feb. 26, 2002.

67. Candy out, granola in. *Down East,* Nov. 2001, citing from the *Bangor Daily News,* p. 21.

68. Wechsler H, Basch C, Zybert P, Shea S. Promoting the selection of low-fat milk in elementary school cafeterias in an inner-city Latino community: Evaluation of an intervention. *American Journal of Public Health,* 1998;88:427.

69. Hayasaki E. Schools to end soda sales. *Los Angeles Times,* Aug. 28, 2002; Canter M, Hudley-Hayes G. LA's fat and fizzy campuses. Health should trump money: curtail soda sales at public schools. *Los Angeles Times,* Aug. 26, 2002.

70. Brownell KD, Ludwig DS. Fighting obesity and the food lobby (Editorial). *The Washington Post,* Jun. 17, 2002.

71. French SA, Story M, Fulkerson JA, Gerlach AF. Food environment in secondary schools: A la carte, vending machines, food policies and practices. *American Journal of Public Health,* in press.

Chapter 8

1. Siano J. Garages make supersized SUVs even bigger for superrich MVPs. *New York Times,* Aug. 27, 2000, A1.

2. Data from Wendy's, Burger King, and McDonald's websites. Accessed Dec. 11, 2002. 2,000 calories per day was used as the reference day's intake, as was 64 grams of fat.

3. Spake A. A fat nation. *U.S. News & World Report,* Aug. 19, 2002.

4. Fast Food's Most Decadent Burger Arrives at Jack in the Box® Restaurants. Jack in the Box corporate website. Press release from Apr. 13, 2001. Available at www.jackinthebox.com/pressroom/pressreleases/pr.php?UID =17&Year=2001. Accessed Dec. 11, 2002.

5. *Arizona Republic.* We are what we eat—big: Time to start downsizing our supersize appetites. Jun. 14, 2001, B8.

6. Lipid Clinic News: Just Supersize It. Available at www.ohsu.edu/som-lipid/vol151/super.htm. Accessed Oct. 11, 2001.

7. Young LR, Nestle M. The contribution of expanding portion sizes to the U.S. obesity epidemic. *American Journal of Public Health,* 2002;92:246–249.

8. *Arizona Republic.* We are what we eat—big: Time to start downsizing our supersize appetites. Jun. 14, 2001, B8.

9. Avila J. Supersizing of America: As portions become bigger, so do our waistlines. NBC Nightly News Health, Aug. 20, 2000. Available at www.msnbc.com/news/616763.asp?cp1=1. Accessed Oct. 11, 2001.

10. Rozin P, Kabnick K, Pete E, Fischler C, Shields C. The ecology of eating: Part of the French paradox results from lower food intake in French than Americans, because of smaller portion sizes. *Psychological Science,* in press.

11. Schwartz MB, Hrabosky JI, Brownell KD. Nutrition analysis of children's meals at fast food and family restaurants. Paper submitted for publication, 2002.

12. American Institute for Cancer Research. As restaurant portions grow, vast majority of Americans still belong to "Clean Plate Club." Survey released Jan. 15, 2001. Available at www.aicr.org. Accessed Dec. 14, 2002.

13. Ello-Martin JA, Roe LS, Meengs JS, Wall DE, Rolls BJ. Increasing the portion size of a unit food increases energy intake. *Appetite,* 2002;39:74.

14. Rolls BJ, Morris EL, Roe LS. Portion size of food affects energy intake in normal-weight and overweight men and women. *American Journal of Clinical Nutrition,* 2002;76:1207–1213.

15. Wansink B. Accounting for taste: Prototypes that predict preference. *Journal of Database Marketing,* 2000;7:308–320.

16. Wansink B. Can package size accelerate usage volume? *Journal of Marketing,* 1996;60:1–14; Wansink B. Accounting for taste: Prototypes that predict preference. *Journal of Database Marketing,* 2000;7:308–320; Wansink B, Deshpande R. Out of sight, out of mind: The impact of household stockpiling on usage rates. *Marketing Letters,* 1994;5:91–100.

17. Marketing prof's work captures national media attention. University of Illinois release. Available at www.cba.uiuc.edu/insight/spring99/research.htm. Accessed Dec. 14, 2002.

18. Nelson E. Marketers push single servings and families hungrily dig in. *Wall Street Journal,* Jul. 23, 2002, 1.

19. Ibid.

20. Rolls BJ, Kim S, Fedoroff IC. Effects of drinks sweetened with sucrose or aspartame on hunger, thirst, and food intake in men. *Physiology & Behavior,* 1990;48:19–26.

21. Kral TVE, Roe LS, Meengs JS, Wall DE, Rolls BJ. Increasing the portion size of a packaged snack increases energy intake. *Appetite,* 2002;39:86.

22. Yanovski JA, Yanovski SZ, Sovik KN, Nguyen TT, O'Neil PM, Sebring NG. A prospective study of holiday weight gain. *New England Journal of Medicine,* 2000;342:861–867.

23. Hill JO, Peters JC. Environmental contributions to the obesity epidemic. *Science,* 1998;280:1371–1374.

24. American Institute for Cancer Research. As restaurant portions grow, vast majority of Americans still belong to "Clean Plate Club." Survey released Jan. 15, 2001. Available at www.aicr.org. Accessed Dec. 14, 2002; Calorie Control Council. *Calorie Control Commentary,* Summer/Fall, 2000;22:1. Available at www.caloriecontrol.org/commentarysf00.pdf. Accessed Dec. 14, 2002.

25. American Institute for Cancer Research. As restaurant portions grow, vast majority of Americans still belong to "Clean Plate Club." Survey released Jan. 15, 2001. Available at www.aicr.org. Accessed Dec. 14, 2002.

26. Lansky D, Brownell KD. Estimates of food quantity and calories: errors in self-report among obese patients. *American Journal of Clinical Nutrition,* 1982;35:727–732.

27. American Institute for Cancer Research. As restaurant portions grow, vast majority of Americans still belong to "Clean Plate Club." Survey released Jan. 15, 2001. Available at www.aicr.org. Accessed Dec. 14, 2002.

28. Young LR, Nestle M. The contribution of expanding portion sizes to the U.S. obesity epidemic. *American Journal of Public Health,* 2002;92:246–249.

29. American Institute for Cancer Research. Nutritionists warn public: Portion sizes out of control. Oct. 20, 1999. Available at www.aicr.org/r102099.htm. Accessed Nov. 9, 2001.

30. Rolls BJ, Engell D, Birch LL. Serving portion size influences five-year-old but not three-year-old children's food intakes. *Journal of the American Dietetic Association,* 2000;100:232–234; McConahy KL, Smiciklas-Wright H, Birch LL, Mitchell DC, Picciano MF. Food portions are positively related to energy intake and body weight in early childhood. *Journal of Pediatrics,* 2002;140:340–347.

31. Ordonez J. Hamburger joints call them "heavy users"— but not to their faces. *Wall Street Journal,* Jan. 12, 2000.

32. Information Resources, Inc. At the checkout: Big sales for big products. *Wall Street Journal,* Oct. 12, 1993, B1; Berry E. Pricing tactics and the search for profits. *Advertising Forum,* 1983;4:12–13, 71–72.

33. Brody JE. Avoiding confusion on serving size is key to food pyramid. *New York Times,* April 13, 1999, F6.

Chapter 9

1. Blaylock J, Smallwood D, Kassel K, Variyam J, Aldrich L. Economics, food choices, and nutrition. Agricultural Outlook Forum 1999. Economic Research Service, U.S. Department of Agriculture, 1999. Available at www.usda.gov/agency/oce/waob/outlook99/speeches/027/blaylock.txt. Accessed Nov. 29, 2002.

2. Pollan M. *The Botany of Desire*. New York: Random House, 2001; Scott JC. *Seeing Like a State: How Certain Schemes to Improve the Human Condition Have Failed*. New Haven: Yale University Press, 1998; Lappe FM, Lappe A. *Hope's Edge: The Next Diet for a Small Planet*. New York: Tarcher/Putnam, 2002.

3. Nestle M. *Food Politics: How the Food Industry Influences Nutrition and Health*. Berkeley, CA: University of California Press, 2002; Sims LS. *The Politics of Fat: Food and Nutrition Policy in America*. Armonk, New York: M.E. Sharpe, 1988.

4. Philipson T. The worldwide growth in obesity: an economic research agenda. *Health Economics*, 2001;10:1–7; Lakdawalla D, Philipson T. The growth of obesity and technological change: A theoretical and empirical examination. Working paper No. 8946, National Bureau of Economic Research. Cambridge, MA: National Bureau of Economic Research, May 2002; Philipson TJ, Posner RA. The long-run growth in obesity as a function of technological change. Working paper No. 7423, National Bureau of Economic Research. Cambridge, MA: National Bureau of Economic Research, Nov. 1999.

5. Lakdawalla D, Philipson T. The growth of obesity and technological change: A theoretical and empirical examination. Working paper No. 8946, National Bureau of Economic Research. Cambridge, MA: National Bureau of Economic Research, May, 2002.

6. *Food Marketing Institute and Prevention Magazine*. Shopping for health. Report prepared by Parkwood Research Associates, 1995.

7. The price of eating well in Niagara. Regional Niagara Press Release. Available at http://regional.niagara.on.ca/media.2000/sep25-00.html. Accessed Dec. 13, 2002.

8. Che J, Chen J. Food insecurity in Canadian households. Health Reports, Health Statistics Division, Statistics Canada. Catalog no. 82-003-XPE, Vol. 12, 11–22. Available at www.statcan.ca/english/indepth/82-003/feature/hrab2001012004s0a01.htm. Accessed Aug. 15, 2001; *Dieticians of Canada*. The cost of eating in BC: The challenge of healthy eating on a low income. Oct. 2001.

9. Frazao E, Allshouse J. Size and growth of nutritionally improved foods market. *Agricultural Information Bulletin* No. 723. Economic Research Service, U.S. Dept. of Agriculture, 1996.

10. McAllister M, Baghurst K, Record S. Financial costs of healthful eating: A comparison of three different approaches. *Journal of Nutrition Education*, 1994;26:131–139.

11. McDonald's Mickey D's Dollar Menu. Available at www.mytownmcdonalds.com/DOLLAR percent20 MENU.htm. Accessed Dec. 1, 2002; Burger King 99¢ BK Value Menu. Available at www.burgerking.com/val-uemenu/value_menu.html. Accessed Dec. 1, 2002.

12. Information Resources, Inc. At the checkout: Big sales for big products. *Wall Street Journal*, Oct. 12, 1993, B1; Berry E. Pricing tactics and the search for profits. *Advertising Forum*, 1983;4:12–13, 71–72.

13. National Alliance for Nutrition and Activity. From wallet to waistline: The hidden costs of super sizing. Report issued in June 2002. Available at www.cspinet.org/new/pdf/final_price_study.pdf. Accessed Dec. 12, 2002.

14. Reidpath DD, Burns C, Garrard J, Mahoney M, Townsend M. An ecological study of the relationship between social and environmental determinants of obesity. *Health Place*, 2002:8;141–145.

15. Poulter S, Hale B. Poor families priced out of a healthy diet. *Daily Mail*, Oct. 24, 2001. Available at www.thefooddoctor.co.uk/pricedout.htm. Accessed Dec. 13, 2001.

16. Morland K, Wing S, Diez Roux A, Poole C. Neighborhood characteristics associated with the location of food stores and food service places. *American Journal of Preventive Medicine*, 2002;22:23–29.

17. Martin K. Food security and community: Putting the pieces together. Hartford Food System, 2001.

18. Winnie M. Will Hartford re-store itself? *Seedling: Newsletter of the Hartford Food System*, Summer, 2002.

19. Morland K, Wing S, Roux AD. The contextual effect of the local food environment on residents' diets: The Atherosclerosis Risk in Communities Study. *American Journal of Public Health*, 2002;92:1761–1787.

20. Shaffer A. The persistence of L.A.'s grocery gap: The need for a new food policy and approach to market development. Report from the Center for Food and Justice, Occidental College, May 28, 2002. Available at http://departments.oxy.edu/uepi/cfj/resources/supermarkets02.pdf. Accessed Dec. 8, 2002; Supermarket shortage still plagues inner-city Los Angeles ten years after the 1992 riots, new report shows. Press release from Occidental College, May 21, 2002. Available at www.oxy.edu/oxy/news/articles/020631-supermarket.html. Accessed Dec. 8, 2002.

21. Morland K, Wing S, Roux AD. The contextual effect of the local food environment on residents' diets: The Atherosclerosis Risk in Communities Study. *American Journal of Public Health*, 2002;92:1761–1787; Duenwald M. Good health is linked to grocer. *New York Times*, Nov. 12, 2002.

22. BBC News. Poorer children miss out on healthy food. Dec. 13, 2001. Available at http://news.bbc.co.uk/hi/english/uk/newid_1707000/1707636.stm. Accessed Dec. 15, 2001.

23. Wilde PE, McNamara PE, Ranney CK. The effect on dietary quality of participation in the food stamp and WIC programs. *Food Assistance and Nutrition Research Report*, 2000; No. 9. Available at http://ers.usda.gov/publications/Fanrr9. Accessed Nov. 28, 2002.

24. Besharov DJ. We're feeding the poor as if they're starving. *The Washington Post*, 2002, Dec. 8, B01.

25. Besharov DJ, Germanis P. *Rethinking WIC: An Evaluation of the Women, Infants, and Children Program.* American Enterprise Institute: Washington, DC, 2001.

26. Besharov DJ. We're feeding the poor as if they're starving. *The Washington Post*, 2002, Dec. 8, B01.

27. Zigler E, Muenchow S. *Head Start: The Inside Story of America's Most Successful Educational Experiment.* New York: Basic Books, 1992.

28. Zigler E, Styfco SJ. *Head Start and Beyond: A National Plan for Extended Childhood Education.* New Haven, CT: Yale University Press, 1993.

29. Philipson TJ, Posner RA. The long-run growth in obesity as a function of technological change. Working paper No. 7423, National Bureau of Economic Research. Cambridge, MA: National Bureau of Economic Research, Nov. 1999.

30. Parks SE, Housemann RA, Brownson RC. Differential correlates of physical activity in urban and rural adults of various socioeconomic backgrounds in the United States. *Journal of Epidemiology and Community Health*, 2003;57:29–35.

31. Foodmakers indulge cravings with more fatty products. *New Haven Register*, May 9, 2000, D1.

32. E-mail correspondence with Rosemary Deahl, CEO and Founder of Heart Wise restaurants, Dec. 7, 2002.

33. Stein J. Fitness chains step outside familiar territory. *Los Angeles Times*, Nov. 25, 2002.

34. Brownell K. Get slim with higher taxes. *New York Times*, Dec. 15, 1994, A29; Battle EK, Brownell KD. Confronting a rising tide of eating disorders and obesity: Treatment vs. prevention and policy. *Addictive Behaviors*, 1997;21:755–765; Horgen KB, Brownell KD. Confronting the toxic environment: Environmental, public health actions in a world crisis. In TA Wadden & AJ Stunkard (Eds) *Handbook of Obesity Treatment.* New York: Guilford, 2002, pp. 95–106.

35. Warner KE. Cigarette taxation: Doing good by doing well. *Journal of Public Health Policy*, 1984;5:312–319; Ransen MK, Chaloupka FJ, Nguyen SN. Global and regional estimates of the effectiveness and cost-effectiveness of price increases and other tobacco control policies. *Nicotine and Tobacco Research*, 2002;4:311–319.

36. Jacobson MF, Brownell KD. Small taxes on soft drinks and snack foods to promote health. *American Journal of Public Health*, 2000;90:854–857.

37. Boroughs D, Collins S. The ten worst economic moves. *U.S. News and World Report*, Jan. 27, 1992, 54; Molpus M. Prepared testimony of Manly Molpus, President and Chief Executive Officer of the Grocery Manufacturers of America, Inc., before the House Agricultural Committee, Subcommittee of Department Operations and Nutrition. May 17, 1995; Lucas G. Capitol food fight. *San Francisco Chronicle*, Aug. 3, 1991, A16; Vellinga, M. Snack tax crumbles Tuesday: State to suffer big bite. *Sacramento Bee*, Nov. 28, 1992, A1; Lozano C. Tax bite's sour aftertaste. *Los Angeles Times*, Jul, 23, 1991, B1.

38. California. *Daily Report for Executives*, Jan. 1993, 5.

39. Boroughs D, Collins S. The ten worst economic moves. *U.S. News and World Report*, Jan. 27, 1992, 54.

40. Harrison D. Empty Frito-Lay plant awaits change in political tastes. *Baltimore Business Journal*, 1993;10:11.

41. Maryland Comptroller of the Treasury. How are sales of food taxed in Maryland? Available at www.comp.state.md.us/business/taxtips/bustip05.asp. Accessed Apr. 26, 2000.

42. Grocery Manufacturers of America. Public Policy Update. Maine repeals snack tax; Governor signs measure into law. May 2, 2000. Available at www.gmabrands.com/pubpolicy/buzz/pp_update/2000/0502.pdf. Accessed Jan. 18, 2002.

43. Snack Food Association News Release. SFA hails Maine legislature's commitment to snack tax repeal as Secretary of State approves citizen initiative petitions. Available at www.sfa .org/PRMESnackTax.htm. Accessed Jan. 18, 2002.

44. Office of the Chief Financial Officer. DC ends the snack tax. Jun. 1, 2001. Available at www.cfo .washingtondc.gov/services/tax/news/2001/june/06_01_01.shtm. Accessed Jan. 18, 2002.

45. Garry M. To tax or not to tax? California's Proposition 163 would repeal the snack tax. *Progressive Grocer*, 1992;7:10; Harrison D. Empty Frito-Lay plant awaits change in political tastes. *Baltimore Business Journal*, 1993;10:11.

46. Oliver JE, Lee T. Public opinion and the politics of America's obesity epidemic. Paper submitted to the *American Journal of Political Science*. Available at http://ksgnotes1.harvard.edu/Research/wpaper.nsf/rwp/RWP02-017/$File/rwp02_017_lee.pdf. Accessed Nov. 16, 2002.

47. Olson BH. Attitudes toward obesity. Abstract submitted for Experimental Biology annual meeting, 2002. Author is at Michigan State University.

48. Bruskin-Goldring Research, telephone survey. Washington, DC: Center for Science in the Public Interest, 1999.

49. National Snack Food Association website. Available at www.sfa.org/SFABrochure.htm#Intro. Accessed Nov. 19, 2002.

50. Jacobson MF, Brownell KD. Small taxes on soft drinks and snack foods to promote health. *American Journal of Public Health*, 2000;90:854–857.

51. Horgen K, Brownell K. Policy change as a means for reducing the prevalence and impact of alcoholism, smoking, and obesity. In Miller W, Heather N. *Treating Addictive Behaviors* (2nd Ed). New York: Plenum, 1998, pp. 105–118.

52. Lewit EM. U.S. tobacco taxes: Behavioral effects and policy implications. *British Journal of Addiction*, 1989;84:1217–1235; Cummings KM, Sciandra R. The public health benefit of increasing tobacco taxes in New York State. *New York State Journal of Medicine*, April 1990, 174–175; Flewelling RL, Kenney E, Elder JP, Pierce J, Johnson M, Bal DG. First-year impact of the 1989 California cigarette tax increase on cigarette consumption. *American Journal of Public Health*, 1992;82: 867–869; Ranson MK, Chaloupka FJ, Nguyen SN. Global and regional estimates of the effectiveness and cost-effectiveness of price increases and other tobacco control policies. *Nicotine and Tobacco Research*, 2002;4:311–319.

53. French SA, Jeffery RW, Story M, Breitlow KK, Baxter JS, Hanna P, Snyder MP. Pricing and promotion effects on low-fat vending snack purchases: the CHIPS study. *American Journal of Public Health*, 2001;91:112–117; French SA, Jeffery RW, Story M, Hannan P, Snyder MP. A pricing strategy to promote low-fat snack choices through vending machines. *American Journal of Public Health*, 1997;87:849–851; Hannan P, French SA, Story M, Fulkerson JA. A pricing strategy to promote sales of lower fat foods in high school cafeterias: acceptability and sensitivity analysis. *American Journal of Health Promotion*, 2002;17:1–6.

54. Horgen KB, Brownell KD. Comparison of price change and health message interventions in promoting healthy food choices. *Health Psychology*, 2002;21:505–512.

55. Shaffer A. The persistence of L.A.'s grocery gap: The need for a new food policy and approach to market development. Report from the Center for Food and Justice, Occidental College, May 28, 2002. Available at http://departments.oxy.edu/uepi/cfj/resources/supermarkets02.pdf. Accessed Dec. 8, 2002.

56. Ibid.

57. Besharov DJ, Germanis P. *Rethinking WIC: An Evaluation of the Women, Infants, and Children Program.* American Enterprise Institute: Washington, DC, 2001; Besharov DJ. We're feeding the poor as if they're starving. *The Washington Post*, 2002, Dec. 8, B01.

58. We are grateful to Edward Zigler of Yale University and Douglas Besharov of the American Enterprise Institute and University of Maryland for input on Head Start and WIC programs.

59. Reger B, Wootan MG, Booth-Butterfield S, Smith H. 1 percent or less: a community-based nutrition campaign. *Public Health Reports*, 1998;113:410–419; Reger B, Wootan MG, Booth-Butterfield S. Using mass media to promote healthy eating: a community-based demonstration project. *Preventive Medicine*, 1999;29:414–421.

60. Jacobson MF, Brownell KD. Small taxes on soft drinks and snack foods to promote health. *American Journal of Public Health*, 2000;90:854–857.

Chapter 10

1. Brownell KD, Ludwig DS. Fighting obesity and the food lobby. *The Washington Post*, Jun. 9, 2002, B07.

2. Testimony of Lisa Katic on behalf of the Grocery Manufacturers of America (GMA) to the Senate Committee on Health, Education, Labor and Pensions, May 21, 2002. Available at www.gmabrands.com/news/docs/Testimony.cfm?DocID=956&. Accessed Jun. 19, 2002.

3. National Soft Drink Association website. Available at www.nsda.org/about/whatisnsda.html. Accessed Jun. 19, 2002.

4. Nestle M. *Food Politics: How the Food Industry Influences Nutrition and Health.* Berkeley, CA: University of California Press, 2002; Sims LS. *The Politics of Fat: Food and Nutrition Policy in America.* Armonk, New York: M.E. Sharpe, 1988.

5. The Espy probe: Key stories. *The Washington Post*, Dec. 1998. Available at http://jobs.washingtonpost.com/wp-srv/politics/special/counsels/espy.htm. Accessed Dec. 20, 2002.

6. U.S. Department of Agriculture. Press release, Oct. 15, 2002. Available at www.usda.gov/news/releases/2002/10/hhs.htm. Accessed Dec. 20, 2002.

7. Olson E. Fighting fat by going to the source. *New York Times*, Nov. 17, 2000.

8. Grocery Manufacturers of American (GMA). Top administration officials brief GMA board. GMA website. Available at www.gmabrands.com/news/docs/NewsRelease.cfm?DocID=1028&. Accessed Nov. 17, 2002.

9. Kersh R, Morone J. How the personal becomes political: Prohibitions, public health and obesity. *Studies in American Political Development*, 2002:16:162–175; Kersh R, Morone J. The politics of obesity: Seven steps to government action. *Health Affairs*, 2002;21:142–153; Morone J. *Hellfire Nation*. New Haven, CT: Yale University Press, 2003.

10. Kersh R, Morone J. How the personal becomes political: Prohibitions, public health and obesity. *Studies in American Political Development*, 2002:16:162–175.

11. Ritch WA, Begay ME. Strange bedfellows: The history of collaboration between the Massachusetts Restaurant Association and the tobacco industry. *American Journal of Public Health,* 2001;91:598–603.

12. Kessler DA. *A Question of Intent: A Great American Battle with a Deadly Industry.* New York: Public Affairs, 2002.

13. Warner KE. Tobacco industry scientific advisors: serving society or selling cigarettes? *American Journal of Public Health,* 1991;81:839–842; Neuman M, Bitton A, Glantz S. Tobacco industry strategies for influencing European Community tobacco advertising legislation. *Lancet,* 2002;359:1323–1330; Mekemson C, Glantz SA. How the tobacco industry built its relationship with Hollywood. *Tobacco Control,* 2002;11(Suppl):181–191.

14. Nestle M. *Food Politics: How the Food Industry Influences Nutrition and Health.* Berkeley, CA: University of California Press, 2002.

15. Website of Tobacco.org. Available at www.tobacco.org/Documents/dd/ddfrankstatement.html. Accessed Dec. 20, 2002.

16. Testimony of Lisa Katic on behalf of the Grocery Manufacturers of America (GMA) to the Senate Committee on Health, Education, Labor, and Pensions, May 21, 2002. Available at www.gmabrands.com/news/docs/Testimony.cfm?DocID=956&. Accessed Jun. 19, 2002.

17. National Soft Drink Association website. Available at www.nsda.org/softdrinks/CSDHealth/Nutrition/NutritionPR/Consumption43.html. Accessed Jun. 19, 2002.

18. Action on Smoking and Health website. Available at www.ash.org.uk/html/conduct/html/trustus.html#_Toc514752783. Accessed Dec. 20, 2002.

19. National Soft Drink Association website. Available at www.nsda.org/softdrinks/CSDHealth/Index.html. Accessed Jun. 19, 2002.

20. Tobacco.org website. Available at www.tobacco.org/Documents/dd/ddbasebusiness.html. Accessed Dec. 21, 2002.

21. Hilts PJ. *Smoke Screen: The Truth Behind the Tobacco Industry Cover-up.* Reading, MA: Addison-Wesley, 1996, p. 98.

22. Horovitz B. McDonald's rediscovers its future with kids. *USA Today,* Apr. 18, 1997.

23. Warner KE. What's a cigarette company to do? *American Journal of Public Health,* 2002;92:897–900.

24. Frito-Lay (PepsiCo) press release. Frito-Lay eliminates trans fats from America's favorite salty snacks: Doritos, Tostitos, and Cheetos. Sep. 24, 2002. Available at www.pepsico.com/news/fritolay/2002/20020924f.shtml. Accessed Dec. 17, 2002.

25. You can eat right at McDonald's (letter to the editor). *Business Week,* Nov. 11, 2002.

26. Testimony of Lisa Katic on behalf of the Grocery Manufacturers of America (GMA) to the Senate Committee on Health, Education, Labor, and Pensions, May 21, 2002. Available at www.gmabrands.com/news/docs/Testimony.cfm?DocID=956&. Accessed Jun. 19, 2002.

27. Nestle M. *Food Politics: How the Food Industry Influences Nutrition and Health.* Berkeley, CA: University of California Press, 2002.

28. Center for Responsive Politics website. Available at www.opensecrets.org. Accessed Jun. 19, 2002.

29. Hastings G, MacFadyen L. A day in the life of an advertising man: Review of internal documents from the UK tobacco industry's principal advertising agencies. *BMJ,* 2000;321:3663–3671.

30. Snack Food Association website. Available at www.sfa.org/SFABrochure.htm#Mission. Accessed Jun. 20, 2002.

31. Severson K. L.A. schools to stop soda sales: district takes cue from Oakland ban. *San Francisco Chronicle,* Aug. 28, 2002, A1.

32. Testimony of Lisa Katic on behalf of the Grocery Manufacturers of America (GMA) to the Senate Committee on Health, Education, Labor, and Pensions, May 21, 2002. Available at www.gmabrands.com/news/docs/Testimony.cfm?DocID=956&. Accessed Jun. 19, 2002.

33. Comments of the National Soft Drink Association on the National Action Plan on Overweight and Obesity. Available at www.nsda.org/softdrinks/CSDHealth/comments.html. Accessed Nov. 26, 2002.

34. Leung S. The flight from fast food. *Wall Street Journal* (Campus Edition), Nov. 11, 2002.

35. Branch S. Food makers get defensive about gains in U.S. obesity. *Wall Street Journal,* Jun. 13, 2002.

36. Testimony of Lisa Katic on behalf of the Grocery Manufacturers of America (GMA) to the Senate Committee on Health, Education, Labor, and Pensions, May 21, 2002. Available at www.gmabrands.com/news/docs/Testimony.cfm?DocID=956&. Accessed Jun. 19, 2002.

37. Sugar Association website. Available at www.sugar.org/newsroom/mfs.html#disease. Accessed Aug. 21, 2002.

38. Fisher JO, Birch LL. Restricting access to palatable foods affects children's behavioral response, food selection, and intake. *American Journal of Clinical Nutrition,* 1999;69:1264–1272.

39. Burita M. Article on the obesity epidemic in *Medical Crossfire,* 2002;4:23–24.

40. Discussion following testimony of Lisa Katic of the Grocery Manufacturers of America (GMA) to the Senate Committee on Health, Education, Labor and Pensions, May 21, 2002. Available at www.fdch.com. Accessed Jul.11, 2002.

41. Burita M. Article on the obesity epidemic in *Medical Crossfire*, 2002;4:23–24.

42. Nestle M. *Food Politics: How the Food Industry Influences Nutrition and Health*. Berkeley, CA: University of California Press, 2002.

43. Letter from attorney Jeffrey Tenenbaum representing the Sugar Association to Marion Nestle of New York University (Mar. 27, 2002), and the letter Nestle wrote to Mr. Tenenbaum in response (Apr. 5, 2002). Both letters available at www.foodpolitics.com. Accessed Aug. 19, 2002.

44. Impropaganda review: A rogues gallery of industry front groups and antienvironment think tanks. PR Watch. Available at www.prwatch.org/improp/ddam.html. Accessed Nov. 26, 2002.

45. Article in *Food Arts* magazine on "Food Cops Run Amok" by R Berman, available from Center for Consumer Freedom website. Available at www.consumerfreedom.com/oped_detail.cfm?OPED_ID=123. Accessed Jun. 19, 2002.

46. Center for Consumer Freedom website. Available at www.consumerfreedom.com/ad_campaign.cfm. Accessed Jun. 19, 2002

47. Center for Consumer Freedom website. Available at www.cspinot.com. Accessed Jun. 19, 2002.

48. Center for Consumer Freedom website. Available at www.consumerfreedom.com/oped_detail.cfm?OPED_ID=123. Accessed Jun. 19, 2002.

49. John Banzhaf has a website with considerable information on food company lawsuits. Available at http://banzhaf.net. Accessed Dec. 22, 2002.

50. Jacobson PD, Warner KE. Litigation and public health policy making: the case of tobacco control. *Journal of Health Politics, Policy & Law*, 1999;24:769–804.

51. Ordonez J. Hamburger joints call them "heavy users"—but not to their faces. *Wall Street Journal*, Jan. 12, 2000.

52. We are grateful to James Morone of Brown University for input on this topic.

53. Brownell KD, Ludwig DS. Fighting obesity and the food lobby. *The Washington Post*, Jun. 9, 2002, B07.

Chapter 11

1. Kersh R, Morone J. How the personal becomes political: Prohibitions, public health and obesity. *Studies in American Political Development*, 2002:16:162–175; Kersh R, Morone J. The politics of obesity: Seven steps to government action. *Health Affairs*, 2002;21:142–153; Morone J. *Hellfire Nation*. New Haven, CT: Yale University Press, 2003.

2. Oliver JE, Lee T. Public opinion and the politics of America's obesity epidemic. Paper submitted to the *American Journal of Political Science*. Available at http://ksgnotes1.harvard.edu/Research/wpaper.nsf/rwp/RWP02-017/$File/rwp02_017_lee.pdf. Accessed Nov. 16, 2002.

3. International Food Information Council website. Available at www.ific.org. Accessed Dec. 26, 2002.

4. Egan T. In bid to improve nutrition, schools expel soda and chips. *New York Times*, May 20, 2002: A1.

5. Break for Coke plant OK'd. *Times Picayune*, May 21, 1993, C1; Louisiana Act 203 (1993).

6. Horovitz B. McDonald's going after the small fry. *USA Today*, Oct. 8, 1998, 3B.

7. Rolls BJ. The role of energy density in the overconsumption of fat. *Journal of Nutrition*, 2000;130 (2S Suppl):268S–271S; Rolls BJ. *The Volumetrics Weight Control Plan: Feel Full on Fewer Calories*. New York: HarperCollins, 2000; Pereira MA, Ludwig DS. Dietary fiber and body-weight regulation: Observations and mechanisms. *Pediatric Clinics of North America*, 2001:48:969–980; Kimm SY. The role of dietary fiber in the development and treatment of childhood obesity. *Pediatrics*, 1995;96:1010–1014.

8. Dietz WH, Gortmaker SL. Preventing obesity in children and adolescents. *Annual Review of Public Health*, 2001;22:337–353; Dietz WH. Strategies for a national nutrition and physical activity effort to prevent chronic diseases. Paper submitted for publication.

9. Dietz WH. Breast-feeding may help prevent childhood overweight. *JAMA*, 2001;285:2506–2507; Hediger ML, Overpeck MD, Kuczmarski RJ, Ruan WJ. Association between infant breast-feeding and overweight in young children. *JAMA*, 2001;285:2453–2460; Gillman MW, Rifas-Shiman SL, Camargo CA Jr., Berkey CS, Frazier AL, Rockett HR, Field AE, Colditz GA. Risk of overweight among adolescents who were breast-fed as infants. *JAMA*, 2001;285:2461–2467.

10. Rooney BL, Schauberger CW. Excess pregnancy weight gain and long-term obesity: one decade later. *Obstetrics & Gynecology*, 2002;100:245–252.

11. Robinson TN. Reducing children's television viewing to prevent obesity: a randomized controlled trial. *JAMA*, 1999;282:1561–1567; Dietz WH. The obesity epidemic in young children. Reduce television viewing

and promote playing. *BMJ*, 2001;322:313–314; Dietz WH, Gortmaker SL. Preventing obesity in children and adolescents. *Annual Review of Public Health*, 2001;22:337–353.

12. Car 54, where's your ad? *Christian Science Monitor*, Nov. 6, 2002; Commercial Alert website. Available at www.commrecialalert.org. Accessed Dec. 26, 2002.

13. Center for Science in the Public Interest. What's at stake: Tell the Smithsonian to say no to McDonald's junk food. CSPA website, available at http://actionnetwork.org/campaign/Smithsoniansaynotojunkfood2/explanation. Accessed Aug. 8, 2002.

14. Cram P, Nallamothu BK, Fendrick AM, Saint S. Fast-food franchises in hospitals. *JAMA*, 2002;287:2945–2946.

15. Betty Crocker website. Available at www.bettycrocker.com/prodandpromo/partners/part.asp. Accessed Aug. 8, 2002.

16. Jacoby J. The bullies' next target: junk food. *Boston Globe*, Nov. 12, 1998.

17. Who's next? (editorial). *Wall Street Journal*, Apr. 22, 1998, a22.

18. National Smokers Alliance website. Available at www.speakup.org. Accessed Jan. 16, 1999.

19. Center for Consumer Freedom website. Available at www.consumerfreedom.com/oped_detail.cfm?OPED_ID=123. Accessed Jun. 19, 2002.

20. Ahmad S. Is it time for a twinkie tax? *U.S. News and World Report*, Dec. 29, 1997.

21. Rosin H. The fat tax: Is it really such a crazy idea? *The New Republic*, May 18, 1998.

22. Goodman E. A weighty case against Big Macs. *Boston Globe*, Dec. 12, 2002.

23. Selling to—and selling out—children. *The Lancet*, 2002;360:959.

24. Rossner S. Obesity: The disease of the 21st century. *International Journal of Obesity and Related Metabolic Disorders*, 2002; 26 (Suppl 4):S2–S4.

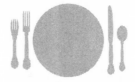

INDEX